9th Edition

NEUROANATOMY
IN CLINICAL CONTEXT

An Atlas of
Structures,
Sections,
Systems,
and Syndromes

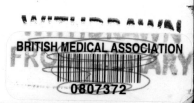

9th Edition
NEUROANATOMY
IN CLINICAL CONTEXT

An Atlas of
Structures,
Sections,
Systems,
and Syndromes

Duane E. Haines, Ph.D., F.A.A.A.S., F.A.A.A.

Professor, Department of Neurobiology and Anatomy and Professor, Department of Neurology,
Wake Forest School of Medicine, Winston-Salem, NC
And
Professor Emeritus, Department of Neurobiology and Anatomical Sciences and Professor, Departments
of Neurology and of Neurosurgery, The University of Mississippi Medical Center, Jackson, MS

Illustrators: M. P. Schenk, BS, MSMI, CMI, FAMI and W. K. Cunningham, BA, MSMI
Computer Graphics: C. P. Runyan, BS
Photographers: G. W. Armstrong, RBP; R.W. Gray, BA
Typist: L. K. Boyd

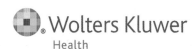
Wolters Kluwer
Health

Philadelphia · Baltimore · New York · London
Buenos Aires · Hong Kong · Sydney · Tokyo

Acquisitions Editor: Crystal Taylor
Product Manager: Jennifer Verbiar
Marketing Manager: Joy Fisher-Williams
Senior Production Project Manager: Bridgett Dougherty
Manufacturing Manager: Margie Orzech
Designer: Stephen Druding
Compositor: Aptara, Inc.

First Edition, 1983	
Second Edition, 1987	Portuguese Translation, 1991
Third Edition, 1991	
Fourth Edition, 1995	Japanese Translation, First Japanese Edition, 1996; Chinese (Taiwan) Translation, 1997
Fifth Edition, 2000	Japanese Translation, Second Japanese Edition, 2000; Chinese (Beijing) Translation, 2002; Chinese (Nanjing) Translation 2002
Sixth Edition, 2004	Brazilian Translation, 2006; Japanese Translation, Third Japanese Edition, 2005
Seventh Edition, 2008	Chinese (Taiwan) Translation, 2010; Russian Translation, 2008; Korean Translation, 2008
Eighth Edition, 2012	Spanish Translation, 2012; Japanese Translation, Fourth Japanese Edition, 2013

Library of Congress Cataloging-in-Publication Data

Haines, Duane E., author.
[Neuroanatomy]
Neuroanatomy in clinical context : an atlas of structures, sections, systems, and syndromes /
Duane E. Haines; illustrators, M.P. Schenk, W.K. Cunningham; computer graphics, C.P.
Runyan; photographers, G.W. Armstrong, R.W. Gray; typist, L.K. Boyd.—Ninth edition.
    p. ; cm.
Preceded by Neuroanatomy / Duane E. Haines. 8th ed. c2012.
Includes bibliographical references and index.
   ISBN 978-1-4698-3202-9 (paperback)
I. Title.
[DNLM: 1. Central Nervous System—anatomy & histology—Atlases. WL 17]
QM451
611'.8—dc23
                                                              2013044480

DISCLAIMER
Care has been taken to confirm the accuracy of the information present and to describe generally accepted practices. However, the authors, editors, and publisher are not responsible for errors or omissions or for any consequences from application of the information in this book and make no warranty, expressed or implied, with respect to the currency, completeness, or accuracy of the contents of the publication. Application of this information in a particular situation remains the professional responsibility of the practitioner; the clinical treatments described and recommended may not be considered absolute and universal recommendations.

The authors, editors, and publisher have exerted every effort to ensure that drug selection and dosage set forth in this text are in accordance with the current recommendations and practice at the time of publication. However, in view of ongoing research, changes in government regulations, and the constant flow of information relating to drug therapy and drug reactions, the reader is urged to check the package insert for each drug for any change in indications and dosage and for added warnings and precautions. This is particularly important when the recommended agent is a new or infrequently employed drug.

Some drugs and medical devices presented in this publication have Food and Drug Administration (FDA) clearance for limited use in restricted research settings. It is the responsibility of the health care provider to ascertain the FDA status of each drug or device planned for use in their clinical practice.

To purchase additional copies of this book, call our customer service department at (800) 638-3030 or fax orders to (301) 223-2320. International customers should call (301) 223-2300.

Visit Lippincott Williams & Wilkins on the Internet: http://www.lww.com. Lippincott Williams & Wilkins customer service representatives are available from 8:30 am to 6:00 pm, EST.

Preface to the Ninth Edition

The first edition of this book contained several unique features, one of which was a particular emphasis on clinical correlations. This approach was one of several guiding principles that were followed through subsequent editions. By the seventh and eighth editions, many figure descriptions contained over 50% clinical information.

The Ninth Edition continues and improves the approach of emphasizing clinical relevance. Clinical content has been revised and increased throughout all chapters, and an all-new chapter on herniation syndromes has been added, all while maintaining an appropriate level of relevant neuroanatomical detail. Recognizing this continuing, and expanded, emphasis on clinically relevant neurobiology, the title has been modified to *Neuroanatomy in Clinical Context* to more accurately reflect these important long-term features of this Atlas. The subtitle, *An Atlas of Structures, Sections, Systems, and Syndromes,* has also been slightly modified to reflect the past and continuing emphasis on syndromes as well as the addition of new syndromes describing brain herniations and disc extrusions.

This new edition of *Neuroanatomy in Clinical Context* continues to: (1) provide a sound anatomical base for integrating neurobiological and clinical concepts; (2) introduce new text, MRI, CT, and artwork that emphasize information and concepts that are encountered in the clinical setting; (3) utilize contemporary clinical and basic science terminology; and (4) emphasize neuroscience information, concepts, and images that collectively constitute a comprehensive overview of systems neurobiology. In addition, the revision of existing pages, the addition of new pages in some chapters, and the inclusion of a new chapter on herniations, have resulted in an increase in the number of MRI, CT, CTA, and angiograms from about 260 to over 380. Understanding systems neurobiology is an absolutely essential element in the successful diagnosis and treatment of the neurologically compromised patient.

Many comments, suggestions, insights, and ideas from my colleagues, medical students, residents, and graduate students have been factored into the modifications in this new edition; their candor is greatly appreciated. While minor corrections, or changes, have been made on almost every page, the major improvements and new information introduced in the Ninth Edition of *Neuroanatomy in Clinical Context* are as follows:

First, all clinical information throughout the Atlas appears in a light blue screen. This: (1) makes it very easy to identify any and all clinical comments, or examples, on every page; (2) does not reduce clinical concepts by trying to compress them into small summary boxes; (3) keeps all clinical correlations and information in their proper neuroanatomical context; and (4) emphasizes the overall amount—and relevance—of the clinical information presented in this Atlas. This approach allows the user to proceed from a basic point to a clinical point or from a clinical point to a basic point, without a break in the flow of information, or the need to go to a different page. This greatly expedites the learning process.

Second, all gross spinal cord and brain images in Chapters 2 and 3 now appear in color. In some cases, original specimens were rephotographed; in other situations, new specimens were used that clearly reflected the orientation and view of the original black/white image. Also, a couple of new images are introduced. A special effort was made to present color images of the best quality as reasonably possible. Generally speaking, these color images follow the same sequence, are of the same views, and correlate with the same vascular illustrations as in the previous edition.

Third, brain herniation is ubiquitous in cases of trauma to the head that results in an increase in intracranial pressure. Sulci and cisterns may be obliterated, and the brain may be extruded from one compartment into another. Herniation may be silent or, more likely, may result in deficits reflecting the particular brain region damaged. Herniation syndromes have elegant anatomical correlates; in most of these cases, there is a close correlation between the brain structures injured and the deficits experienced by the patient. Recognizing the intimate relationship between function and structure, a new and succinct chapter on "Herniation Syndromes" (Chapter 9) is introduced. It is placed at this location since a mastery of systems neurobiology (from Chapter 8) will greatly expedite an understanding of the clinical implications of a herniation be it of the brain or of an intervertebral disc.

Fourth, the existing color coronal forebrain images in Chapter 6 and the axial and sagittal brain images in Chapter 7 were replaced with new high-quality versions of the same pictures. This was accomplished by making high-resolution scans of the original glass slides and processing them to emphasize clarity and detail.

Fifth, the color images of the spinal cord and the brainstem in Chapter 6, although previously scanned from original glass slides, have been carefully revised and reprocessed for further detail and clarity. In addition, a new cross section has been added to illustrate the fact that the trochlear nucleus, decussation of the superior cerebellar peduncle, substantia nigra, and the crus cerebri are characteristic features in a cross section of the brainstem at the level of the inferior colliculus.

Sixth, the two line drawings that illustrate the functional components of spinal cord and brainstem nuclei that previously appeared at the beginning of Chapter 8 have been revised, recolorized, and now appear as the introductory two pages for Chapter 6. The revised color scheme emphasizes the concept of four functional components (although information on the traditional seven functional components is still included), an approach that is more in line with contemporary developmental studies. The content of these two pages relates directly to spinal cord and brainstem nuclei that are shown on subsequent pages in Chapter 6 beginning with Figures 6-3A and B. A version of the longitudinal overview (Figure 6-2) also appears next to each stained section (e.g., Figure 6-3B) with only the nuclei at that specific level indicated and labeled. The spinal and brainstem nuclei in the line drawings at each level in Chapter 6 (e.g., Figure 6-3A) have been revised to match the color plate of the repositioned overview. This allows the user to easily identify the nuclei at that level, their functional component, and their continuity with other related nuclei of comparable function above and below that particular level.

Seventh, many other minor adjustments have been made throughout; these include, labeling changes and/or corrections, adding and/or relocating CT and MRI (both normal and abnormal) for a better correlation, clarifying clinical and neuroanatomical information, stressing a better correlation between structure and function, **bolding** key terms while retaining *italics* for emphasis of important points, and integrating tidbits of information that are encountered in the initial educational experience and that certainly energize the learning opportunity.

Two further issues figured prominently in this new edition. *First*, the question of whether, or not, to use eponyms in their possessive form. To paraphrase one of my clinical colleagues, "Parkinson did not die of his disease (so-called 'Parkinson' disease); he died of a stroke. It was never his own personal disease." There are rare exceptions, such as Lou Gehrig disease, but the point is well taken. McKusick (1998a,b) also has made compelling arguments in support of using the nonpossessive form of eponyms. However, it is acknowledged that views differ on this question—much like debating how many angels can dance on the head of a pin. Consultation with my neurology and neurosurgery colleagues, the style adopted by *Dorland's Illustrated Medical Dictionary* (2012) and *Stedman's Medical Dictionary* (2006), a review of some of the more comprehensive neurology texts (e.g., Rowland and Pedley, 2010; Ropper and Samuels, 2009), the standards established in the *Council of Biology Editors Manual for Authors, Editors, and Publishers* (1994), and the *American Medical Association's Manual of Style* (2007) clearly indicate an overwhelming preference for the nonpossessive form. Recognizing that many users of this book will enter clinical training, it was deemed appropriate to encourage a contemporary approach. Consequently, the nonpossessive form of the eponym is used.

The *second* issue concerns use of the most up-to-date anatomical terminology. With the publication of *Terminologia Anatomica* (Thieme, New York, 1998), a new official international list of anatomical terms for neuroanatomy is available. This new publication, having been adopted by the International Federation of Associations of Anatomists, supersedes *all* previous terminology lists. Every effort has been made to incorporate any applicable new or modified terms into this book. In addition, the well-reasoned modification in the Edinger-Westphal terminology that reflects its functional characteristics is also adapted for this Atlas (Kozicz et al., 2011). The Edinger-Westphal complex consists of an Edinger-Westphal preganglionic nucleus (EWpg) that projects specially to the ciliary ganglion and a Edinger-Westphal centrally projecting nucleus (EWcp) that projects to a variety of targets including the spinal cord, spinal trigeminal, cuneate, gracile, facial, inferior olivary, and parabrachial nuclei, and to the reticular formation, but does not project to the ciliary ganglion.

Lastly, the pagination of the Ninth Edition has been slightly modified to accommodate changes which have increased integration, introduced significant new clinical correlates and images, repositioned a few images to enhance learning opportunities and the overall flow of information, and to accommodate new pages and a new chapter on herniation syndromes. A sampling of Q&As are included in this print version with a much larger sample available online through thePoint. All the Q&As have been revised and updated to assist the user in practicing his or her level of understanding, comprehension, and competence.

Duane E. Haines
Jackson, Mississippi
Winston-Salem, North Carolina

References

Council of Biology Editions Style Manual Committee. *Scientific Style and Format—The CBE Manual for Authors, Editors, and Publishers.* 6th ed. Cambridge: Cambridge University Press; 1994.

Dorland's Illustrated Medical Dictionary. 32nd ed. Philadelphia, PA: Saunders/Elsevier; 2012.

Federative Committee on Anatomical Terminology. *Terminologia Anatomica.* New York, NY: Thieme; 1998.

Iverson C, Christiansen S, Flanagin A, et al. *American Medical Association Manual of Style—A Guide for Authors and Editors.* 10th ed. New York, NY: Oxford University Press; 2007.

Kozicz T, Bittencourt JC, May PJ, et al. The Edinger-Westphal nucleus: A historical, structural, and functional perspective on a dichotomous terminology. *J Comp Neurol.* 2011;519(8):1413–1434.

McKusick VA. On the naming of clinical disorders, with particular reference to eponyms. *Medicine (Baltimore).* 1998a;77(1):1–2.

McKusick VA. *Mendelian Inheritance in Man: A Catalog of Human Genes and Genetic Disorders.* 12th ed. Baltimore, MD: The Johns Hopkins University Press; 1998b.

Ropper AH, Samuels MA. *Adams and Victor's Principles of Neurology.* 9th ed. New York, NY: McGraw-Hill Companies, Inc.; 2009.

Rowland LP, Pedley TA. *Merritt's Neurology.* 12th ed. Baltimore, MD: Lippincott Williams & Wilkins; 2010.

Stedman's Medical Dictionary. 28th ed. Philadelphia, PA: Lippincott Williams & Wilkins; 2006.

Acknowledgments

My basic science colleagues in the Department of Neurobiology and Anatomical Sciences (Dr. Michael Lehman, chair) and my clinical colleagues in the Department of Neurology (Dr. Alex Auchus, chair) and the Department of Neurosurgery (Dr. H. Louis Harkey, chair), all at The University of Mississippi Medical Center, have been very gracious in offering suggestions and comments, both great and small, on the revisions for this Ninth Edition. I especially appreciate their patience with my repeated inquiries, also great and small. Their kindness and outstanding cooperation has directly contributed to the educational usefulness of this document.

The modifications in this Ninth Edition focus on improving the integration of basic science concepts with the realities of their clinical applications, and offer several new innovations that make the learning of, and the transition between, basic science and clinical concepts easier, more fluid, and seamless. The color coding of all clinical information throughout the text, addition of new clinically relevant information and examples, and the upgrading of contemporary anatomical and clinical concepts and terms are but some examples.

A special thank you is due the following individuals: Drs. Bishnu Sapkota and David Sinclair (Neurology); Drs. Robert McGuire and William McCluskey (Orthopedics); Drs. Louis Harkey and Andy Parent (Neurosurgery); Dr. Alan Sinning, Mr. Ken Sullivan, and graduate student Mr. Martin O. Bohlen (Neurobiology and Anatomical Sciences); medical students Ms. Kelly Brister and Mr. Jarrett R. Morgan (for their help with a laminectomy); Dr. Tim McCowan (Radiology); Dr. Jonathan Wisco (UCLA, for a great idea that was used in modified format); Drs. Amy Jones and Bridgett Jones (Resident graduates); and Drs. Kim Simpson and Jim Lynch (Neurobiology and Anatomical Sciences). Their contributions included locating particular cases, extensively reviewing new and extant clinical text, unfettered access to radiological images, reviewing the previous edition for changes (the Joneses), assisting with new brain and spinal dissections, and for responding to numerous general inquiries. I have also greatly appreciated the high quality of my interaction with the Residents in Neurology and Neurosurgery. The cooperation with all of the above was a significant, and important aspect of getting this Ninth Edition done. There has been a long history of excellent cooperation and cross talk between all of these clinical departments and Neurology and Anatomical Sciences.

The reviewers commissioned by LWW were: Pheobe Askie, Onita Bhattasali, Dr. Charles Hubscher, Douglas James, Dr. Pétur H. Petersen, Dr. Johannes van Loon, and Dr. Stephney Whillier. Their time and energy represented an essential element in this new edition.

Modifications, both great and small, to the existing artwork and labeling scheme, and the generation of many new renderings, tables, and compiling plates, were the work of Mr. Michael Schenk (Director of Biomedical Illustration Services) and Mr. Walter (Kyle) Cunningham

(Medical Illustrator). Mr. Chuck Runyan (Biomedical Photography) patiently cleaned and adjusted brightness, color, and contrast to improve the color images of the stained sections in Chapters 6 and 7. Mr. Bill Armstrong (Manager of Biomedical Photography) and Mr. Robert W. Gray (Biomedical Photography) photographed new brain and spinal cord specimens for this edition. I am enormously appreciative of the time, energy, dedication, and professionalism of these individuals to create the best possible images, photographs, artwork, and finished plates for this new edition. Their interest in going the extra mile to "get it perfect," and their outstanding cooperation (and, I might add, patience) with the author, is greatly appreciated. They are not only skilled professionals but also great friends. Ms. Lisa Boyd, who has helped me on several editions, provided important typing assistance.

Over the years, many colleagues, friends, and students (now faculty or medical/dental practitioners) have made many helpful comments. They are again acknowledged here, because these earlier suggestions continue to influence this book: Drs. A. Agmon, A. Alqueza, B. Anderson, C. Anderson, R. Baisden, S. Baldwin, R. Borke, P. A. Brewer, A. S. Bristol, Patricia Brown, Paul Brown, A. Butler, T. Castro, B. Chronister, C. Constantinidis, A. Craig, J. L. Culberson, P. DeVasto, V. Devisetty, E. Dietrichs, L. Ehrlichman, J. Evans, E. M. Fallon, B. Falls, C. Forehand, R. Frederickson, G. C. Gaik, E. Garcis-Rill, G. Grunwald, B. Hallas, T. Imig, J. King, J. A. Kmiec, P. S. Lacy, A. Lamperti, G. R. Leichnetz, E. Levine, R. C. S. Lin, J. C. Lynch, T. McGraw-Ferguson, G. F. Martin, A. Miam, G. A. Mihailoff, M. V. Mishra, B. G. Mollon, R. L. Norman, R. E. Papka, A. N. Perry, K. Peusner, C. Phelps, B. Puder, H. J. Ralston, J. Rho, L. T. Robertson, D. Rosene, A. Rosenquist, I. Ross, J. D. Schlag, M. Schwartz, J. Scott, V. Seybold, L. Simmons, K. L. Simpson, A. Singh, D. Smith, S. Stensaas, C. Stefan, D. G. Thielemann, M. Thomadaki, S. Thomas, M. Tomblyn, J. A. Tucker, D. Tolbert, F. Walberg, S. Walkley, M. Woodruff, M. Wyss, R. Yezierski, and A. Y. Zubkov. I have greatly appreciated their comments and suggestions. The stained sections used in this Atlas are from the teaching collection in the Department of Neurobiology and Anatomy at West Virginia University School of Medicine. The author, who was on the faculty at WVU from 1973–1985, expresses his appreciation to Mr. Bruce Palmer, Professional Technologist at WVU, for providing high-resolution scans of selected existing sections for use in this new Edition. These scans were further processed by Mr. Chuck Runyan.

This Ninth Edition would not have been possible without the interest and support of the publisher, Lippincott Williams & Wilkins. I want to express thanks to my editors, Crystal Taylor (Acquisitions Editor), Catherine Noonan (Associate Product Manager), Joy Fisher-Williams (Marketing Manager), Bridgett Dougherty (Senior Production Project Manager), Amanda Ingold (Editorial Assistant), and especially Kelly Horvath (Freelance Editor) for their encouragement, continuing interest, and confidence in this project. Their cooperation has given me the opportunity to make the improvements seen herein.

Lastly, but clearly not least, I want to express a special thanks to my wife, Gretchen. The significant changes made in this edition required attention to many, and multiple, details. She carefully and critically reviewed the text, patiently listened to more neurobiology than she could have ever imagined, and gleefully informed me about rules of grammar and punctuation that I am not sure I even knew existed. I gladly dedicate this Ninth Edition to Gretchen.

Table of Contents

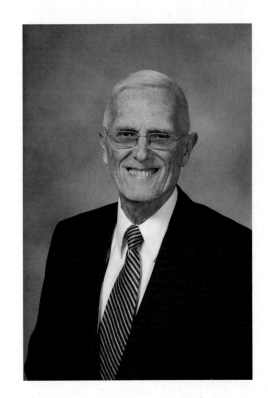

Duane E. Haines, Ph.D.

Recipient of the 2008 Henry Gray/Elsevier Distinguished Educator Award from The American Association of Anatomists

Elected a Fellow of the American Association of Anatomists and a Fellow of the American Association for the Advancement of Science

Recipient of the 2010 Alpha Omega Alpha Robert J. Glaser Distinguished Teacher Award from AOA and The Association of American Medical Colleges

Neuroanatomy Consultant for Stedman's Medical Dictionary and for Dorland's Illustrated Medical Dictionary

Introduction and User's Guide

This new edition of *Neuroanatomy in Clinical Context* continues to emphasize brain anatomy in a clinically relevant format. This includes: (1) correlating the central nervous system (CNS) anatomy with magnetic resonance images (MRIs) and computed tomography (CT) throughout, and making these latter images available to teach basic neurobiology; (2) introducing numerous clinical terms, phrases, and examples in their proper context; (3) highlighting cerebrovascular anatomy and selected variations, all with clinical examples; (4) emphasizing regional brain anatomy, internal vascular territories throughout the CNS, and the myriad deficits resulting from vascular lesions as broadly defined; and (5) presenting an extensive treatment of systems neurobiology that integrates pathways, connections, blood supply, and deficits at all levels of the neural axis.

A major innovation in this new edition is the presentation of all clinical information in a light blue screen throughout the text. This: (1) makes it very easy to identify any and all clinical comments, or examples; (2) does not reduce clinical concepts to small summary boxes; (3) keeps all clinical correlations and information in their proper context; and (4) emphasizes the overall amount—and relevance—of the clinical information presented. This approach allows the user to proceed from a basic point to a clinical point or from a clinical point to a basic point, without a break in the flow of information, or the need to go to a different page.

The opportunity to view, study, and understand CNS anatomy in both **Anatomical** and **Clinical Orientations** continues to be provided, and emphasized. The style of presentation, sequence of topics (from external CNS anatomy, to internal details, to regions, to systems), and emphasis on clinical application expedite learning and understanding that will be eminently useful in the clinical years. This approach allows for learning concepts in a basic neurobiologic setting that can be seamlessly transferred to, and applied within, the clinical environment. A focused approach in this new edition is to continue the emphasis on integration of basic science with clinical application.

Recognizing that about 50% of intracranial events that result in neurological deficits are vascular in nature, as broadly defined, vascular anatomy, distribution territories, and vascular patterns and variations thereof are covered in appropriate detail. These related topics, and their clinical correlations are discussed and illustrated, to varying degrees, with computed tomography angiography (CTA), magnetic resonance angiography (MRA), and magnetic resonance venography (MRV) *in all chapters*. Recognizing vascular patterns, territories, variations, and the appearance of extravasated blood is central to a successful diagnosis.

A thorough knowledge and understanding of systems, reflexes, pathways, their blood supply, and the results of lesions thereof, are essential to diagnosis of the neurologically compromised patient. All of these topics are covered in this new edition. Put simply, the deficits seen in many patients who present with neurologic consequences are *a direct reflection of damage to functional systems* that convey information from the periphery to targets in the brainstem or forebrain, or centrally generated signals that convey information that influences motor activity. A thorough knowledge of systems neurobiology (sensory and motor pathways, spinal and brainstem reflexes) is absolutely essential. A concurrent understanding of the appearance and relationships of brain regions in MRI and CT is an integral part of the diagnostic effort. Systems traverse regions; it is not possible to become competent in one and not the other.

Frequent cross-references are included (figure and page number) to allow easy integration between chapters. In addition, the number of images (CT, CTA, MRI, MRA, MRV, angiograms, and venograms) has been increased from about 260 to more than 390 in this new edition. The use of these images in a contemporary educational setting is absolutely essential for preparing the student for the realities of the clinical experience. In the clinical years, the student will not be studying gross brain or stained slices, but will rely almost exclusively on CT, MRI, or variations on these modalities. The goal is to give students the knowledge base and skills needed to excel in the clinical environment.

Imaging the Brain (CT and MRI)

Imaging the brain in vivo is now commonplace for the patient with neurological deficits. With this in mind, it is appropriate to make a few general comments on these imaging techniques and what is routinely seen, or best seen, in each. For details, consult sources such as Buxton,[1] Grossman,[2] Harnsberger et al.,[3] Lee et al.,[4] or Osborn et al.[5]

Computed Tomography (CT)

In CT, the patient is passed between a source of x-rays and a series of detectors. Tissue density is measured by the effects of x-rays on atoms within the tissue as x-rays pass through the tissue. Atoms of higher number have a greater ability to attenuate (stop) x-rays, whereas those with lower numbers are less able to attenuate x-rays. The various attenuation intensities are computerized into numbers (Hounsfield units or CT numbers). Bone is given the value of +1,000 and is white, whereas air is given a value of −1,000 and is black. In this respect, a lesion or defect in a CT that is **hyperdense** is shifted toward the appearance of bone; it is more white. For example, acute subarachnoid blood in CT is **hyperdense** to the surrounding brain; it is more white than the brain and is shifted more to the appearance of bone (Figure 1-1). A lesion in CT that is **hypodense** is shifted toward the appearance of air or cerebrospinal fluid; it is more black than the surrounding brain (Figure 1-2). In this example, the territory of the middle cerebral artery is *hypodense* (Figure 1-2). **Isodense** in CT refers to a condition in which the lesion and the surrounding brain have textures and/or shades of gray that are essentially the same. Iso- is Greek for equal: "equal density." Extravascular blood, an enhanced tumor, fat, the brain (gray and white matter), and cerebrospinal fluid form an intervening continuum from white to black. In general, Table 1-1 summarizes the white to black intensities seen for selected tissues in CT.

The advantages of CT are: (1) it is done rapidly, which is especially important in trauma; (2) it clearly shows acute and subacute hemorrhages into the meningeal spaces and brain; (3) it is especially useful for children in trauma cases; (4) it shows bone (and skull fractures) to advantage; and (5) it is less expensive than MRI. The disadvantages of CT are: (1) it does not clearly show acute or subacute infarcts or ischemia, or brain edema;

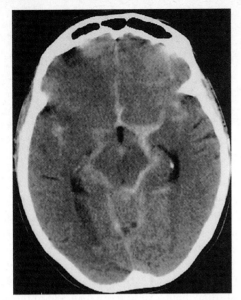

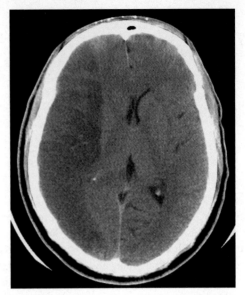

1-1 CT in the axial plane of a patient with subarachnoid hemorrhage. Bone is white, acute blood (white) outlines the subarachnoid space, brain is gray, and cerebrospinal fluid in the third and lateral ventricles is black.

1-2 Axial CT showing a hypodense area within the territory of the middle cerebellar artery on the right side of the patient. This is indicative of a lesion in this region which would result in substantive deficits.

(2) it does not clearly differentiate white from gray matter within the brain nearly as well as MRI; and (3) it exposes the patient to ionizing radiation.

Magnetic Resonance Imaging (MRI)

The tissues of the body contain proportionately large amounts of protons (hydrogen). Protons have a positive nucleus, a shell of negative electrons, and a north and south pole; they function like tiny spinning bar magnets. Normally, these atoms are arranged randomly in relation to each other because of the constantly changing magnetic field produced by the electrons. MRI uses this characteristic of protons to generate images of the brain and body.

When radio waves are sent in short bursts into the magnet containing the patient, they are called a radiofrequency pulse (RP). This pulse may vary in strength. When the frequency of the RP matches the frequency of the spinning proton, the proton will absorb energy from the radio wave (resonance). The effect is twofold. First, the magnetic effects of some protons are canceled out; second, the magnetic effects and energy levels in others are increased. When the RP is turned off, the relaxed protons release energy (an "echo") that is received by a coil and computed into an image of that part of the body.

The two major types of MRI images (MRI/T1 and MRI/T2) are related to the effect of RP on protons and the reactions of these protons (relaxation) when the RP is turned off. In general, those canceled-out protons return slowly to their original magnetic strength. The image constructed from this time constant is called T1 (Figure 1-3). On the other hand, those protons that achieved a higher-energy level (were not canceled out) lose

their energy more rapidly as they return to their original state; the image constructed from this time constant is T2 (Figure 1-4). The creation of a T1-weighted image versus a T2-weighted image is based on a variation in the times used to receive the "echo" from the relaxed protons.

The terms **hyperintense, hypointense,** and **isointense** apply to T1- and T2-weighted MRI. **Hyperintense** in T1 is a shift toward the appearance of fat, which is white in the normal patient; a hyperintense lesion in T1 is more white than the surrounding brain (Figure 1-5A; Table 1-2). A meningioma, and the surrounding edematous areas, are **hyperintense:** more white than the surrounding brain (Figure 1-5A). In T2, **hyperintense** is a shift toward the appearance of cerebrospinal fluid, which is also white in the normal individual (Figure 1-4); a hyperintense condition in T2 is also more white than the surrounding brain (Table 1-2). **Hypointense** in both T1 and T2 is a shift toward the appearance of air or bone in the normal patient; this is a shift to more black than the surrounding brain. In this example, there are **hypointense** areas (**arrows**) adjacent to the lateral ventricles in the frontal and occipital areas (Figure 1-5B). **Isointense** refers to a situation in which a lesion and the surrounding brain have shades of gray and/or textures that are basically the same. In this example of a pituitary tumor in a T1 MRI, the color and texture of the tumor is essentially the same as the surrounding brain; it is **isointense** (Figure 1-5C). **Iso-** is Greek for equal: "equal intensity."

Table 1-2 summarizes the white to black intensities seen in MRI images that are T1-weighted versus T2-weighted. It should be emphasized that a

Table 1-1 The Brain and Related Structures in CT

STRUCTURE/FLUID/SPACE	GRAY SCALE
Bone, acute blood	Very white
Enhanced tumor	Very white
Subacute blood	Light gray
Muscle	Light gray
Gray matter	Light gray
White matter	Medium gray
Cerebrospinal fluid	Medium gray to black
Air, fat	Very black

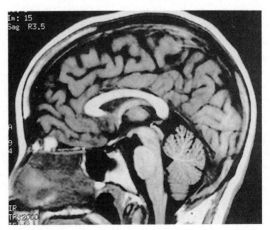

1-3 A sagittal T1-weighted MRI. Brain is gray, and cerebrospinal fluid is black.

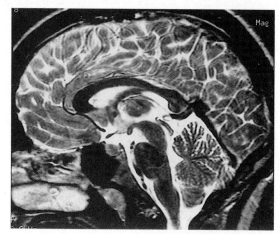

1-4 A sagittal T2-weighted MRI. Brain is gray, blood vessels frequently appear black, and cerebrospinal fluid is white.

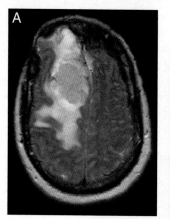

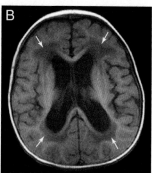

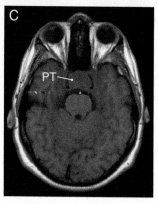

1-5 Axial MRIs showing a hyperintense lesion, meningioma, and edema (**A**), hypointense areas in the white matter of the hemisphere (**B, arrows**), and a pituitary tumor (PT) that is isointense (**C**).

number of variations on these two general MRI themes are routinely seen in the clinical environment.

The advantages of MRI are: (1) it can be manipulated to visualize a wide variety of abnormalities or abnormal states within the brain; and (2) it can show great detail of the brain in normal and abnormal states. The disadvantages of MRI are: (1) it does not show acute or subacute subarachnoid hemorrhage or hemorrhage into the substance of the brain in any detail; (2) it takes much longer to do and, therefore, is not useful in acute situations or in some types of trauma; (3) it is comparatively more expensive than CT; and (4) the scan is extremely loud and may require sedation in children. The ensuing discussion briefly outlines the salient features of individual chapters.

Chapter 2

This chapter presents: (1) the gross anatomy of the spinal cord and its principal arteries; and (2) the external morphology of the brain from all views, including the insular cortex, accompanied by MRIs and drawings of the vasculature patterns from the same perspectives. In this new edition, all gross brain images appear in color, two new images have been included but none eliminated, and clinical terminology such as that used for segments of the cerebral vessels (A_1–A_5, M_1–M_4, and P_1–P_4), continues to be emphasized. In addition, new line drawings and accompanying CT that focus on vascular variations that have clinical implications are featured in this chapter.

Table 1-2 The Brain and Related Structures in MRI

NORMAL	T1	T2
Bone	Very black	Very black
Air	Very black	Very black
Muscle	Dark gray	Dark gray
White matter	Light gray	Dark gray
Gray matter	Dark gray	Light gray
Fat	White	Gray
Cerebrospinal fluid	Very black	Very white
ABNORMAL	T1	T2
Edema	Dark gray	Light gray to white
Tumor	Variable	Variable
Enhanced tumor	White	(Rarely done)
Acute infarct	Dark gray	Light gray to white
Subacute infarct	Dark gray	Light gray to white
Acute ischemia	Dark gray	Light gray to white
Subacute ischemia	Dark gray	Light gray to white

Chapter 3

This chapter focuses on: (1) the relationships of cranial nerves; (2) their exits from the brainstem; (3) their appearance in representative MRI; and (4) examples of cranial nerve deficits seen in cases with lesions of the brainstem. All of the gross brain images showing the positions of cranial nerves now appear in color and minor corrections have been made in Table 3-1. The detailed cross-reference to other sections or pages in the Atlas where additional cranial nerve information is found was also revised. The figure descriptions were updated to increase their clinical value and relevance.

Chapter 4

The structure of the meninges, and their appearance in MRI or CT, is affected by a wide variety of events such as infections (meningitis), trauma, vascular incidents (epidural, subdural, subarachnoid hemorrhage), and tumor (meningioma) all of which are featured in this chapter. In addition, they are a central element in cases of increased intracranial pressure and consequent herniation. The size, shape, and relations of the ventricular system are clearly correlated with the distribution of intraventricular blood, and tumors of the choroid plexus; all of which are illustrated and described in this chapter. New clinical correlations have been added and all figure descriptions updated.

Chapter 5

The general morphology of the forebrain and brainstem is continued into the two sections of Chapter 5. A major improvement in this chapter is the replacement of all black/white photographs with comparable color images in the same coronal and axial planes and at the same general levels in each plane. A second change was to colorize the orientation drawings (upper left on each page) and to orient the axial drawing so as to increase its informational value.

The MRIs have been reorganized, and in several cases new ones inserted, so as to maintain the remarkably close correlation between structures identified in the brain slice and the same structures seen in the corresponding MRIs. The MRI and the brain slice appear on the same page so the correlation can be instantly made. Since brain sections at autopsy or in clinic–pathologic conferences are viewed as unstained specimens, the preference here is to present this material in a format that will most closely parallel what is seen in these clinical settings.

Chapter 6

The improvements made to this chapter are far-reaching, significant, and greatly improve its educational value and clinical emphasis, while retaining the innovations, overall organization, and sequence of earlier editions. Although many minor modifications were made, only the more encompassing are mentioned here.

First, the drawings and text explaining the functional components of the spinal cord and brainstem sensory and motor nuclei have always appeared at the beginning of Chapter 8 as Figures 8-1 and 8-2. Unfortunately, in this location, the succeeding images in Chapter 8 were concerned with neural systems and *not* particularly with the spinal cord or brainstem nuclei.

To redress this matter, these two images were moved to the beginning of Chapter 6, where they now appear as Figures 6-1 and 6-2. In this new location, their content, sensory and motor nuclei of the spinal cord and brainstem, *relate directly to, and correlate with*, the structures shown on the succeeding 25 or so pages regarding *all levels of the spinal cord and brainstem*. This new location recognizes the functional and structural relatedness to the information on the immediately following pages of this chapter.

Second, concurrent with relocating these images to Figures 6-1 and 6-2, both drawings were recolored based on newer thinking in developmental biology. The traditional view of *seven* functional components has been supplemented with a more contemporary view that these seven may be condensed into *four* functional components. To this end, the color coding has been simplified to four colors that correspond with the four functional components. However, the text and figure labels explaining the *traditional* and *contemporary versions* are both presented so that the user may adopt/adapt whichever view works best in a given educational setting. Both the traditional and contemporary views are correct, to a large extent interchangeable, and useful.

Third, relocating the functional component images to Chapter 6 allowed for one of these images to be used, in a slightly modified format, on all spinal cord and brainstem images in this chapter. A version of Figure 6-2 was placed next to the stained image on the right-hand page (e.g., 6-4B), a line placed thereon representing the level of that specific cross section, and only those nuclei were labeled (in this case, spinal cord) that appear at this particular level (Figure 1-6). This approach was used on all spinal cord and brainstem levels in Chapter 6 and allows the user to easily visualize the relationships and continuity of functionally related cell columns at any level.

Fourth, the revised color palate was also used on the line drawings of the spinal cord and brainstem for all sensory and motor nuclei. For example, the line drawing in Figure 6-4A (facing 6-4B) now matches the overall color scheme (Figure 1-6). Consequently, the color of the spinal cord and brainstem sensory and motor nuclei on all left-hand pages is consistent throughout. All color coding matches in all drawings and at all levels of detail from Figure 6-3A to 6-28B throughout Chapter 6.

Fifth, the following structures are characteristic found at the level of a cross section through the inferior colliculus: the nuclei of the inferior colliculus, the trochlear nucleus, the decussation of the superior cerebellar peduncle, and caudal parts of the substantia nigra. A set of pages (line drawing and stained section) was added that illustrates these relationships.

Sixth, the color images of the spinal cord and brainstem in Chapter 6 had previously been scanned from the original glass slide; for this new edition these images were reprocessed to improve clarity and detail. The

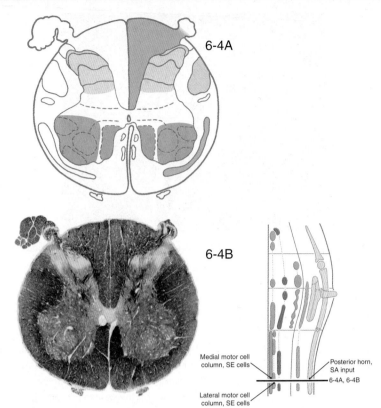

6-4A

6-4B

Medial motor cell
column, SE cells

Lateral motor cell
column, SE cells

Posterior horn,
SA input
6-4A, 6-4B

1-6 A stained section of the lumbar spinal cord (lower) and the overview on spinal cord and brainstem cell columns showing the level of this section and of the line drawing on the facing page. For convenience only, these examples from 6-4A and 6-4B are reduced here to fit in a single column.

color images of the coronal sections of the forebrain in Chapter 6 were replaced with high-resolution color scans of original glass slides and then processed to bring out the best detail and clarity possible.

Innovations that were introduced in recent editions that integrated clinical with anatomical information, that provided options for viewing images in a format consistent with that seen in the clinical environment, and that stressed the clinical relevance and applicability of basic neurobiology are further emphasized in this new edition. First, the ability to flip an image from an **Anatomical Orientation** to a **Clinical Orientation** places everything in the image (line drawing or stained section) into a clinical format: (1) the images match exactly the corresponding MRI or CT, (2) the image has right and left sides, and (3) the topography of all tracts and nuclei in flipped images matches that as seen in CT or MRI. All images in Chapter 6 that can be flipped to a **Clinical Orientation** are identified by this symbol in the lower left of the image.

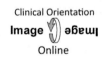

Clinical Orientation

Image ⟳ əɓɐɯı

Online

Understanding the brain and its internal structures in Clinical Orientation is absolutely essential to successful diagnosis. Second, the inherent value of viewing brain anatomy and line drawings in a Clinical Orientation is stressed throughout this chapter, particularly in relation to somatotopy, vascular supply and territories, clinical examples, and the MRI or CT, most of which are featured on the same page as the line drawing or stained section. Third, the color keys have been revised to reflect the modified color palate for the sensory and motor nuclei of the spinal cord and brainstem. Fourth, continuity from **Anatomical Orientation** to **Clinical Orientation** is again illustrated in a series of line drawings and MRI and CT on odd numbered pages showing spinal cord and brainstem levels (Figure 1-7). This new edition continues to utilize CT cisternograms as an integral part of the learning experience (Figure 1-8).

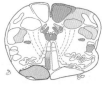
Anatomical orientation

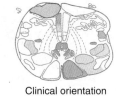
Clinical orientation

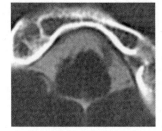

Py
ML
PO
ALS
SpTTr +
SpTNu
NuCu
NuGr
HyNu

MRI, T1-weighted image   MRI, T2-weighted image

CT cisternogram

1-7   An example of the brainstem showing anatomical and clinical orientations at about the caudal one-third of the medulla and the corresponding T1-weighted MRI (with especially important structures labeled), T2-MRI, and CT cisternogram. The abbreviations are keyed to the full label on the facing page in Chapter 6. For additional examples and details of brainstem and spinal cord, see Chapter 6.

Chapter 7

The arrangement of pages in this chapter remains the same as in previous editions: axial brain images in color and the corresponding axial MRI are on left-hand pages and sagittal brain images in color and the corresponding sagittal MRI are on right-hand pages. The heavy red line on the axial images (odd numbered Figures 7-1 to 7-9) indicates the plane of section of the sagittal image on the facing page; similarly, the heavy red line on the sagittal images (even numbered Figures 7-2 to 7-10) indicates the plane of section of the axial image on the facing page. Correlations between stained slices and between structures in MRI can be easily made.

A significant new improvement in this chapter is that high-resolution scans of the original stained sections mounted on glass slides were made and carefully processed for clarity and detail. This resulted in images of high quality in which internal detail is enhanced and anatomical relationships of all structures are more apparent.

The ability to compare different planes of section (stained section and MRI) on facing pages allows the user to build a three-dimensional view of a variety of internal structures in images that are commonly available in the clinical environment. However, these images can also be viewed as an axial series (all left-hand pages) or a sagittal series (all right-hand pages). Educational flexibility is inherent within these arrangements.

Chapter 8

This chapter illustrates a wide variety of clinically relevant CNS tracts/pathways in both **Anatomical and Clinical Orientations**, includes 15 illustrations of pathways of spinal and brainstem reflexes that may be tested during a comprehensive neurological examination, and contains

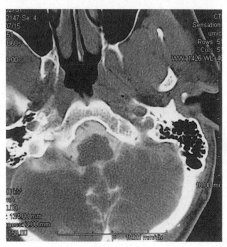

1-8   CT of a patient following injection of a radiopaque contrast media into the lumbar cistern. In this example, at the medullary level (a cisternogram), neural structures appear gray and the subarachnoid space appears light.

literally dozens of clinical correlations or examples. The following features enhance the user's comprehension of information and concepts that are directly relevant to diagnosing the impaired patient. *First,* inclusion of comprehensive pathways in an atlas format allows for the learning of clinically relevant concepts in a variety of settings: lecture, laboratory, self-study, small group, and during clinical rotations. *Second,* pathways that are most important to developing diagnostic skills are presented in **Anatomical** and **Clinical Orientations** which show: (1) its origin, extent, course, and termination; (2) **laterality**, an enormously important clinical concept; (3) position throughout the neural axis and its decussation, if applicable; (4) somatotopy within tracts; and (5) the blood supply at all levels. *Third,* a brief summary of the principal neuroactive substances associated with many pathways, whether they result in excitation (+) or inhibition (–) at their receptor sites, and deficits that may correlate with the loss of particular neurotransmitters is included. *Fourth,* clinical correlations accompany each pathway drawing; these describe deficits, lesions, clinical terminology, and laterality of deficits at different levels of the pathway. In toto, the drawings in Chapter 8 provide a maximal amount of clinically relevant information; each in a single easy-to-follow illustration.

Interspersed within this chapter are 13 sets (26 pages) of illustrations presented in **Clinical Orientation** that immediately follow, and complement, the corresponding pathway presented in **Anatomical Orientation** (Figures 1-9 and 1-10). These clinical illustrations overlay MRIs, focus on cranial nerves and long tracts that are especially important to the diagnosis of the impaired patient. This approach recognizes that in some educational settings pathways are taught anatomically, while in others the emphasis is on a Clinical Orientation; both approaches are accommodated in this atlas. It is, however, important to emphasize that when viewing MRI or CT of a patient compromised by neurologic lesion or disease, *all of the internal brain anatomy and all tracts, including their somatotopy, are seen in a* **Clinical Orientation**. It is absolutely essential that the user *recognize and understand this fact of clinical reality.*

Since *all* possible pathways that may be taught in a given neurobiology course cannot be anticipated, flexibility is designed into this chapter. The last figure in each section is a blank master drawing that follows the same format as the preceding figures. These may be used for learning, review, practicing pathways, in an instructional setting, and as a substrate for examination questions.

Chapter 9

This new chapter on **Herniation Syndromes: Brain and Spinal Discs** illustrates, in more than 60 new line drawings, MRIs, and CT scans, the

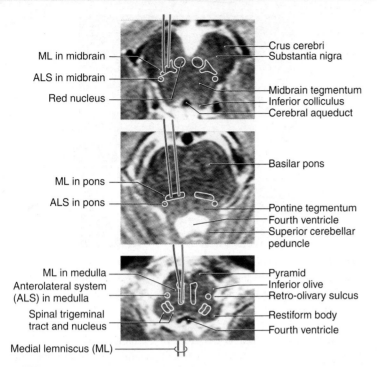

ML in midbrain

ALS in midbrain

Red nucleus

Crus cerebri
Substantia nigra

Midbrain tegmentum
Inferior colliculus
Cerebral aqueduct

Basilar pons

ML in pons

ALS in pons

Pontine tegmentum
Fourth ventricle
Superior cerebellar
peduncle

ML in medulla
Anterolateral system
(ALS) in medulla

Spinal trigeminal
tract and nucleus

Medial lemniscus (ML)

Pyramid
Inferior olive
Retro-olivary sulcus

Restiform body
Fourth ventricle

1-9 The medulla, pons, and midbrain portions of the posterior column-medial lemniscus pathway (see Figure 8-3A for the entire pathway) superimposed on MRI and shown in a *Clinical Orientation*. For convenience only, this example from Figure 8-3A is reduced here to fit in a single column.

close correlation between structures damaged resultant to a herniation and the predictable deficits. There are elegant, and in many situations, remarkably precise correlations between the deficits experienced by the patient and the structures damaged in herniation syndromes; in some cases the deficits accurately predict the type and location of the herniation. Recognizing that brain herniations share general features in common with intervertebral disc extrusions, selected spinal cord syndromes are included to offer a more complete picture of this general phenomenon.

There is a finite amount of space in the cranial cavity; small space-taking events may temporarily be accommodated, while large and especially rapidly occurring events are not tolerated. Anything that compromises this finite amount of space, such as a tumor, hemorrhagic event, brain edema, or any of a number of other causes, may result in increased intracranial pressure (ICP) and a cascade of events that leads to herniation of the brain from one location/compartment to another; these are commonly called *herniation syndromes*. A herniation may be silent with deficits to follow later, or may result in sudden and potentially catastrophic deficits; in some cases, and if untreated, death may follow within minutes.

Increased ICP may be signaled by effacement of sulci or cisterns or a shift in brain structures that may be subtle, particularly in an isodense CT, or obvious as in an edematous tumor. Once evidence of ICP has been determined, a course of treatment is put in motion to guard against further deterioration.

Chapter 10

This chapter contains a series of angiograms (arterial and venous phases), MRA images, and MRV images. The angiograms are shown in lateral and anterior–posterior projections—some as standard views with corresponding digital subtraction images. MRA and MRV technology are noninvasive methods that allow for the visualization of arteries (MRA) and veins and venous sinuses (MRV). However, there are many situations when both arteries and veins are seen with either method. Use of MRA and MRV is commonplace, and this technology is an important diagnostic tool.

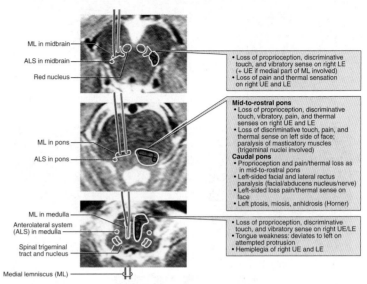

ML in midbrain
ALS in midbrain
Red nucleus

- Loss of proprioception, discriminative touch, and vibratory sense on right LE (+ UE if medial part of ML involved)
- Loss of pain and thermal sensation on right UE and LE

Mid-to-rostral pons
- Loss of proprioception, discriminative touch, vibratory, pain, and thermal senses on right UE and LE
- Loss of discriminative touch, pain, and thermal sense on left side of face; paralysis of masticatory muscles (trigeminal nuclei involved)
Caudal pons
- Proprioception and pain/thermal loss as in mid-to-rostral pons
- Left-sided facial and lateral rectus paralysis (facial/abducens nucleus/nerve)
- Left-sided loss pain/thermal sense on face
- Left ptosis, miosis, anhidrosis (Horner)

ML in pons
ALS in pons

ML in medulla
Anterolateral system
(ALS) in medulla
Spinal trigeminal
tract and nucleus

- Loss of proprioception, discriminative touch, and vibratory sense on right UE/LE
- Tongue weakness: deviates to left on attempted protrusion
- Hemiplegia of right UE and LE

Medial lemniscus (ML)

1-10 The medulla, pons, and midbrain portions of the posterior column-medial lemniscus pathway (see Figure 8-3B for the entire pathway) superimposed on MRI in a *Clinical Orientation*, with lesions and corresponding deficits at representative levels. For convenience only, this example from Figure 8-3B is reduced here to fit in a single column.

Chapter 11

The questions and corresponding answers of Chapter 11 recognize that examinations are an essential part of the educational process and that these elements should prepare, as much as reasonably possible, the user for future needs and expectations. Many are prepared as a patient vignette and in the USMLE Step-1 style (single best answer) which emphasize: (1) anatomical and clinical correlations; (2) application of basic neurobiology concepts to clinical practice; (3) integration of regional neurobiology, systems neurobiology, neurovascular patterns, and disease processes; and (4) the topographical maps within motor and sensory systems as related to lesions of tracts, nuclei, and the cerebral cortex.

While generally grouped by chapter, questions may draw on information from more than one chapter thus reflecting the reality of many major examinations. Correct answers are given, incorrect answers are explained, and page references are given for more detail. A sampling of questions and answers is provided in this chapter with a total of over 300 provided online. While not exhaustive, these questions represent a broad range of clinically relevant topics.

References

1. Buxton RB. *Introduction to Functional Magnetic Resonance Imaging, Principles and Techniques.* Cambridge, UK: Cambridge University Press; 2002.
2. Grossman CB. *Magnetic Resonance Imaging and Computed Tomography of the Head and Spine.* 2nd ed. Baltimore, MD: Williams & Wilkins; 1996.
3. Harnsberger HR, Osborn AG, Macdonald AJ, et al. *Diagnostic and Surgical Imaging Anatomy: Brain, Head & Neck, Spine.* Salt Lake City, UT: Amirsys Publishing Inc; 2011.
4. Lee SH, Rao KCVG, Zimmerman RA. *Cranial MRI and CT.* 4th ed. New York, NY: McGraw-Hill Health Professions Division; 1999.
5. Osborn AG, Salzman KL, Barkovich AJ, et al. *Diagnostic Imaging: Brain,* 2nd ed. Salt Lake City, UT: Amirsys Publishing Inc.; 2010.

Q&A for this chapter is available online on **thePoint**

External Morphology of the Central Nervous System 2

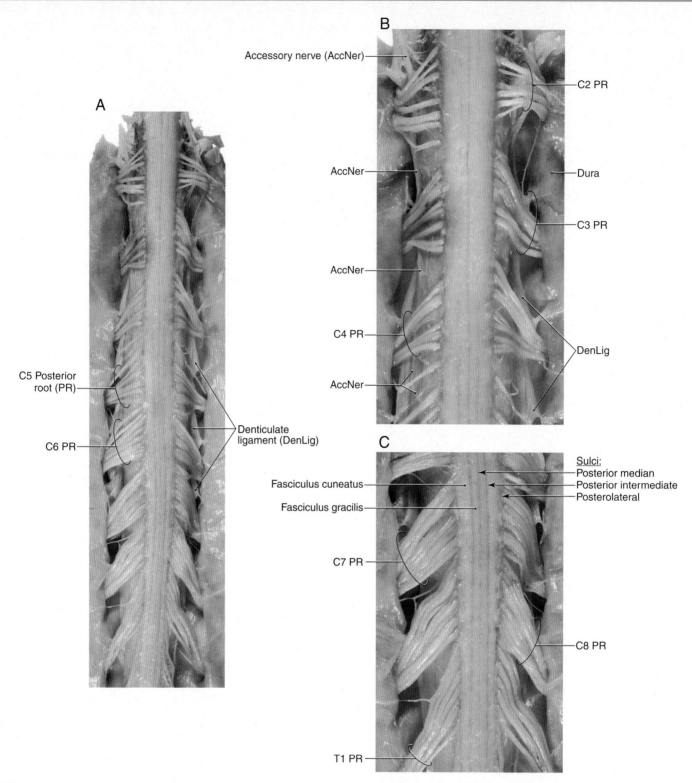

2-1 Overview of a posterior aspect of the spinal cord from C2–T1 (**A**) and details from the same specimen showing the C2–C4 and C7–T1 levels (**B, C**). The **denticulate ligaments** anchor the spinal cord within the dural sac; they are pial tissue sheets that extend laterally to attach to the arachnoid on the inner surface of the dura. The **accessory nerve** courses between the anterior and posterior roots (**B**) and the posterior surface of the cord clearly shows structures and sulci characteristic of the posterior column system (**C**).

Posterior and **anterior spinal medullary arteries** accompany their respective roots (Figure 2-3 on facing page) and the radicular arteries supply their respective roots. The posterior spinal artery is located

medial to the posterior root entry zone and the anterior spinal artery is in the anterior median sulcus (Figure 2-3 on facing page).

Radiculopathy results from spinal nerve root damage. The most common causes are **intervertebral disc disease/protrusion** or **spondylolysis**, and the main symptoms are *pain radiating in a root or dermatomal distribution, weakness,* and **hyporeflexia** of the muscles served by the affected root. The discs most commonly involved at cervical (C) and lumbar (L) levels are C6–C7 (65%–70%), C5–C6 (16%–20%), L4–L5 (40%–45%), and L5–S1 (40%–45%). Thoracic disc problems are rare, well under 1% of all disc protrusions. For additional information on spinal disc extrusions, see Chapter 9.

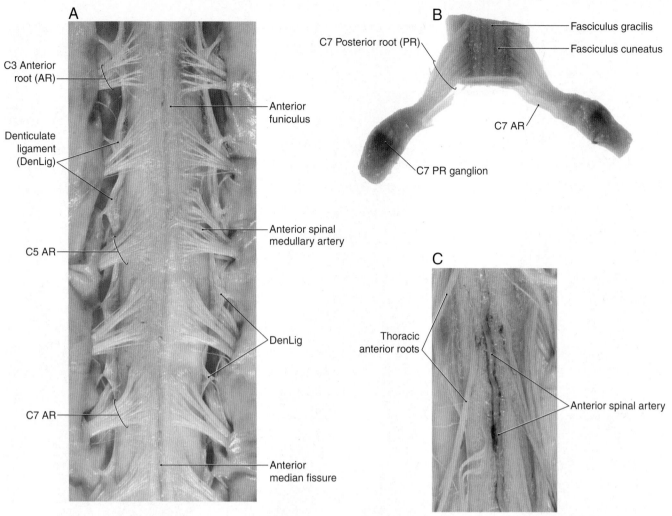

A

C3 Anterior root (AR)

Denticulate ligament (DenLig)

C5 AR

C7 AR

Anterior funiculus

Anterior spinal medullary artery

DenLig

Anterior median fissure

B

C7 Posterior root (PR)

Fasciculus gracilis

Fasciculus cuneatus

C7 AR

C7 PR ganglion

C

Thoracic anterior roots

Anterior spinal artery

2-2 Anterior aspect of the spinal cord from C3–C7 (**A**), the C7 segment showing the **posterior** and **anterior roots** and the **posterior root ganglion** (**B**), and a view of the anterior surface at thoracic levels showing the **anterior spinal artery** and the comparatively diminutive size of the thoracic roots (**C**).

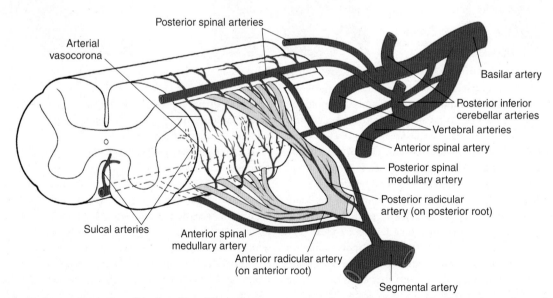

Posterior spinal arteries

Arterial vasocorona

Basilar artery

Posterior inferior cerebellar arteries

Vertebral arteries

Anterior spinal artery

Posterior spinal medullary artery

Posterior radicular artery (on posterior root)

Sulcal arteries

Anterior spinal medullary artery

Anterior radicular artery (on anterior root)

Segmental artery

2-3 Semi-diagrammatic representation showing the origin and general location of principal arteries supplying the spinal cord. The **anterior and posterior radicular arteries** arise at every spinal level and serve their respective roots and ganglia. The **anterior and posterior spinal medullary arteries** (also called **medullary feeder arteries** or **segmental medullary arteries**) arise at intermittent levels and serve to augment the blood supply to the spinal cord. The **artery of Adamkiewicz** is an unusually large spinal medullary artery arising usually on the left in low thoracic or upper lumbar levels (T9–L1). The arterial vasocorona is a diffuse anastomotic plexus covering the cord surface.

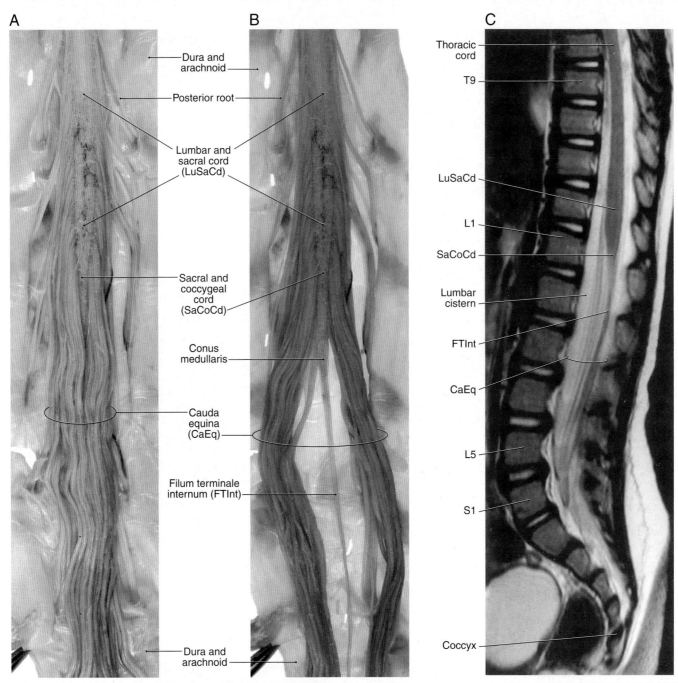

A

- Dura and arachnoid
- Posterior root
- Lumbar and sacral cord (LuSaCd)
- Sacral and coccygeal cord (SaCoCd)
- Conus medullaris
- Cauda equina (CaEq)
- Filum terminale internum (FTInt)
- Dura and arachnoid

B

C

- Thoracic cord
- T9
- LuSaCd
- L1
- SaCoCd
- Lumbar cistern
- FTInt
- CaEq
- L5
- S1
- Coccyx

2-4 Overall posterior (**A, B**) and sagittal MRI (**C**, T2-weighted) views of the **lower thoracic, lumbar, sacral,** and **coccygeal spinal cord segments** and the **cauda equina.** The dura and arachnoid are retracted in **A** and **B.** The cauda equina is shown in situ in **A,** and in **B** the nerve roots of the cauda equina have been spread laterally to expose the **conus medullaris** and **filum terminale internum.** This latter structure is also called the **pial part of the filum terminale.** See Figures 6-3 and 6-4 on pp. 98–99 for cross-sectional views of the cauda equina.

In the sagittal MRI (**C**), the lower portions of the cord, the filum terminale internum, and cauda equina are clearly seen. In addition, the intervertebral discs and the bodies of the vertebrae are clear. The **lumbar cistern** is an enlarged part of the **subarachnoid space** caudal to the end of the spinal cord. This space contains the anterior and posterior roots from the lower part of the spinal cord that collectively form the cauda equina. The filum terminale internum also descends from the conus medullaris through the lumbar cistern to attach to the inner surface of the dural sac. The **dural sac** ends at about the level of the S2 vertebra and is attached to the coccyx by the **filum terminale externum**

(also see Figure 4-1 on p. 59). A **lumbar puncture** is made by inserting a large-gauge needle (18–22 gauge) between the L4 and L5 (preferred) vertebrae or the L3 and L4 vertebrae and retrieving a sample of **cerebrospinal fluid** from the lumbar cistern. This sample may be used for a number of diagnostic procedures.

A **cauda equina syndrome** may be seen when an extruded disc (L4–L5 more common level) that impinges on the cauda equina or in patients with tumor, trauma, or other conditions that damage these nerve roots. The symptoms are usually bilateral and may include: 1) significant **weakness (paraplegia** is a possible outcome) and hypo- or areflexia of the lower extremity; 2) **saddle anesthesia** (commonly seen), which presents as sensory deficits on the buttocks, medial and posterior aspects of thighs, genitalia and anus, and perineum; 3) **urinary retention** (commonly seen) or **incontinence, decreased sphincter tone,** and **fecal incontinence;** and 4) **decrease in sexual function** (may appear later if cause is left untreated). Although sensory loss is common, these patients may or may not experience low back pain or **sciatica.**

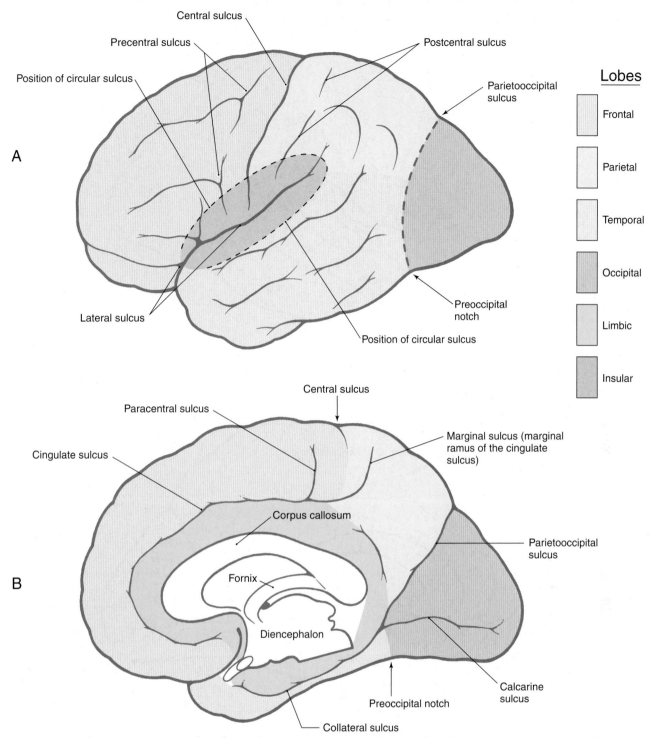

2-5 Lateral (**A**) and medial (**B**) views of the cerebral hemisphere showing the landmarks used to divide the cortex into its main lobes.

On the lateral aspect, the central sulcus (of Rolando) separates frontal and parietal lobes. The lateral sulcus (of Sylvius) forms the border between frontal and temporal lobes. The occipital lobe is located caudal to an arbitrary line drawn between the terminus of the parietooccipital sulcus and the preoccipital notch. A horizontal line drawn from approximately the upper two-thirds of the lateral fissure to the rostral edge of the occipital lobe represents the border between parietal and temporal lobes. The insular cortex (see also Figures 2-40 to 2-42 on pp. 36–37) is located internal to the lateral sulcus in the general area that is shaded gray (**A**). This part of the cortex is made up of long and short gyri that are separated from each other by the central sulcus of the insula. The insula, as a whole, is separated from the adjacent portions of the frontal, parietal, and temporal opercula by the circular sulcus. This sulcus is generally located at the circumference of the gray area (**A**); see also Figures 2-40 to 2-42 on pp. 36–37.

On the medial aspect, the **cingulate sulcus** separates medial portions of frontal and parietal lobes from the **limbic lobe**. An imaginary continuation of the central sulcus intersects with the cingulate sulcus and forms the border between frontal and parietal lobes. The parietooccipital sulcus and an arbitrary continuation of this line to the preoccipital notch separate the parietal, limbic, and temporal lobes from the occipital lobe.

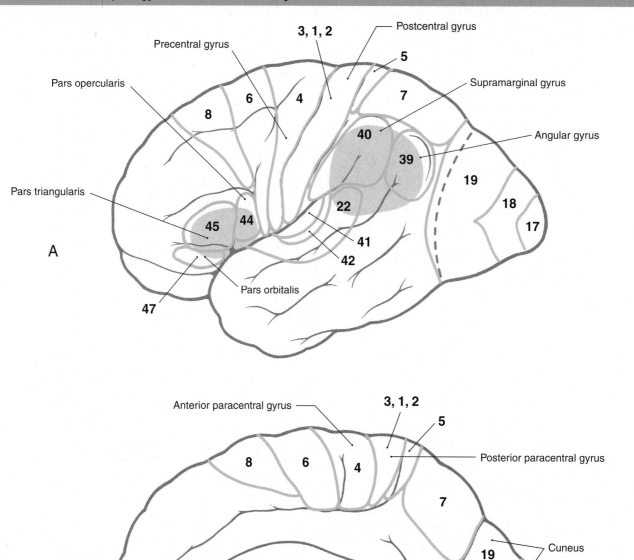

Lateral (**A**) and medial (**B**) views of the cerebral hemisphere showing the more commonly described **Brodmann areas**. In general, **area 4** comprises the primary somatomotor cortex, **areas 3, 1, and 2** the primary somatosensory cortex, and **area 17** the primary visual cortex. **Area 41** is the primary auditory cortex, and the portion of **area 6** in the caudal part of the middle frontal gyrus is generally recognized as the frontal eye field.

The inferior frontal gyrus has three portions: a **pars opercularis**, a **pars triangularis**, and a **pars orbitalis**. A lesion that is located primarily in **areas 44 and 45** (shaded) will give rise to what is called a **Broca aphasia**, also called **motor, expressive, or nonfluent aphasia**. These patients do not have paralysis of the vocal apparatus, but rather have great

difficulty turning ideas into meaningful speech. These patients may have **mutism** or slow, labored speech that consists of familiar single words or short phrases with words left out (telegraphic speech). These patients are well aware of their deficits.

The inferior parietal lobule consists of **supramarginal** (**area 40**) and **angular** (**area 39**) gyri. Lesions in this general area of the cortex (shaded), and sometimes extending into **area 22**, will give rise to what is known as **Wernicke aphasia**, also sometimes called **sensory, receptive, or fluent aphasia**. Patients with a sensory aphasia speak freely and without hesitation, but what is said may make little sense due to the use of inappropriate words at inappropriate places in the sentences (**paraphasia**, or sometimes called **word salad**). These patients may be unaware of their deficits.

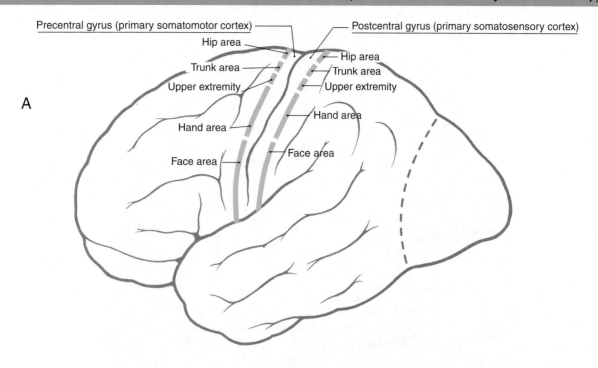

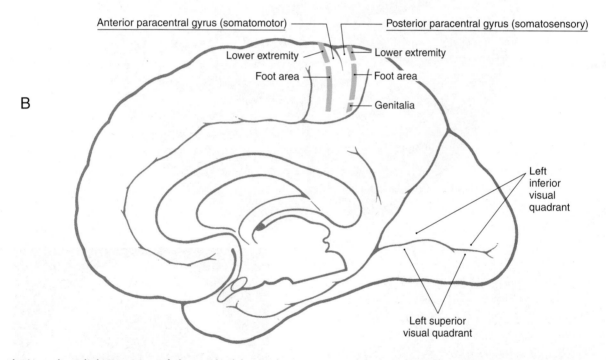

2-7 Lateral (**A**) and medial (**B**) views of the cerebral hemisphere showing the **somatotopic organization** of the **primary somato-motor and somatosensory cortices.** The lower extremity and foot areas are located on medial aspects of the hemisphere in the anterior paracentral (motor) and the posterior paracentral (sensory) gyri. The remaining portions of the body extend from the margin of the hemisphere over the convexity to the lateral sulcus in the precentral and postcentral gyri.

An easy way to remember the somatotopy of these important cortical areas is to divide the precentral and postcentral gyri generally into thirds: a lateral third that represents the face area, a middle third that represents the upper extremity and hand with particular emphasis on the hand, and a medial third that represents the trunk and hip. The rest of the body representation, lower extremity and foot, is on the medial

aspect of the hemisphere in the **anterior** (motor) and **posterior** (sensory) **paracentral gyri.** Lesions of the somatomotor cortex result in motor deficits on the contralateral side of the body, whereas lesions in the somatosensory cortex result in a loss of sensory perception from the contralateral side of the body. The medial surface of the right hemisphere (**B**) illustrates the position of the left portions of the visual field. The inferior visual quadrant is located in the **primary visual cortex** above the calcarine sulcus, whereas the superior visual quadrant is found in the cortex below the calcarine sulcus. Lesions of visual structures caudal to the optic chiasm may result in a **contralateral** (either **left** or **right** based on the side of the lesion) **homonymous hemianopia** or may present in other situations as a **quadrantanopia.**

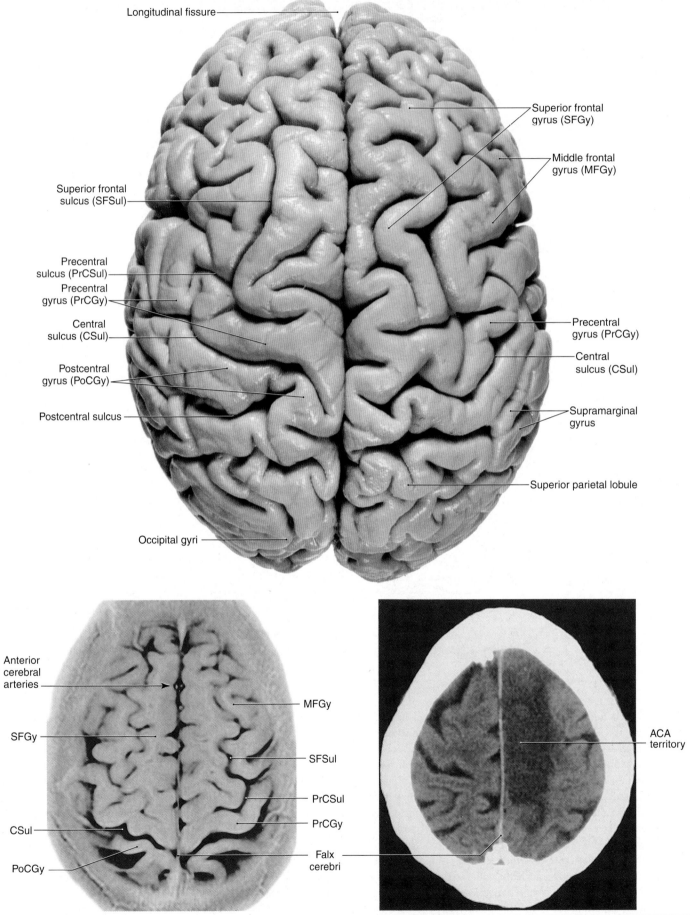

Longitudinal fissure

Superior frontal gyrus (SFGy)

Middle frontal gyrus (MFGy)

Superior frontal sulcus (SFSul)

Precentral sulcus (PrCSul)

Precentral gyrus (PrCGy)

Central sulcus (CSul)

Postcentral gyrus (PoCGy)

Postcentral sulcus

Precentral gyrus (PrCGy)

Central sulcus (CSul)

Supramarginal gyrus

Superior parietal lobule

Occipital gyri

Anterior cerebral arteries

SFGy

CSul

PoCGy

MFGy

SFSul

PrCSul

PrCGy

Falx cerebri

ACA territory

2-8 Superior (dorsal) view of the cerebral hemispheres showing the main gyri and sulci and an MRI (inverted inversion recovery—lower left) and a CT (lower right) identifying structures from the same perspective. Note the area of infarction representing the territory of the anterior cerebral artery (ACA). The infarcted area involves lower extremity, hip, and, possibly, lower trunk cortical areas; because the lesion is in the left hemisphere, the deficits are on the patient's right side.

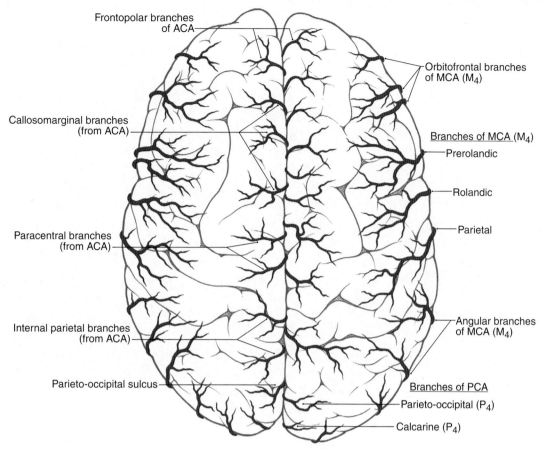

Frontopolar branches of ACA

Orbitofrontal branches of MCA (M₄)

Callosomarginal branches (from ACA)

Branches of MCA (M₄)
Prerolandic

Rolandic

Parietal

Paracentral branches (from ACA)

Internal parietal branches (from ACA)

Angular branches of MCA (M₄)

Parieto-occipital sulcus

Branches of PCA
Parieto-occipital (P₄)

Calcarine (P₄)

2-9 Superior (dorsal) view of the cerebral hemispheres showing the location and general branching patterns of the **anterior (ACA)**, middle **(MCA)**, and **posterior (PCA) cerebral arteries**. Compare the distribution of ACA branches with the infarcted area in Figure 2-8 on the facing page.

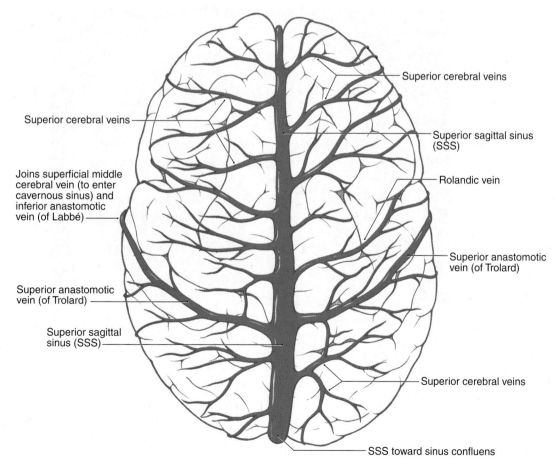

Superior cerebral veins

Superior cerebral veins

Superior sagittal sinus (SSS)

Joins superficial middle cerebral vein (to enter cavernous sinus) and inferior anastomotic vein (of Labbé)

Rolandic vein

Superior anastomotic vein (of Trolard)

Superior anastomotic vein (of Trolard)

Superior sagittal sinus (SSS)

Superior cerebral veins

SSS toward sinus confluens

2-10 Superior (dorsal) view of the cerebral hemispheres showing the location of the **superior sagittal sinus** and the locations and general branching patterns of **veins**. See Figures 10-4 and 10-5 (pp. 313–314) for comparable angiograms (venous phase) of the superior sagittal sinus.

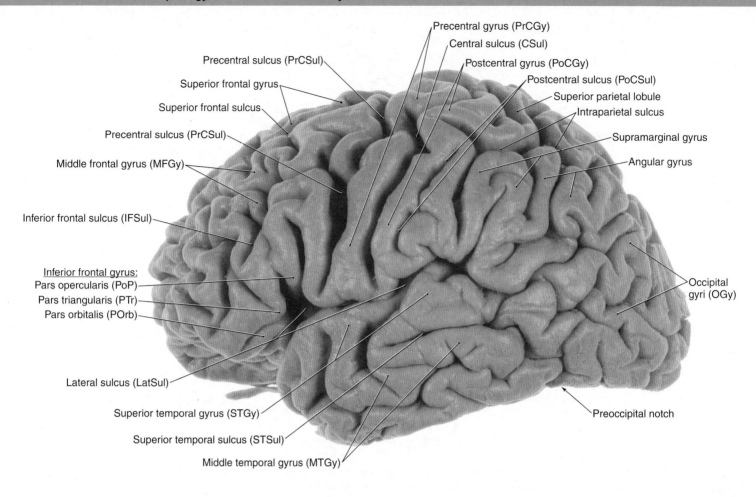

Precentral gyrus (PrCGy)
Central sulcus (CSul)
Precentral sulcus (PrCSul)
Postcentral gyrus (PoCGy)
Superior frontal gyrus
Postcentral sulcus (PoCSul)
Superior frontal sulcus
Superior parietal lobule
Intraparietal sulcus
Precentral sulcus (PrCSul)
Supramarginal gyrus
Middle frontal gyrus (MFGy)
Angular gyrus
Inferior frontal sulcus (IFSul)

Inferior frontal gyrus:
Pars opercularis (PoP)
Pars triangularis (PTr)
Pars orbitalis (POrb)
Occipital gyri (OGy)

Lateral sulcus (LatSul)
Preoccipital notch
Superior temporal gyrus (STGy)
Superior temporal sulcus (STSul)
Middle temporal gyrus (MTGy)

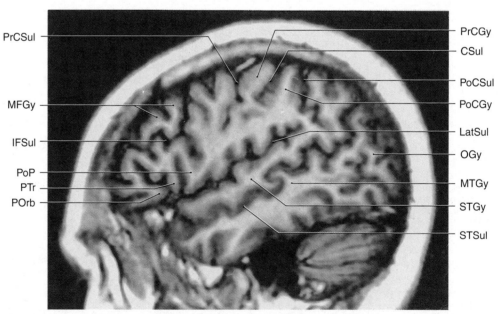

PrCSul
PrCGy
CSul
MFGy
PoCSul
PoCGy
IFSul
LatSul
OGy
PoP
PTr
MTGy
POrb
STGy
STSul

2-11 Lateral view of the left cerebral hemisphere showing the principal gyri and sulci and a T1 MRI on which many of these structures can be identified from the same perspective. Especially important cortical areas are the **precentral** and **postcentral gryi** (primary **somatomotor** and **somatosensory cortex,** respectively, for the body, excluding the lower extremity), the parts of the **inferior frontal gyrus** (partes opercularis, triangularis, and orbitalis), and the **supramarginal** and **angular gyri** that collectively form the **inferior parietal lobule.** The **frontal eye field** is located primarily in the caudal area of the middle frontal gyrus adjacent to the precentral gyrus.

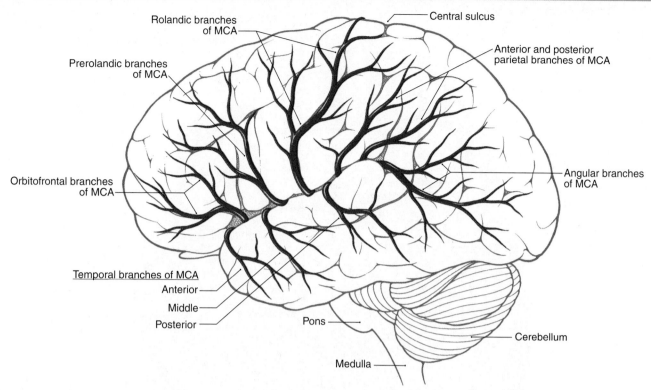

2-12 Lateral view of the left cerebral hemisphere showing the branching pattern of the middle cerebral artery. The **middle cerebral artery** initially branches in the depths of the lateral sulcus (as M_2 and M_3 **segments**: see Figures 2-41 and 2-42 on p. 37); these branches, when seen on the surface of the hemisphere, represent the M_4 **segment**. The individual branches of the overall M_4 segment are named usually according to their relationship to gyri, sulci, or position on a lobe. Terminal branches of the **posterior** and **anterior cerebral arteries** course over the edges of the temporal and occipital lobes, and parietal and frontal lobes, respectively (see Figure 2-9 on p. 15). See Figure 10-1 (p. 310) for a comparable angiogram of the middle and anterior cerebral arteries.

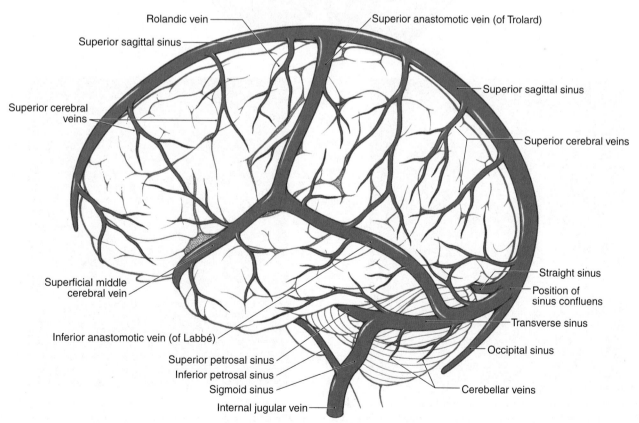

2-13 Lateral view of the left cerebral hemisphere showing the locations of **sinuses** and the locations and general branching patterns of **veins**. Communication between veins and sinuses or between sinuses also is indicated. See Figures 10-2 (p. 311) and 10-11 (p. 320) for comparable angiogram and MRV of the sinuses and superficial veins.

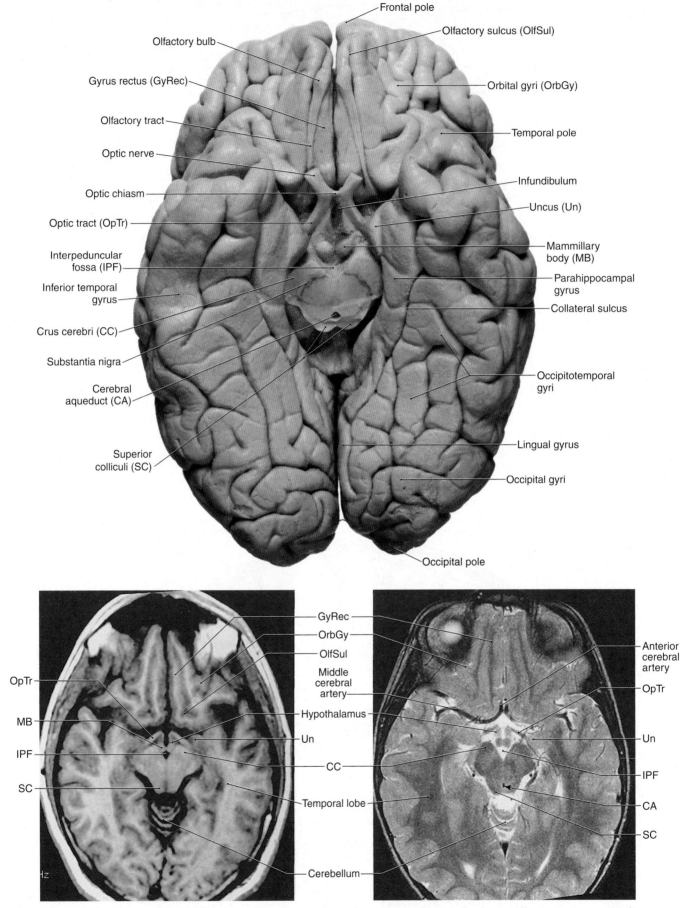

Frontal pole

Olfactory bulb

Olfactory sulcus (OlfSul)

Gyrus rectus (GyRec)

Orbital gyri (OrbGy)

Olfactory tract

Temporal pole

Optic nerve

Infundibulum

Optic chiasm

Uncus (Un)

Optic tract (OpTr)

Mammillary body (MB)

Interpeduncular fossa (IPF)

Parahippocampal gyrus

Inferior temporal gyrus

Collateral sulcus

Crus cerebri (CC)

Substantia nigra

Occipitotemporal gyri

Cerebral aqueduct (CA)

Superior colliculi (SC)

Lingual gyrus

Occipital gyri

Occipital pole

GyRec

OrbGy

OlfSul

Anterior cerebral artery

Middle cerebral artery

OpTr

MB

Hypothalamus

OpTr

IPF

Un

Un

SC

CC

IPF

Temporal lobe

CA

SC

Cerebellum

2-14 Inferior (ventral) view of the **cerebral hemispheres** and **diencephalon** with the brainstem caudal to midbrain removed and two MRIs (inversion recovery—lower left; T2-weighted—lower right) showing many structures from the same perspective. Note the relationships of the midbrain to surrounding structures (**cerebellum**, medial aspect of the **temporal lobe, uncus** [as related to **uncal herniation**], and **hypothalamus** and **optic tract**) and to the cisterns.

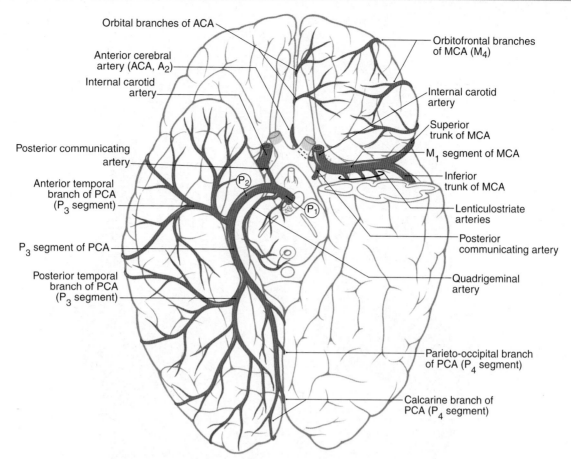

Orbital branches of ACA

Anterior cerebral artery (ACA, A₂)

Internal carotid artery

Posterior communicating artery

Anterior temporal branch of PCA (P₃ segment)

P₃ segment of PCA

Posterior temporal branch of PCA (P₃ segment)

P₂

P₁

Orbitofrontal branches of MCA (M₄)

Internal carotid artery

Superior trunk of MCA

M₁ segment of MCA

Inferior trunk of MCA

Lenticulostriate arteries

Posterior communicating artery

Quadrigeminal artery

Parieto-occipital branch of PCA (P₄ segment)

Calcarine branch of PCA (P₄ segment)

2-15 Inferior (ventral) view of the cerebral hemisphere, with the brainstem removed, showing **segments P₁–P₄** of the **posterior cerebral artery (PCA)**, a small portion of the anterior cerebral artery, and the initial branching of the **M₁ segment** of the **middle cerebral artery** into superior and inferior trunks. The correlation between the superior and inferior trunks of the MCA and segments **M₂–M₄** are shown in Figure 2-42 on p. 37.

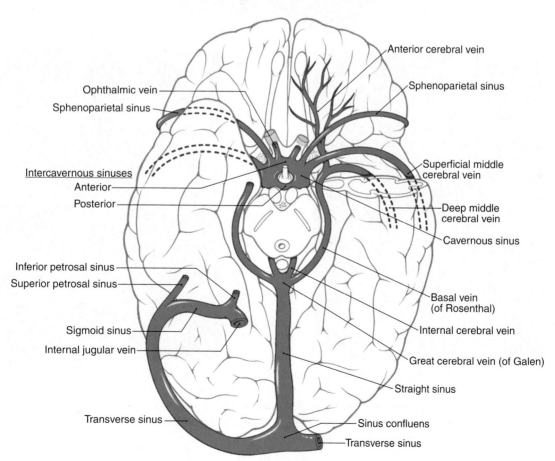

Ophthalmic vein

Sphenoparietal sinus

Intercavernous sinuses
Anterior
Posterior

Inferior petrosal sinus

Superior petrosal sinus

Sigmoid sinus

Internal jugular vein

Transverse sinus

Anterior cerebral vein

Sphenoparietal sinus

Superficial middle cerebral vein

Deep middle cerebral vein

Cavernous sinus

Basal vein (of Rosenthal)

Internal cerebral vein

Great cerebral vein (of Galen)

Straight sinus

Sinus confluens

Transverse sinus

2-16 Inferior (ventral) view of the cerebral hemisphere, with the brainstem removed, showing the relationships of the main sinuses and the **anterior cerebral vein**, the **deep middle cerebral vein**, and the **superficial middle cerebral vein.** See Figures 10-5 (p. 314), 10-9 (p. 318), and 10-11 (p. 320) for comparable views of these veins and sinuses.

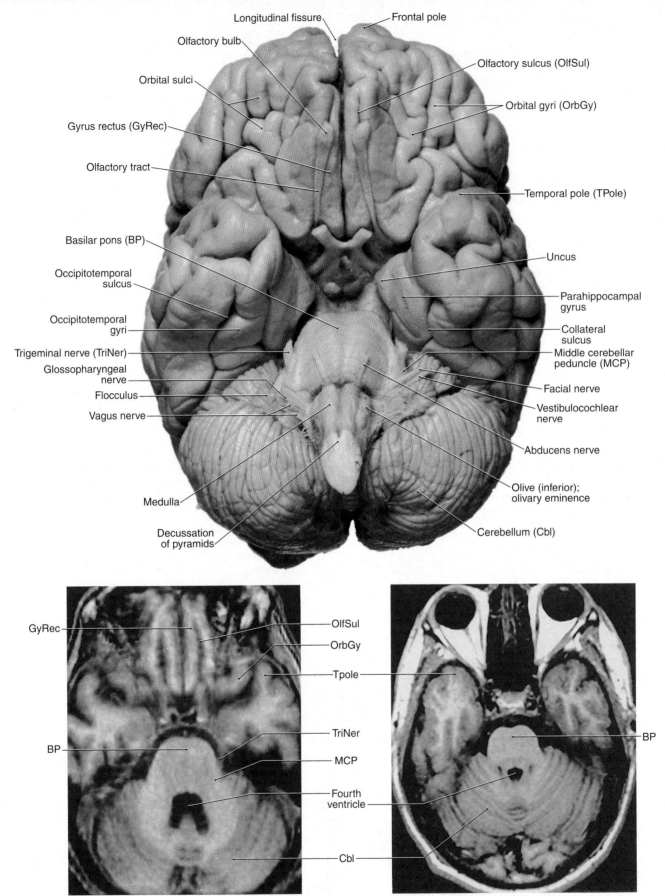

Longitudinal fissure

Olfactory bulb

Orbital sulci

Gyrus rectus (GyRec)

Olfactory tract

Basilar pons (BP)

Occipitotemporal sulcus

Occipitotemporal gyri

Trigeminal nerve (TriNer)

Glossopharyngeal nerve

Flocculus

Vagus nerve

Medulla

Decussation of pyramids

Frontal pole

Olfactory sulcus (OlfSul)

Orbital gyri (OrbGy)

Temporal pole (TPole)

Uncus

Parahippocampal gyrus

Collateral sulcus

Middle cerebellar peduncle (MCP)

Facial nerve

Vestibulocochlear nerve

Abducens nerve

Olive (inferior); olivary eminence

Cerebellum (Cbl)

GyRec

BP

OlfSul

OrbGy

Tpole

TriNer

MCP

Fourth ventricle

Cbl

BP

2-17 Inferior (ventral) view of the **cerebral hemispheres, dien-cephalon, brainstem,** and **cerebellum,** and two MRIs (both T1-weighted images) that show structures from the same perspec-tive. Note the slight differences in the sizes of the **fourth ventricle.** The larger space seen in the right MRI is representative of a slightly lower axial plane through the pons when compared to the left MRI, which represents a slightly more superior plane. The latter is bor-dered by the **superior cerebellar peduncles.** A detailed view of the inferior (ventral) aspect of the brainstem is seen in Figure 2-20 on p. 22.

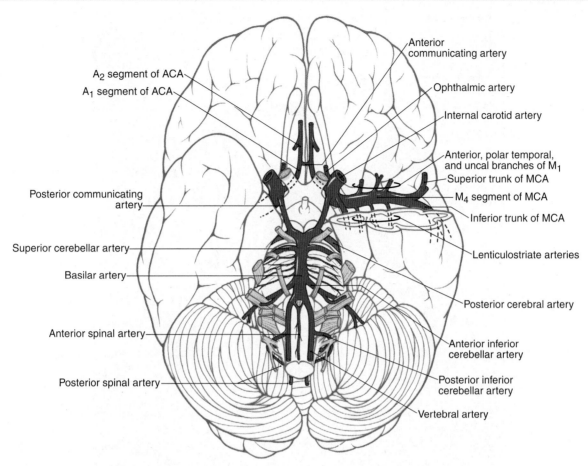

2-18 Inferior (ventral) view of the **cerebral hemispheres, diencephalon, brainstem,** and **cerebellum,** which shows the arterial patterns created by the **internal carotid** and **vertebrobasilar systems.** Note the **cerebral arterial circle** (of Willis). Details of the cerebral arterial circle and the vertebrobasilar arterial pattern are shown in Figure 2-21 on p. 23. See Figure 10-9 and 10-10 (pp. 318–319) for comparable MRAs of the cerebral arterial circle and its major branches.

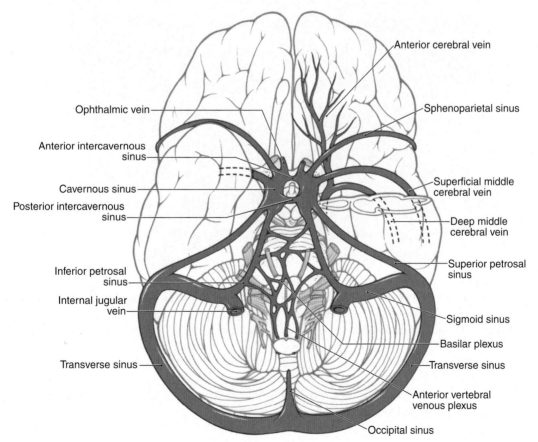

2-19 Inferior (ventral) view of the **cerebral hemispheres, diencephalon, brainstem,** and **cerebellum** showing the locations and relationships of **principal sinuses and veins.** Compare this figure with Figure 2-16 (p. 19).

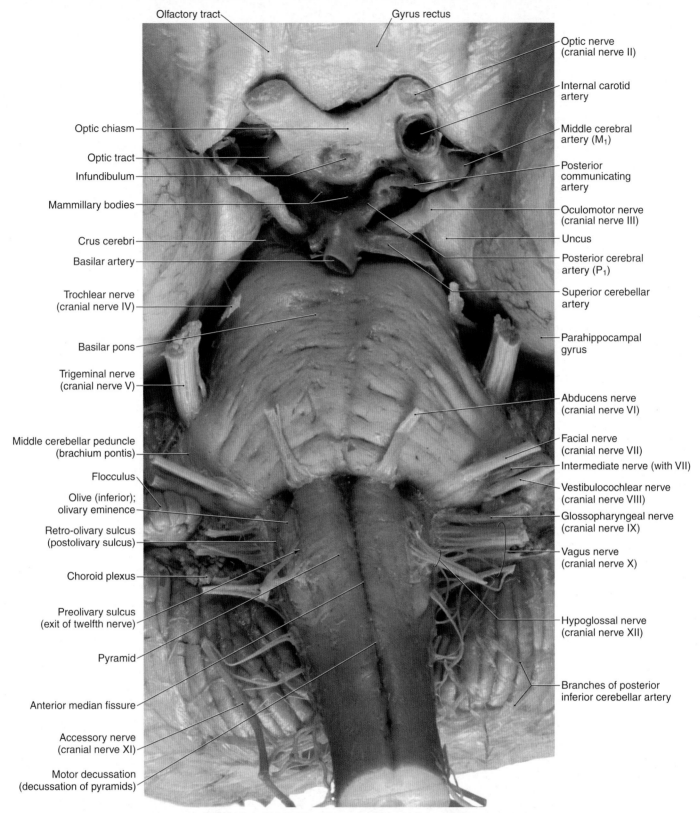

Olfactory tract

Gyrus rectus

Optic chiasm

Optic tract

Infundibulum

Mammillary bodies

Crus cerebri

Basilar artery

Trochlear nerve
(cranial nerve IV)

Basilar pons

Trigeminal nerve
(cranial nerve V)

Middle cerebellar peduncle
(brachium pontis)

Flocculus

Olive (inferior);
olivary eminence

Retro-olivary sulcus
(postolivary sulcus)

Choroid plexus

Preolivary sulcus
(exit of twelfth nerve)

Pyramid

Anterior median fissure

Accessory nerve
(cranial nerve XI)

Motor decussation
(decussation of pyramids)

Optic nerve
(cranial nerve II)

Internal carotid
artery

Middle cerebral
artery (M_1)

Posterior
communicating
artery

Oculomotor nerve
(cranial nerve III)

Uncus

Posterior cerebral
artery (P_1)

Superior cerebellar
artery

Parahippocampal
gyrus

Abducens nerve
(cranial nerve VI)

Facial nerve
(cranial nerve VII)

Intermediate nerve (with VII)

Vestibulocochlear nerve
(cranial nerve VIII)

Glossopharyngeal nerve
(cranial nerve IX)

Vagus nerve
(cranial nerve X)

Hypoglossal nerve
(cranial nerve XII)

Branches of posterior
inferior cerebellar artery

2-20 Detailed view of the inferior (ventral) aspect of the **diencephalon** and **brainstem** with particular emphasis on exit and/or entrance points of cranial nerves (CNs II–XII) and the general relationships of the **optic nerve, chiasm, and tract.** Note an important relationship: *the oculomotor nerve exits between the superior cerebellar and the posterior cerebral (P_1 segment of PCA) arteries.* In this location, it is susceptible to damage from **aneurysms arising from the basilar bifurcation or from the posterior communicating artery/PCA intersection.** Such lesions give rise to deficits (seen individually or in combinations) characteristic of third nerve injury, such as **dilated pupil, loss of most eye movement,** and **diplopia.** Other important relationships also include the cranial nerves of the **pons–medulla junction** (VI, VII, VIII) and the cranial nerves associated with the **cerebellopontine angle** (VII, VIII, IX, X). In this view, it is easy to appreciate the fact that cranial nerves VI–XII occupy a compact area at the caudal aspect of the pons and lateral medulla. Lesions in this area may result in a variety of cranial nerve, and potentially additional, deficits.

Vessels
Structures

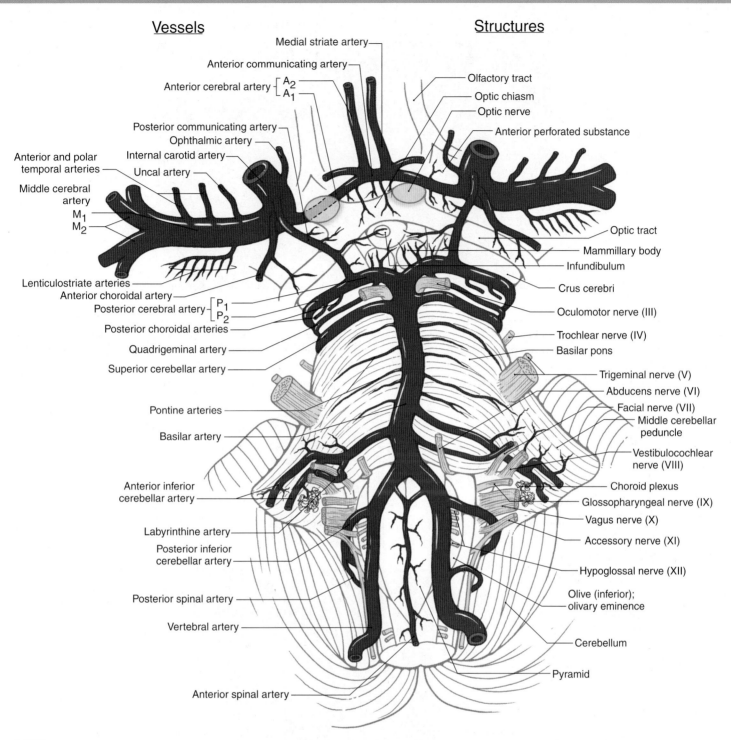

Medial striate artery

Anterior communicating artery

Anterior cerebral artery $\begin{bmatrix} A_2 \\ A_1 \end{bmatrix}$

Posterior communicating artery

Ophthalmic artery

Internal carotid artery

Anterior and polar temporal arteries

Uncal artery

Middle cerebral artery

M_1
M_2

Lenticulostriate arteries

Anterior choroidal artery

Posterior cerebral artery $\begin{bmatrix} P_1 \\ P_2 \end{bmatrix}$

Posterior choroidal arteries

Quadrigeminal artery

Superior cerebellar artery

Pontine arteries

Basilar artery

Anterior inferior cerebellar artery

Labyrinthine artery

Posterior inferior cerebellar artery

Posterior spinal artery

Vertebral artery

Anterior spinal artery

Olfactory tract

Optic chiasm

Optic nerve

Anterior perforated substance

Optic tract

Mammillary body

Infundibulum

Crus cerebri

Oculomotor nerve (III)

Trochlear nerve (IV)

Basilar pons

Trigeminal nerve (V)

Abducens nerve (VI)

Facial nerve (VII)

Middle cerebellar peduncle

Vestibulocochlear nerve (VIII)

Choroid plexus

Glossopharyngeal nerve (IX)

Vagus nerve (X)

Accessory nerve (XI)

Hypoglossal nerve (XII)

Olive (inferior); olivary eminence

Cerebellum

Pyramid

2-21 Inferior (ventral) view of the brainstem showing the relationship of brain structures and cranial nerves to the arteries forming the **vertebrobasilar system** and the **cerebral arterial circle (of Willis)**. The **posterior spinal artery** usually originates from the **posterior inferior cerebellar artery** (left, about 75% of cases), but it may arise from the **vertebral artery** (right, about 25% of individuals). Although the **labyrinthine artery** may occasionally branch from the basilar (right, about 15% of the time), it most frequently originates from the **anterior inferior cerebellar artery** (left, about 85% of cases).

Many vessels that arise ventrally course around the brainstem to serve dorsal structures. The **anterior cerebral artery** consists of A_1 (between the internal carotid bifurcation and the anterior communicating artery) and segments A_2–A_5, which are distal to the **anterior**

communicating artery (see Figure 10-3 on p. 312 for details). Lateral to the **internal carotid bifurcation** is the M_1 **segment** of the middle cerebral artery (MCA), which usually divides into superior and inferior trunks that continue as the M_2 **segments** (branches) on the insular cortex. The M_3 **branches** of the MCA are those located on the inner surface of the opercula, and the M_4 **branches** are located on the lateral aspect of the hemisphere (see Figure 2-42 on p. 37).

Between the **basilar bifurcation** and the **posterior communicating artery** is the P_1 **segment** of the posterior cerebral artery; P_2 is between the posterior communicator and the first temporal branches and P_3–P_4 are distal to this segment. See Figures 10-9, 10-10, and 10-12 (pp. 318, 319, and 321) for comparable MRA of the cerebral arterial circle and vertebrobasilar system. See Figure 4-10 on p. 68 for the blood supply of the choroid plexus.

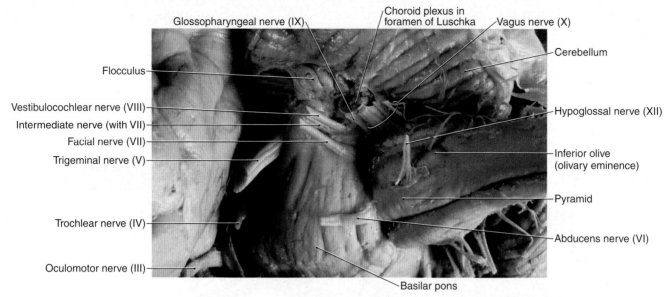

Glossopharyngeal nerve (IX)
Choroid plexus in foramen of Luschka
Vagus nerve (X)
Cerebellum
Flocculus
Vestibulocochlear nerve (VIII)
Intermediate nerve (with VII)
Facial nerve (VII)
Trigeminal nerve (V)
Hypoglossal nerve (XII)
Inferior olive (olivary eminence)
Pyramid
Trochlear nerve (IV)
Abducens nerve (VI)
Oculomotor nerve (III)
Basilar pons

2-22 Lateral view of the left side of the brainstem where the inferior aspects of the cerebellum, medulla, and pons converge; this area is commonly called the **cerebellopontine angle (CPA)**. The cranial nerves (CNs) related to the CPA in decreasing order, based on the deficits seen following lesion/tumors in the CPA, are CNs VII, VIII; less so IX, X, and XI. Although not technically a nerve of the CPA, especially large lesions (generally larger than 2.0 cm) in this area may extend forward and involve CN V with appropriate sensory deficits. **Vestibular schwannoma** is the most common CPA lesion (about 85%) with **meningioma** a distant second at about 5%–10%.

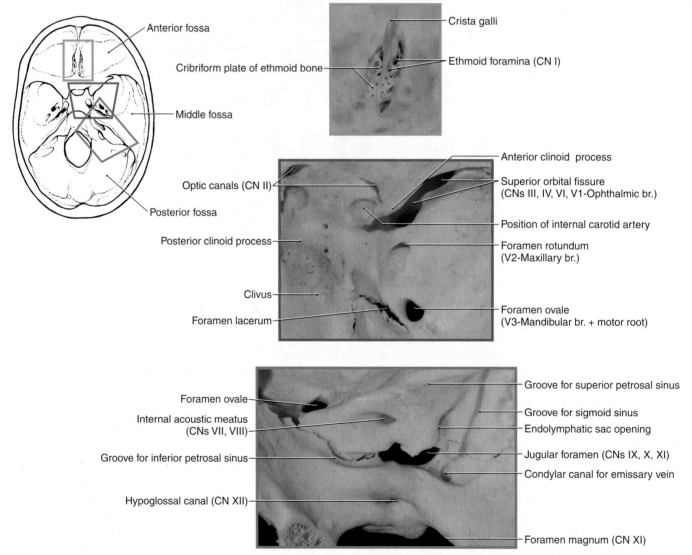

Anterior fossa
Crista galli
Cribriform plate of ethmoid bone
Ethmoid foramina (CN I)
Middle fossa

Anterior clinoid process
Optic canals (CN II)
Superior orbital fissure (CNs III, IV, VI, V1-Ophthalmic br.)
Position of internal carotid artery
Posterior fossa
Posterior clinoid process
Foramen rotundum (V2-Maxillary br.)
Clivus
Foramen lacerum
Foramen ovale (V3-Mandibular br. + motor root)

Foramen ovale
Groove for superior petrosal sinus
Internal acoustic meatus (CNs VII, VIII)
Groove for sigmoid sinus
Endolymphatic sac opening
Groove for inferior petrosal sinus
Jugular foramen (CNs IX, X, XI)
Condylar canal for emissary vein
Hypoglossal canal (CN XII)
Foramen magnum (CN XI)

2-23 Views of the internal aspects of the skull with particular emphasis on the foramina through which the cranial nerves pass. The color boxes on the drawing of the skull base correlate with the color outline of each of the detailed views. Correlate the cranial nerves as seen in Figure 2-22 (above) with their respective foramina. Examples of lesions generally associated with the contents of foramina include **tumors of the jugular foramen** (mainly CNs IX, X, and XI) and **vestibular schwannoma** (mainly CNs VII and VIII). **Meningiomas** of the skull base may involve a number of cranial nerves in different combinations.

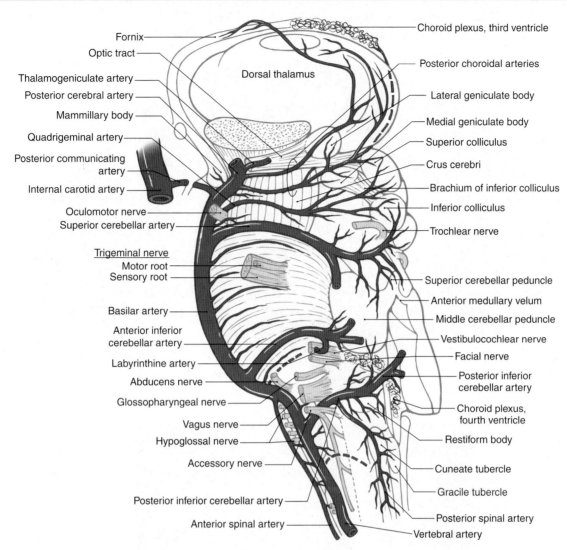

Fornix

Optic tract

Thalamogeniculate artery

Posterior cerebral artery

Mammillary body

Quadrigeminal artery

Posterior communicating artery

Internal carotid artery

Oculomotor nerve

Superior cerebellar artery

Trigeminal nerve
Motor root
Sensory root

Basilar artery

Anterior inferior cerebellar artery

Labyrinthine artery

Abducens nerve

Glossopharyngeal nerve

Vagus nerve

Hypoglossal nerve

Accessory nerve

Posterior inferior cerebellar artery

Anterior spinal artery

Dorsal thalamus

Choroid plexus, third ventricle

Posterior choroidal arteries

Lateral geniculate body

Medial geniculate body

Superior colliculus

Crus cerebri

Brachium of inferior colliculus

Inferior colliculus

Trochlear nerve

Superior cerebellar peduncle

Anterior medullary velum

Middle cerebellar peduncle

Vestibulocochlear nerve

Facial nerve

Posterior inferior cerebellar artery

Choroid plexus, fourth ventricle

Restiform body

Cuneate tubercle

Gracile tubercle

Posterior spinal artery

Vertebral artery

2-24 Lateral view of the left side of the **brainstem** and **thalamus** showing the relationship of structures and cranial nerves to arteries. Arteries that serve dorsal structures originate from ventrally located parent vessels. The approximate positions of the **posterior spinal** and **labyrinthine arteries,** when they originate from the **vertebral** and **basilar arteries,** respectively, are shown as dashed lines. Compare with Figure 2-22 on the facing page. See Figure 10-7 (p. 316) for comparable angiogram of the **vertebrobasilar system.** See Figure 4-10 on p. 68 for another view of the blood supply to the choroid plexus of the third and fourth ventricles.

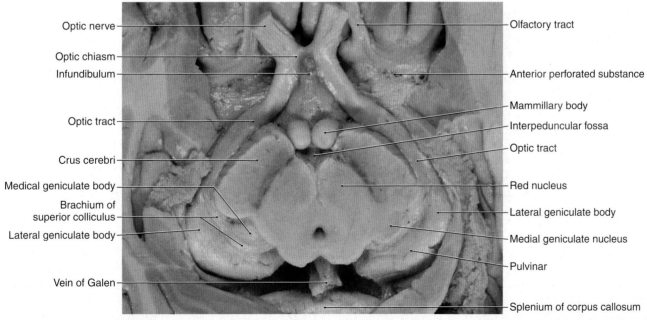

Optic nerve

Optic chiasm

Infundibulum

Optic tract

Crus cerebri

Medical geniculate body

Brachium of superior colliculus

Lateral geniculate body

Vein of Galen

Olfactory tract

Anterior perforated substance

Mammillary body

Interpeduncular fossa

Optic tract

Red nucleus

Lateral geniculate body

Medial geniculate nucleus

Pulvinar

Splenium of corpus callosum

2-25 Inferior (ventral) view of the diencephalon and a cross section of the midbrain at the level of the **midbrain–diencephalon junction.** Note the structures of the hypothalamus, those related to cranial nerve II, and the close relationship of the optic tract to the crus cerebri and lateral geniculate body. Also note the characteristic position of the brachium of the superior colliculus to the medial geniculate body/nucleus. Deficits of the **anterior choroidal artery syndrome** include a **contralateral hemiplegia** (crus cerebri damage) and a **contralateral hemianopia** (optic tract damage).

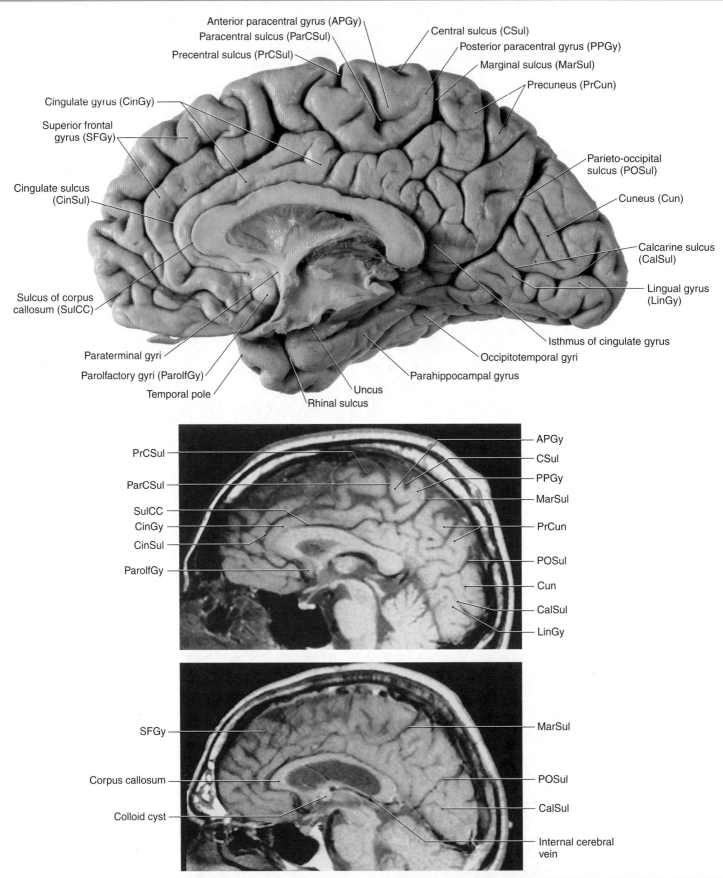

Anterior paracentral gyrus (APGy)
Paracentral sulcus (ParCSul)
Precentral sulcus (PrCSul)
Central sulcus (CSul)
Posterior paracentral gyrus (PPGy)
Marginal sulcus (MarSul)
Precuneus (PrCun)
Cingulate gyrus (CinGy)
Superior frontal gyrus (SFGy)
Parieto-occipital sulcus (POSul)
Cingulate sulcus (CinSul)
Cuneus (Cun)
Calcarine sulcus (CalSul)
Sulcus of corpus callosum (SulCC)
Lingual gyrus (LinGy)
Paraterminal gyri
Isthmus of cingulate gyrus
Parolfactory gyri (ParolfGy)
Occipitotemporal gyri
Temporal pole
Parahippocampal gyrus
Uncus
Rhinal sulcus

PrCSul
APGy
CSul
ParCSul
PPGy
MarSul
SulCC
CinGy
PrCun
CinSul
ParolfGy
POSul
Cun
CalSul
LinGy

SFGy
MarSul

Corpus callosum
POSul
CalSul
Colloid cyst
Internal cerebral vein

2-26 Midsagittal view of the right **cerebral hemisphere** and **diencephalon**, with brainstem removed, showing the main gyri and sulci and two MRIs (both T1-weighted images) showing these structures from the same perspective. The lower MRI is from a patient with a small **colloid cyst** in the interventricular foramen. When compared with the upper MRI, note the **enlarged lateral ventricle with** resultant **thinning of the corpus callosum.**

A **colloid cyst** (colloid tumor) is a congenital growth usually discovered in adult life once the flow of CSF through the interventricular foramina is compromised (**obstructive hydrocephalus**). The patient may have **headache, unsteady gait, weakness of the lower extremities, visual** or **somatosensory disorders**, and/or personality changes or **confusion.** Treatment is usually by surgical removal.

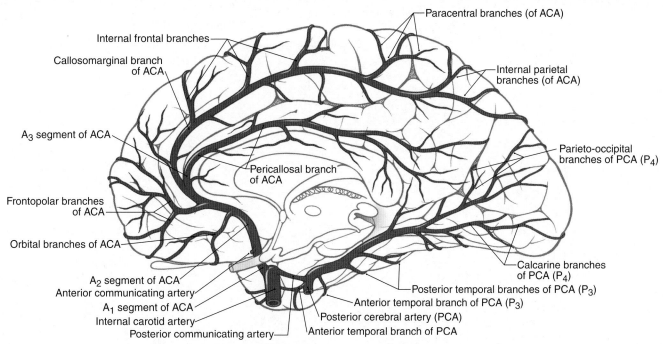

Paracentral branches (of ACA)

Internal frontal branches

Callosomarginal branch of ACA

Internal parietal branches (of ACA)

A_3 segment of ACA

Pericallosal branch of ACA

Parieto-occipital branches of PCA (P_4)

Frontopolar branches of ACA

Orbital branches of ACA

Calcarine branches of PCA (P_4)

A_2 segment of ACA

Posterior temporal branches of PCA (P_3)

Anterior communicating artery

Anterior temporal branch of PCA (P_3)

A_1 segment of ACA

Posterior cerebral artery (PCA)

Internal carotid artery

Posterior communicating artery

Anterior temporal branch of PCA

2-27 Midsagittal view of the right **cerebral hemisphere** and **diencephalon** showing the locations and branching patterns of **anterior (ACA)** and **posterior (PCA) cerebral arteries**. The positions of gyri and sulci can be extrapolated from Figure 2-26 (facing page). Terminal branches of the **anterior cerebral artery** arch laterally over the edge of the hemisphere to serve medial regions of the frontal and parietal lobes, and the same relationship is maintained for the occipital and temporal lobes by branches of the **posterior cerebral artery**. The ACA is made up of segments A_1 (precommunicating), A_2 (infracallosal), A_3 (precallosal), and $A_4 + A_5$ (supracallosal + postcallosal). See Figures 10-1 (p. 310) and 10-7 (p. 316) for comparable angiograms of anterior and posterior cerebral arteries.

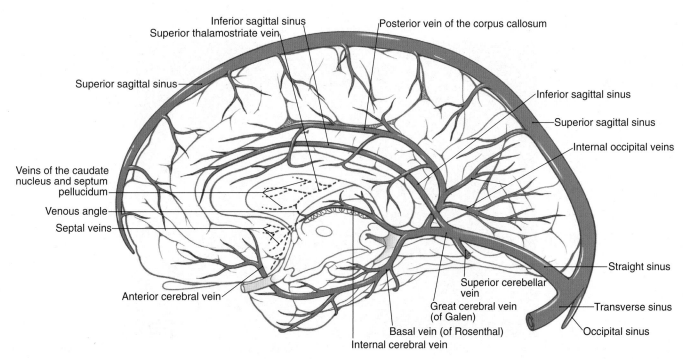

Inferior sagittal sinus

Superior thalamostriate vein

Posterior vein of the corpus callosum

Superior sagittal sinus

Inferior sagittal sinus

Superior sagittal sinus

Internal occipital veins

Veins of the caudate nucleus and septum pellucidum

Venous angle

Septal veins

Straight sinus

Superior cerebellar vein

Anterior cerebral vein

Great cerebral vein (of Galen)

Transverse sinus

Basal vein (of Rosenthal)

Occipital sinus

Internal cerebral vein

2-28 Midsagittal view of the right **cerebral hemisphere** and **diencephalon** showing the locations and relationships of sinuses and the locations and general branching patterns of veins. The continuation of the **superior thalamostriate vein** (also called the terminal vein due to its proximity to the stria terminalis) with the **internal cerebral vein** is the **venous angle**. See Figures 10-2 (p. 311) and 10-11 (p. 320) for comparable angiogram (venous phase) and MRV showing veins and sinuses.

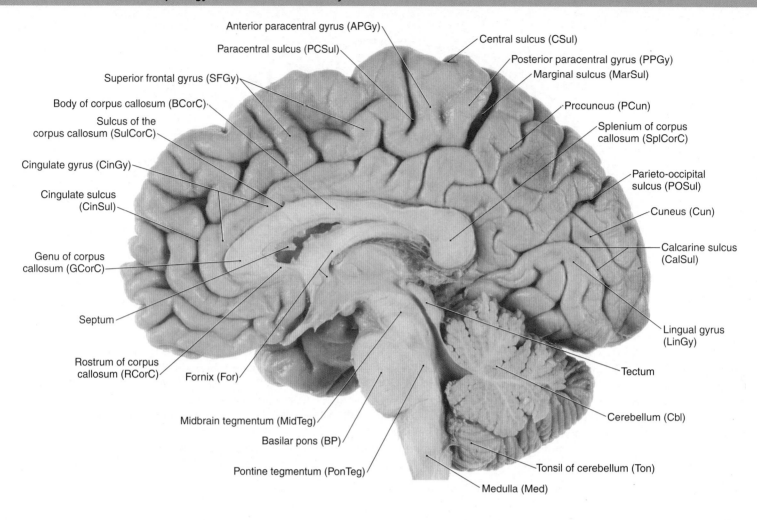

Anterior paracentral gyrus (APGy)
Paracentral sulcus (PCSul)
Superior frontal gyrus (SFGy)
Body of corpus callosum (BCorC)
Sulcus of the corpus callosum (SulCorC)
Cingulate gyrus (CinGy)
Cingulate sulcus (CinSul)
Genu of corpus callosum (GCorC)
Septum
Rostrum of corpus callosum (RCorC)
Fornix (For)
Midbrain tegmentum (MidTeg)
Basilar pons (BP)
Pontine tegmentum (PonTeg)

Central sulcus (CSul)
Posterior paracentral gyrus (PPGy)
Marginal sulcus (MarSul)
Precuneus (PCun)
Splenium of corpus callosum (SplCorC)
Parieto-occipital sulcus (POSul)
Cuneus (Cun)
Calcarine sulcus (CalSul)
Lingual gyrus (LinGy)
Tectum
Cerebellum (Cbl)
Tonsil of cerebellum (Ton)
Medulla (Med)

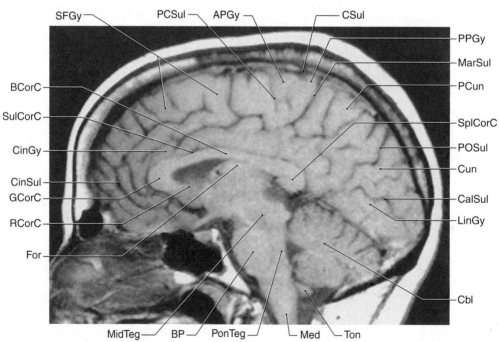

SFGy
PCSul
APGy
CSul
PPGy
MarSul
PCun
BCorC
SulCorC
CinGy
CinSul
GCorC
RCorC
For
SplCorC
POSul
Cun
CalSul
LinGy
Cbl
MidTeg
BP
PonTeg
Med
Ton

2-29 A midsagittal view of the right **cerebral hemisphere** and **diencephalon** with the brainstem and cerebellum in situ. The MRI (T1-weighted image) shows many brain structures from the same perspective. Important cortical relationships in this view include the **cingulate, parietooccipital,** and **calcarine sulci;** the **primary visual cortex** is located on either bank of the calcarine sulcus. The cingulate gyrus, medial aspect of the superior frontal gyrus, and precuneus occupy much of the medial surface of the hemisphere. Note that the medial terminus of the central sulcus is above the splenium of the corpus callosum. This clearly illustrates the fact that the **primary somatomotor** (anterior paracentral gyrus) and **somatosensory** (posterior paracentral gyrus) cortices for the lower extremity are located somewhat caudally on the medial aspect of the hemisphere.

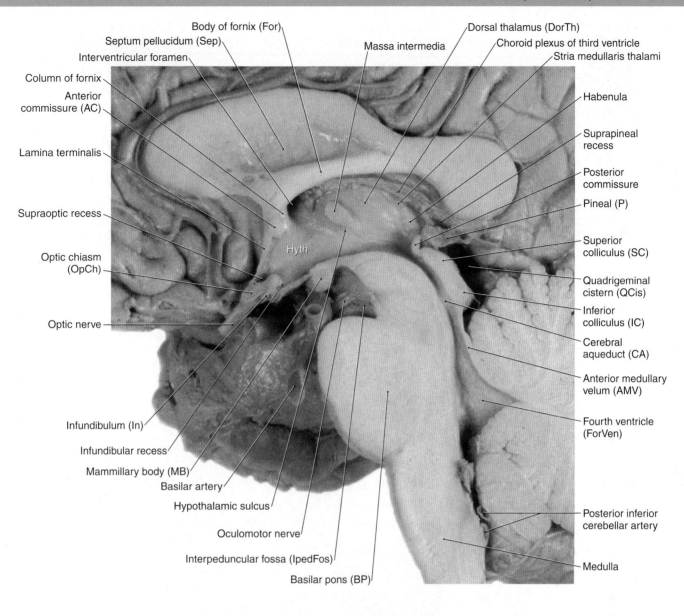

Body of fornix (For)
Septum pellucidum (Sep)
Interventricular foramen
Column of fornix
Anterior commissure (AC)
Lamina terminalis
Supraoptic recess
Optic chiasm (OpCh)
Optic nerve
Infundibulum (In)
Infundibular recess
Mammillary body (MB)
Basilar artery
Hypothalamic sulcus
Oculomotor nerve
Interpeduncular fossa (IpedFos)
Basilar pons (BP)

Massa intermedia
Hyth

Dorsal thalamus (DorTh)
Choroid plexus of third ventricle
Stria medullaris thalami
Habenula
Suprapineal recess
Posterior commissure
Pineal (P)
Superior colliculus (SC)
Quadrigeminal cistern (QCis)
Inferior colliculus (IC)
Cerebral aqueduct (CA)
Anterior medullary velum (AMV)
Fourth ventricle (ForVen)
Posterior inferior cerebellar artery
Medulla

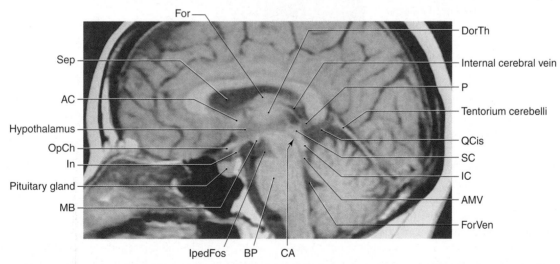

For
Sep
AC
Hypothalamus
OpCh
In
Pituitary gland
MB

IpedFos   BP   CA

DorTh
Internal cerebral vein
P
Tentorium cerebelli
QCis
SC
IC
AMV
ForVen

2-30 A midsagittal view of the right **cerebral hemisphere** and **dien-cephalon** with the brainstem in situ focusing on the details primarily related to the diencephalon and **third ventricle**. The MRI (T1-weighted image) shows these brain structures from the same per-spective. Note the recesses of the third ventricle in the vicinity of the **hypothalamus**, the position of the **lamina terminalis**, and the general relationships of the ventricular system in the midsagittal plane. These relationships are important to understanding images of patients with **subarachnoid hemorrhage** (e.g., see Figure 4-7 on p. 65). Hyth, hypoth-alamus.

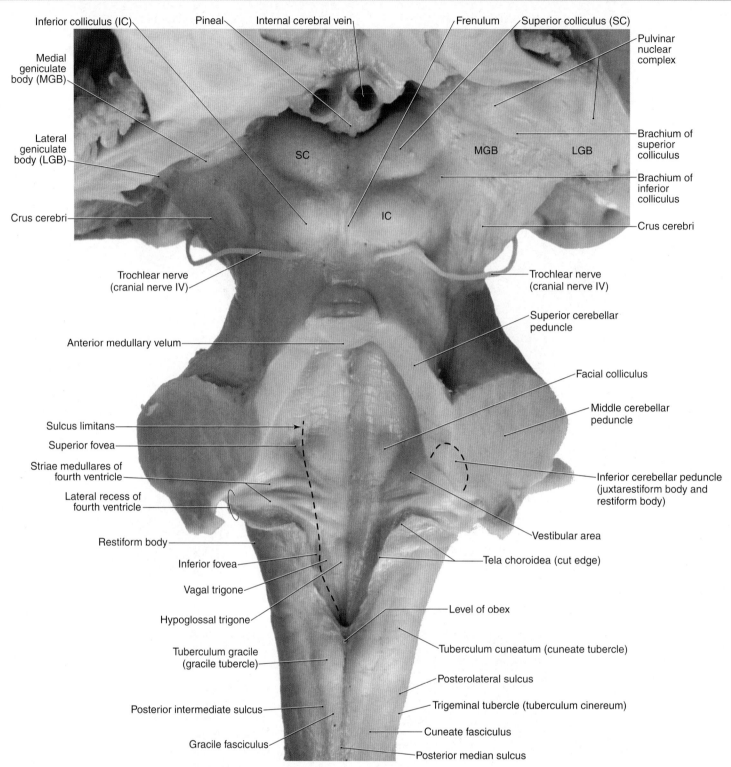

Inferior colliculus (IC)
Pineal
Internal cerebral vein
Frenulum
Superior colliculus (SC)
Pulvinar nuclear complex
Medial geniculate body (MGB)
Lateral geniculate body (LGB)
Brachium of superior colliculus
Brachium of inferior colliculus
Crus cerebri
SC
MGB
LGB
IC
Crus cerebri
Trochlear nerve (cranial nerve IV)
Trochlear nerve (cranial nerve IV)
Superior cerebellar peduncle
Anterior medullary velum
Facial colliculus
Middle cerebellar peduncle
Sulcus limitans
Superior fovea
Striae medullares of fourth ventricle
Lateral recess of fourth ventricle
Inferior cerebellar peduncle (juxtarestiform body and restiform body)
Vestibular area
Restiform body
Tela choroidea (cut edge)
Inferior fovea
Vagal trigone
Level of obex
Hypoglossal trigone
Tuberculum cuneatum (cuneate tubercle)
Tuberculum gracile (gracile tubercle)
Posterolateral sulcus
Posterior intermediate sulcus
Trigeminal tubercle (tuberculum cinereum)
Cuneate fasciculus
Gracile fasciculus
Posterior median sulcus

2-31 Detailed superior (dorsal) view of the **brainstem**, with cerebellum removed, providing a clear view of the **rhomboid fossa** (and floor of the fourth ventricle) and contiguous parts of the caudal **diencephalon.** The dashed line on the left represents the position of the **sulcus limitans** and the area of the **inferior cerebellar peduncle** is shown on the right. This structure is composed of the **restiform body** plus the **juxtarestiform body,** the latter of which contains fibers interconnecting the vestibular area in the lateral floor of the fourth ventricle and cerebellar structures (cortex and nuclei). The

tuberculum cinereum is also called the trigeminal tubercle (tuberculum trigeminale) because it is the surface representation of the spinal trigeminal tract and its underlying nucleus on the lateral aspect of the medulla just caudal to the level of the **obex** (see also Figure 2-32 on the facing page). The **facial colliculus** is formed by the underlying abducens nucleus and internal genu of the facial nerve, the **hypoglossal trigone** by the underlying hypoglossal nucleus, and the **vagal trigone** by the dorsal motor nucleus of the vagal nerve. Also see Figure 2-34 on p. 32.

Vessels

Structures

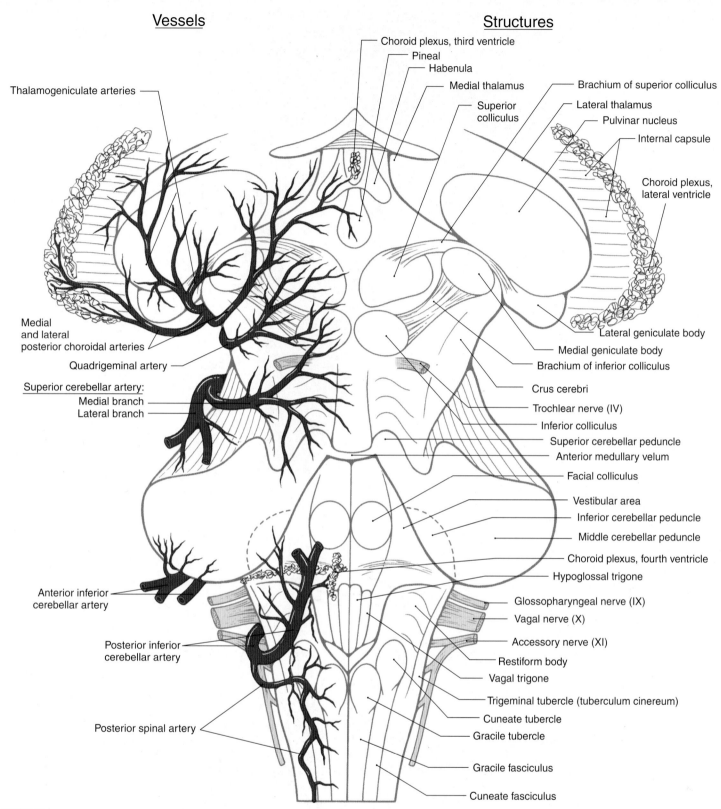

Choroid plexus, third ventricle
Pineal
Habenula
Medial thalamus
Brachium of superior colliculus
Superior colliculus
Lateral thalamus
Pulvinar nucleus
Internal capsule
Thalamogeniculate arteries
Choroid plexus, lateral ventricle
Medial and lateral posterior choroidal arteries
Lateral geniculate body
Medial geniculate body
Quadrigeminal artery
Brachium of inferior colliculus
Crus cerebri
Superior cerebellar artery:
Trochlear nerve (IV)
Medial branch
Inferior colliculus
Lateral branch
Superior cerebellar peduncle
Anterior medullary velum
Facial colliculus
Vestibular area
Inferior cerebellar peduncle
Middle cerebellar peduncle
Choroid plexus, fourth ventricle
Hypoglossal trigone
Anterior inferior cerebellar artery
Glossopharyngeal nerve (IX)
Vagal nerve (X)
Accessory nerve (XI)
Posterior inferior cerebellar artery
Restiform body
Vagal trigone
Trigeminal tubercle (tuberculum cinereum)
Cuneate tubercle
Gracile tubercle
Posterior spinal artery
Gracile fasciculus
Cuneate fasciculus

2-32 Superior (dorsal) view of the **brainstem** and **caudal diencephalon** showing the relationship of structures and some of the cranial nerves to arteries. The vessels shown in this view have originated ventrally and wrapped around the brainstem to gain their dorsal positions. In addition to serving the medulla, branches of the **posterior inferior cerebellar artery** also supply the **choroid plexus** of the fourth ventricle. The **tuberculum cinereum** is also called the **trigeminal tubercle**. For an additional perspective on the blood supply to the choroid plexus of the third and fourth ventricles see Figure 4-10 on p. 68.

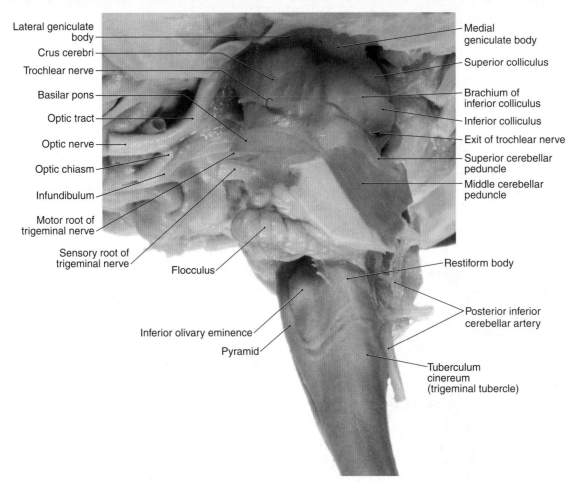

Lateral geniculate body
Crus cerebri
Trochlear nerve
Basilar pons
Optic tract
Optic nerve
Optic chiasm
Infundibulum
Motor root of trigeminal nerve
Sensory root of trigeminal nerve
Flocculus
Inferior olivary eminence
Pyramid

Medial geniculate body
Superior colliculus
Brachium of inferior colliculus
Inferior colliculus
Exit of trochlear nerve
Superior cerebellar peduncle
Middle cerebellar peduncle
Restiform body
Posterior inferior cerebellar artery
Tuberculum cinereum (trigeminal tubercle)

2-33 Lateral view of the left side of the **brainstem** emphasizing structures that are located dorsally and ventrally. Note the several structures, and cranial nerves, seen from this perspective. The cerebellum and portions of the temporal lobe have been removed. Compare with Figure 2-35 on the facing page.

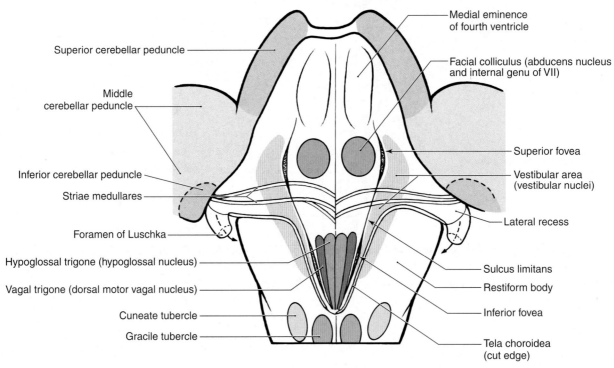

Superior cerebellar peduncle
Middle cerebellar peduncle
Inferior cerebellar peduncle
Striae medullares
Foramen of Luschka
Hypoglossal trigone (hypoglossal nucleus)
Vagal trigone (dorsal motor vagal nucleus)
Cuneate tubercle
Gracile tubercle

Medial eminence of fourth ventricle
Facial colliculus (abducens nucleus and internal genu of VII)
Superior fovea
Vestibular area (vestibular nuclei)
Lateral recess
Sulcus limitans
Restiform body
Inferior fovea
Tela choroidea (cut edge)

2-34 The floor of the fourth ventricle (**rhomboid fossa**) and immediately adjacent structures. The signs and symptoms of lesions in this ventricle may present as deficits representing damage to the **facial colliculus** (sixth nucleus, internal genu of VII), **hypoglossal trigone** (twelfth nucleus), or **vestibular** and possibly **cochlear nuclei**, or may be more global reflecting injury to medullary and pontine centers. The color coding for all structures, other than the cerebellar peduncles, is consistent with that used for the brainstem nuclei in Chapter 6. Also compare with Figure 2-31 on p. 30.

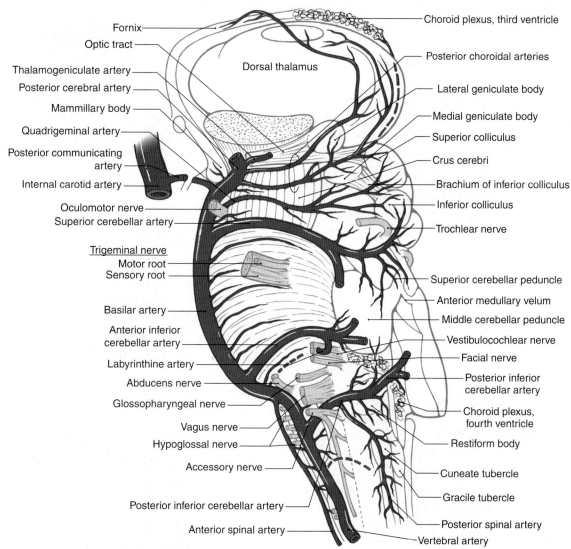

Fornix
Optic tract
Thalamogeniculate artery
Posterior cerebral artery
Mammillary body
Quadrigeminal artery
Posterior communicating artery
Internal carotid artery
Oculomotor nerve
Superior cerebellar artery

Trigeminal nerve
Motor root
Sensory root

Basilar artery
Anterior inferior cerebellar artery
Labyrinthine artery
Abducens nerve
Glossopharyngeal nerve
Vagus nerve
Hypoglossal nerve
Accessory nerve

Posterior inferior cerebellar artery
Anterior spinal artery

Choroid plexus, third ventricle
Dorsal thalamus
Posterior choroidal arteries
Lateral geniculate body
Medial geniculate body
Superior colliculus
Crus cerebri
Brachium of inferior colliculus
Inferior colliculus
Trochlear nerve

Superior cerebellar peduncle
Anterior medullary velum
Middle cerebellar peduncle
Vestibulocochlear nerve
Facial nerve
Posterior inferior cerebellar artery
Choroid plexus, fourth ventricle
Restiform body
Cuneate tubercle
Gracile tubercle
Posterior spinal artery
Vertebral artery

2-35 Lateral view of the **brainstem** and **thalamus,** which shows the relationship of structures and cranial nerves to arteries. The approximate positions of the **labyrinthine** and **posterior spinal arteries,** when they originate from the **basilar** and **vertebral arteries,** respectively, are shown as dashed lines. Arteries that distribute to posterior/dorsal structures originate from the vertebral, basilar, and initial segments of the **posterior cerebral arteries** and arch around the brainstem, or caudal thalamus, to access their targets. From this view, notice the compact nature of the cranial nerves at the pons–medulla junction and the lateral and ventral aspect of the medulla (CNs VI–XII). Compare with Figure 2-33 on the facing page.

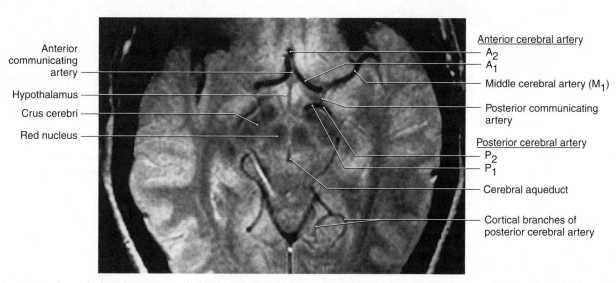

Anterior communicating artery
Hypothalamus
Crus cerebri
Red nucleus

Anterior cerebral artery
A₂
A₁
Middle cerebral artery (M₁)
Posterior communicating artery
Posterior cerebral artery
P₂
P₁
Cerebral aqueduct
Cortical branches of posterior cerebral artery

2-36 An MRI through basal regions of the **hemisphere** and through the **midbrain** showing several major vessels that form part of the **cerebral arterial circle** (of Willis). Compare to Figure 2-21 on p. 23. See Figures 10-9 and 10-10 (pp. 318–319) for comparable MRAs of the cerebral arterial circle.

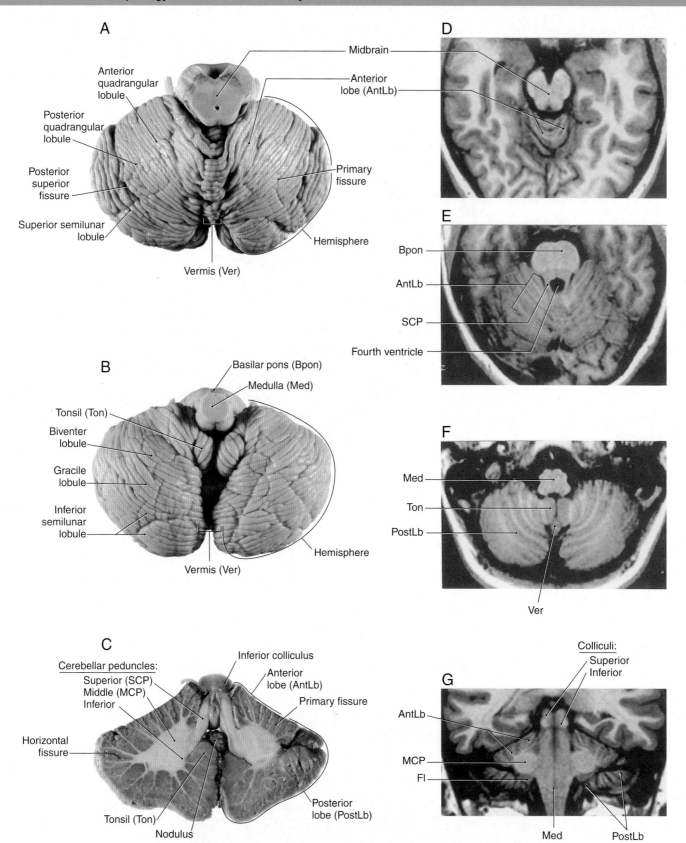

2-37 Rostral (**A,** superior surface), caudal (**B,** inferior surface), and an inferior view (**C,** inferior aspect) of the **cerebellum.**

The view in **C** shows the aspect of the cerebellum that is continuous into the brainstem via **cerebellar peduncles.** The view in **C** correlates with the superior surface of the brainstem (and middle and superior cerebellar peduncles) as shown in Figure 2-31 on p. 30.

Note that the superior view of the cerebellum (**A**) correlates closely with cerebellar structures seen in axial MRIs at comparable levels

(**D, E**). Structures seen on the inferior surface of the cerebellum, such as the **tonsil** (**F**), correlate closely with an axial MRI at a comparable level. In **G**, note the appearance of the margin of the cerebellum, the general appearance and position of the lobes, and the obvious nature of the middle **cerebellar peduncle.** All MRI images are T1-weighted.

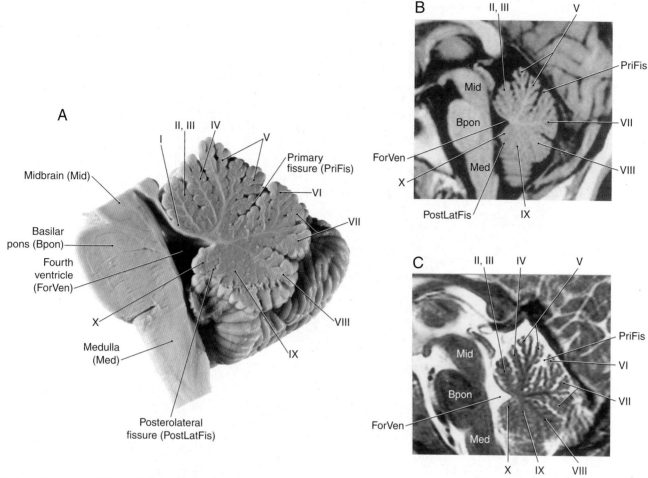

A

Midbrain (Mid)

Basilar
pons (Bpon)

Fourth
ventricle
(ForVen)

X

Medulla
(Med)

I   II, III   IV   V

Primary
fissure (PriFis)

VI

VII

VIII

IX

Posterolateral
fissure (PostLatFis)

B

II, III   V

Mid

Bpon

ForVen

Med

X

PostLatFis   IX

PriFis

VII

VIII

C

II, III   IV   V

Mid

Bpon

ForVen

Med

X   IX   VIII

PriFis

VI

VII

2-38 A median sagittal view of the **cerebellum** (**A**) showing its relationships to the **midbrain, pons,** and **medulla.** This view of the cerebellum also illustrates the two main fissures and the vermis portions of lobules I–X. Designation of these lobules follows the method developed by Larsell.

Lobules I–V are the vermis parts of the **anterior lobe;** lobules VI–IX are the vermis parts of the **posterior lobe;** and lobule X (the nodulus) is the vermis part of the **flocculonodular lobe.** Note the striking similarities between the gross specimen (**A**) and a median sagittal view of the cerebellum in a T1- (**B**) and T2-weighted MRI (**C**).

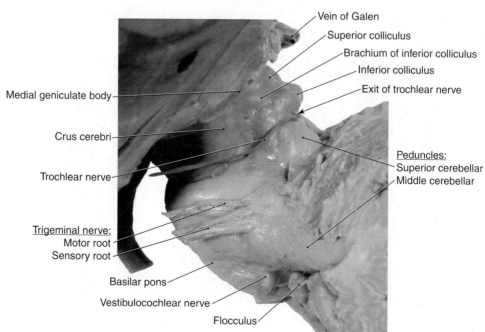

Medial geniculate body

Crus cerebri

Trochlear nerve

Trigeminal nerve:
Motor root
Sensory root

Basilar pons

Vestibulocochlear nerve

Flocculus

Vein of Galen

Superior colliculus

Brachium of inferior colliculus

Inferior colliculus

Exit of trochlear nerve

Peduncles:
Superior cerebellar
Middle cerebellar

2-39 Lateral view of the brainstem showing the **superior** and **inferior colliculi, exit of the trochlear nerve,** and the **crus cerebri.** The exit of the **trigeminal nerve** (motor and sensory roots) differentiates the interface of the **basilar pons** with the **middle cerebellar peduncle.**

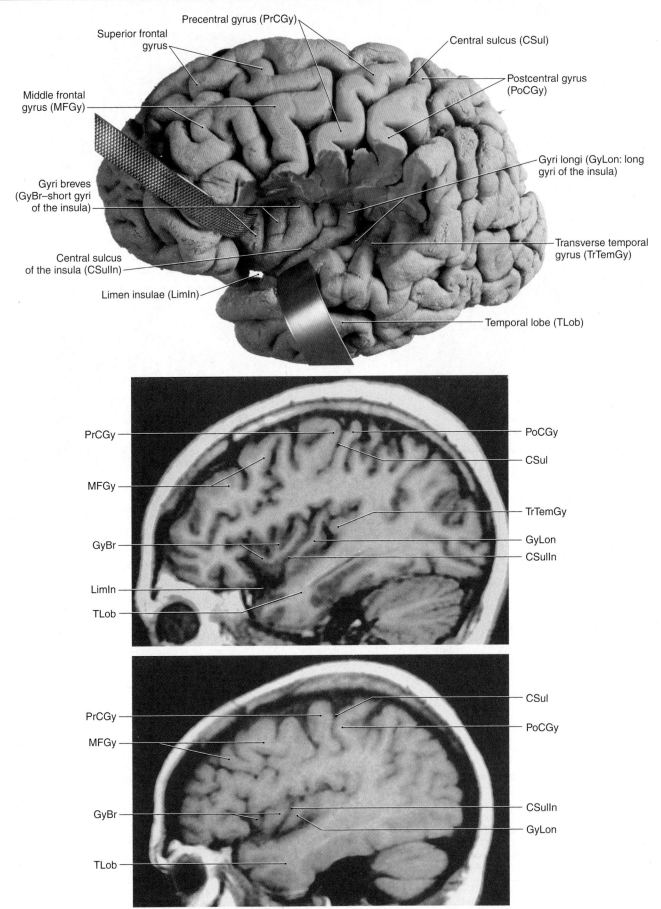

2-40 Lateral view of the left **cerebral hemisphere** with the **frontal** and **parietal opercula** removed and the **temporal operculum** retracted downward exposing the insula. Structures characteristic of the **insular cortex** (including the **long** and **short gyri** and the **central sulcus of the insula**), and immediately adjacent areas, are clearly seen in the two MRIs in the sagittal plane through lateral portions of the hemisphere (inversion recovery—upper; T1-weighted image—lower).

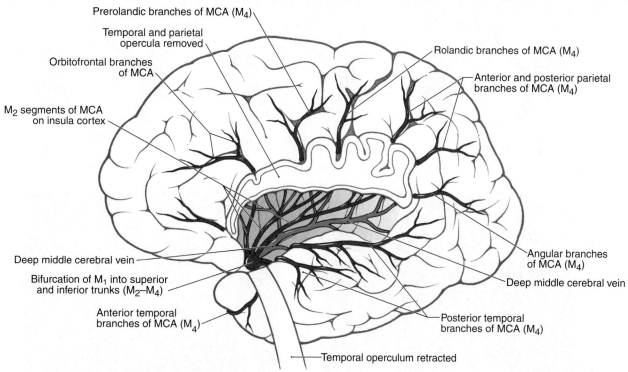

Prerolandic branches of MCA (M₄)

Temporal and parietal
opercula removed

Orbitofrontal branches
of MCA

M₂ segments of MCA
on insula cortex

Deep middle cerebral vein

Bifurcation of M₁ into superior
and inferior trunks (M₂–M₄)

Anterior temporal
branches of MCA (M₄)

Rolandic branches of MCA (M₄)

Anterior and posterior parietal
branches of MCA (M₄)

Angular branches
of MCA (M₄)

Deep middle cerebral vein

Posterior temporal
branches of MCA (M₄)

Temporal operculum retracted

2-41 Lateral view of the left **cerebral hemisphere** showing the pattern of the **middle cerebral artery** (**MCA**) as it branches from **M₁** into **M₂ segments** that pass over the insular cortex. Also shown are the M₄ branches on the surface of the cortex (having exited from the lateral sulcus) and the **deep middle cerebral vein** on the surface of the insula. Compare this view of the vasculature of the insula with the anatomy from the same perspective in Figure 2-40 on the facing page.

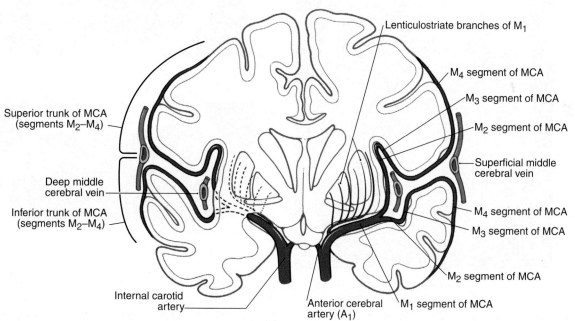

Lenticulostriate branches of M₁

M₄ segment of MCA

M₃ segment of MCA

M₂ segment of MCA

Superficial middle
cerebral vein

Superior trunk of MCA
(segments M₂–M₄)

Deep middle
cerebral vein

Inferior trunk of MCA
(segments M₂–M₄)

Internal carotid
artery

Anterior cerebral
artery (A₁)

M₁ segment of MCA

M₄ segment of MCA

M₃ segment of MCA

M₂ segment of MCA

2-42 Semi-diagrammatic cross-sectional representation of the cerebral hemispheres showing the main arteries and veins related to the **insular cortex**. The **internal carotid artery** branches into the **anterior** and **middle cerebral** (**MCA**) arteries. The first segment of the MCA (**M₁**) passes laterally and diverges into superior and inferior trunks at the **limen insulae** (entrance to the insular cortex). In general, distal branches of the superior trunk course upward and eventually serve the cortex above the lateral sulcus, and distal branches of the inferior trunk course downward to serve the cortex below the lateral sulcus. En route,

these respective branches form the **M₂** (insular part of MCA), **M₃** (opercular part of MCA), and **M₄** (cortical part of MCA) segments, as shown here.

The **deep middle cerebral vein** receives small branches from the area of the insula and joins with the **anterior cerebral vein** to form the **basal vein** (see Figures 2-16 and 2-19 on pp. 19 and 21). The **superficial middle cerebral vein** collects blood from the lateral aspect of the hemisphere and drains into the **cavernous sinus** (see also Figures 2-13, 2-16, and 2-19 on pp. 17, 19, and 21).

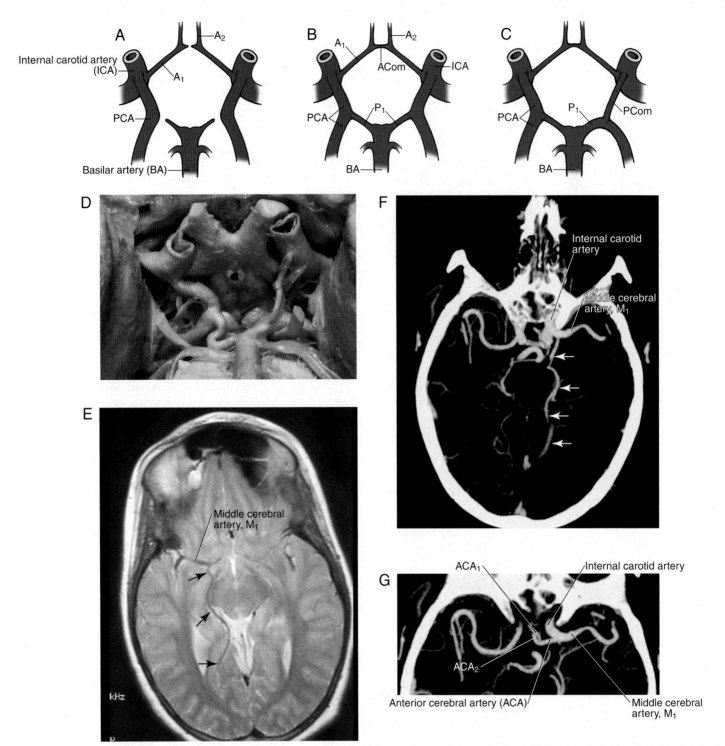

2-43 Early in development, the **posterior cerebral artery** (**PCA**) originates from the **internal carotid artery** (**A**). At this stage, the **cerebral arterial circle** (circle of Willis) is not complete. Vascular sprouts from the basilar artery are growing to meet the PCAs and from the **anterior cerebral arteries** (**ACAs**) to meet on the midline where they will form the **anterior communicating artery** (**ACom**). The initial connection between the basilar artery and the PCA is small (**B**); this will become the adult **P₁ segment**. As development progresses, the initially small P₁ segment enlarges in diameter (to form the major connection between the basilar and the distal PCA, the adult P₁) and the initially large portion of the PCA between the internal carotid artery and the PCA–P₁ junction becomes smaller in diameter (to form the **posterior communicating artery** [**PCom**] of the adult, **C**).

In 22%–25% of adult individuals, the territory served by the PCA is perfused mainly from the internal carotid artery. This is due to the fact that the fetal pattern of the PCA arising from the internal carotid persists into the adult. This is called a **fetal PCA**, or a **persistent fetal PCA**. Examples of a **fetal PCA** are shown here in a specimen (**D**, fetal PCA is on the patient's right, normal pattern on patient's left) and in MRI (**E**, arrows) and CT angiogram (**F**, arrows). Note that in the MRI-T2 (**E**, axial), the PCA can be easily followed from the internal carotid into the occipital lobe (arrows) with no evidence of any substantive connection to a P₁.

A fetal PCA in the adult may coexist with other vascular patterns that deviate from normal. In the axial images in **F and G** (CTA), a **fetal PCA** is present on the patient's left (**F**, arrows) and in the same patient, a single trunk from the left internal carotid artery (**G**) gives origin to both the right and left **anterior cerebral arteries** (**ACA₁** becomes the right ACA; **ACA₂** becomes the left ACA). This is an **azygous** (single or unpaired) **ACA**.

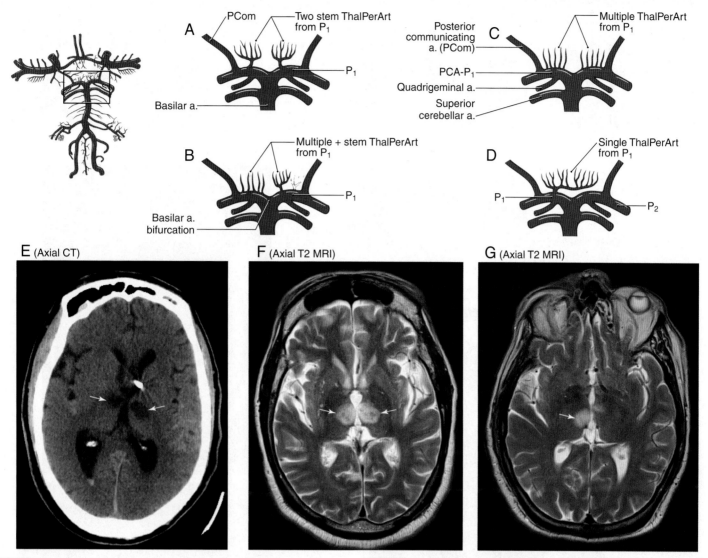

E (Axial CT) F (Axial T2 MRI) G (Axial T2 MRI)

2-44 The **thalamoperforating arteries** (ThalPerArt) arise from the **P₁ segment** of the **posterior cerebral artery** (PCA), the part of the PCA located between the bifurcation of the basilar artery and the junction of the posterior communicating artery with the PCA. This vessel serves primarily the rostral and medial areas of the thalamus that are important synaptic stations in the ascending reticular activating system that influences cortical arousal.

The most common pattern of origin for the thalamoperforating vessels (about 42% of cases) is a single stem artery on each side that branches to serve the thalamus on that side (**A**). One or two single stem vessels on one P₁ with multiple branches from the opposite P₁ (**B**) are seen in about 26% of cases, and small multiple branches from each P₁ (**C**) are the pattern present in about 20% of cases.

The least common, but perhaps most problematic, pattern is when a single stem vessel (sometimes called the **artery of Percheron**) originates from one P₁ and branches to serve both thalami (**D**); this is seen in about 8% of cases. Damage to, or occlusion of, this single stem, or of one stem when there is only one on each side, may adversely affect cortical arousal, consciousness, and contribute to drowsiness, stupor, or coma (**E–G**). In patient **E** (white arrows), a single stem (**D**) was inadvertently trapped during aneurysm surgery, resulting in bilateral lesions (hypodensities in the anterior thalamus in CT). Patient **F** (white arrows) had bilateral strokes in the thalamoperforator territory (hyperintensities in T2, cause unknown); both patients **E** and **F** were comatose post event. A predominately unilateral stroke in this same arterial territory (**G**, hyperintensity in T2 at white arrow) resulted in a patient that was lethargic, in and out of consciousness, and difficult to arouse, but was not comatose.

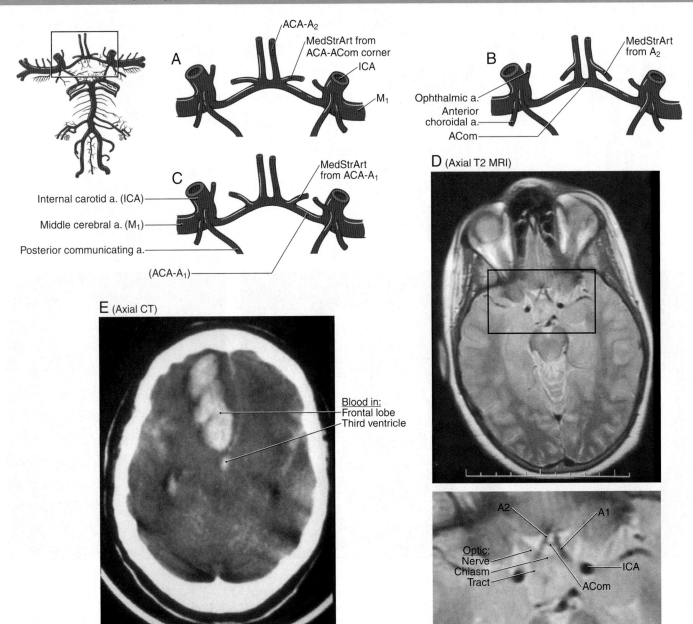

A

ACA-A₂
MedStrArt from
ACA-ACom corner
ICA
M₁

B

MedStrArt
from A₂
Ophthalmic a.
Anterior
choroidal a.
ACom

C

MedStrArt
from ACA-A₁
Internal carotid a. (ICA)
Middle cerebral a. (M₁)
Posterior communicating a.
(ACA-A₁)

D (Axial T2 MRI)

A2   A1
Optic:
Nerve
Chiasm   ICA
Tract   ACom

E (Axial CT)

Blood in:
Frontal lobe
Third ventricle

2-45 The **medial striate artery** (**MedStrArt**), also called the **artery of Heubner**, arises from the **anterior cerebral artery** (**ACA**) in the vicinity of its junction with the **anterior communicating artery** (**ACom**). This intersection is frequently called the "**ACA–ACom corner**" (**A, D**). Structures characteristically found in this area, in addition to the vessels, are the optic nerve, chiasm, and tract, adjacent gyri of the frontal lobe, subarachnoid cisterns (chiasmatic, of the lamina terminalis, interpeduncular), and the lamina terminalis (separating cisterns from the third ventricle) (**D**).

The medial striate artery usually arises from the lateral aspect of the ACA. A large sample of cadaver brains (200) and surgical procedures (375) revealed that about 42% arose from the "corner" (**A**), about 26% from proximal A₂ (**B**), and less than 3% from the distal A₁

(**C**). Recognizing that the origin of the medial striate artery from the ACA may be variable, it is convenient to remember that this vessel usually arises at, or just distal, to the corner. Vascular patterns in this region are highly variable and include azygous (single) or three A₂ segments, both ACAs arising from one side (Figure 2-43G, p. 38), a duplicated or a fenestrated ACom, and occasional asymmetrical origins of its branches.

Aneurysms in this area may arise from the medial aspect of the "corner" or from the branches of the ACom. When an aneurysm at this location ruptures, the extravasated blood may be located in the subarachnoid cisterns in the immediate area, dissect into the frontal lobe, or enter the third ventricle, and ventricular system, through damage to the lamina terminalis (**E**).

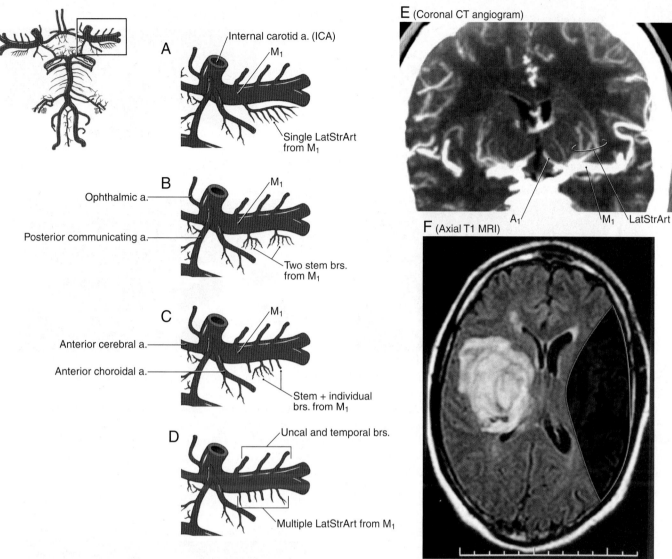

A — Internal carotid a. (ICA) / M₁ / Single LatStrArt from M₁

B — Ophthalmic a. / Posterior communicating a. / M₁ / Two stem brs. from M₁

C — Anterior cerebral a. / Anterior choroidal a. / M₁ / Stem + individual brs. from M₁

D — Uncal and temporal brs. / Multiple LatStrArt from M₁

E (Coronal CT angiogram) — A₁ / M₁ / LatStrArt

F (Axial T1 MRI)

2-46 The **lateral striate arteries (LatStrArt)** are commonly called the **lenticulostriate arteries;** they arise from the M_1 **segment** of the **middle cerebral artery** in three general patterns. About 40% originate as a single stem and then branch into numerous vessels that penetrate the hemisphere via the anterior perforated substance to serve much of the lenticular nucleus and adjacent structures, such as the internal capsule (**A, E**). In approximately 30% of cases, these vessels arise as two stems that divide into numerous penetrating branches (**B**); a variation on this theme is one stem with several direct M_1 branches (**C**). In a similar numbers of cases (about 30%), the lenticulostriate vessels originate as a series of many small arteries directly from the M_1 segment (**D**).

Hemorrhage of the lenticulostriate arteries within the hemisphere, assuming no occlusion of the parent M_1 vessel but with only damage to its branches, results in a lesion within the hemisphere with sparing of the blood supply (the M_1 is patent) to the cerebral cortex (**F**, lesion on right). In contrast, occlusion of the parent vessel, for example the M_1 **segment,** may result in infarction of all territories served by this vessel distal to the obstruction including the basal nuclei, portions of the internal capsule, and all distal cortex (**F,** outline on left).

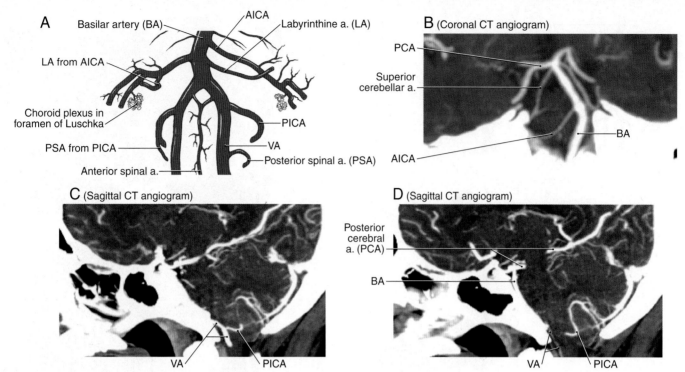

2-47 The **anterior (AICA)** and **posterior (PICA) inferior cerebellar arteries** originate from the **basilar (BA)** and **vertebral arteries (VA)** respectively (**A**). The **AICA** arises from approximately the lower third of the basilar artery in about 75% of patients (**A, B**). In 50%–60% of individuals, it is a single basilar branch on each side, two branches in 20%, and three branches in 20%. The **labyrinthine artery,** an important blood supply to the inner ear, arises from the AICA about 85% of the time and from the basilar in 15% of individuals.

The **PICA** commonly arises as a single branch from each vertebral artery (90% of cases) but is duplicated 6% of the time (**A, C, D: C** and **D** are two different sagittal planes in the same patient to show the continuity of PICA). In 75% of cases, the **posterior spinal artery** is a branch of PICA; about 25% of the time it is a vertebral branch.

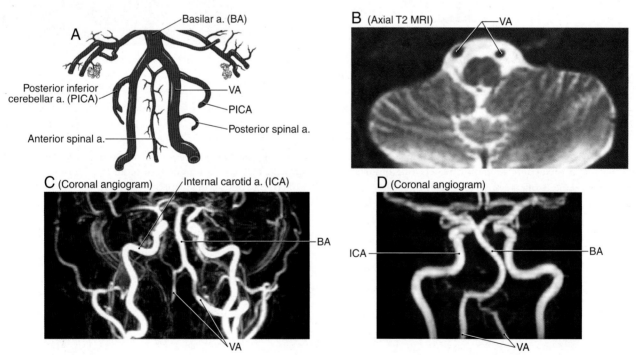

2-48 The **vertebral arteries (VAs)** are generally equal in size in about 25%–30% of cases, or one may be larger than the other (**A, B**). For example, the left vertebral may be slightly larger about 43% of the time (**C**) and the right vertebral in about 33% of cases (**D**). In a minority of individuals, either vertebral artery may be hypoplastic (about 4%–6%; see also Figure 10-12). In less than 1% of cases, the vertebral artery may become the **PICA** on one side; the other vertebral becoming the basilar. Occasionally one of these variations may coexist with a second.

Q&A for this chapter is available online on thePoint

Cranial Nerves

3

Cranial Nerve Deficits in Representative Brainstem Lesions (Figures 3-1 to 3-8)

Table 3-1 Synopsis of Cranial Nerves*

CRANIAL NERVE	COMPONENT(S)	FUNCTION	ATTACHMENT TO BRAIN	ASSOCIATED FORAMEN/FORAMINA	DEFICITS
Olfactory (CN I)	Special sense (SVA/VA)	Sense of smell	Olfactory bulb, olfactory trigone	Ethmoid foramina of cribriform plate	Anosmia, hyposmia, hyperosmia, and olfactory hypesthesia/hyperesthesia
Optic (CN II)	Special sense (SSA/SA)	Vision	Optic chiasm (optic nerve to chiasm to tract)	Optic canal	Blindness, hemianopia, quadrantanopia, and loss of afferent limb corneal reflex (see Figs. on pp. 262–267)
Oculomotor (CN III)	Somatic motor (GSE/SE) Visceral motor (SVE/VE)	Eye movement Pupil constriction	Oculomotor sulcus, medial part of cerebral peduncle With root of CN III	Superior orbital fissure Superior orbital fissure	Paralysis of most eye movement and diplopia (see Figs. on pp. 226–229) Pupillary dilation and loss of efferent limb corneal reflex (see Figs. on pp. 226–229)
Trochlear (CN IV)	Somatic motor (GSE/SE)	Eye movement	Midbrain, caudal to inferior colliculus	Superior orbital fissure	Inability to look down-and-out and diplopia (see Figs. on pp. 226–229)
Trigeminal (CN V)	Somatic sense (GSA/SA) Pharyngeal motor (SVE/SE)	Sensation in face, sinuses, oral cavity, teeth, eyelids, cornea, tongue, forehead, TMJ, and palate (see Figs. on pp. 202–205) Motor to masticatory muscles plus others (see Figs. on pp. 230–233)	Lateral aspect of pons Lateral aspect of pons	Superior orbital fissure (V_1); Foramen rotundum (V_2); Foramen ovale (V_3) Foramen ovale	Loss of sensation on areas of face and in oral cavity served by each division; loss of afferent limb corneal and jaw-jerk reflexes (see Figs. on pp. 202–205) Masticatory muscle weakness/paralysis and loss of efferent limb jaw-jerk reflex (see Figs. on pp. 230–233)
Abducens (CN VI)	Somatic motor (GSE/SE)	Eye movement	Pons–medulla junction (medial location)	Superior orbital fissure	Lateral gaze palsy and diplopia (see Figs. on pp. 226–229)
Facial (CN VII)	Pharyngeal motor (SVE/SE) Visceral motor (GVE/VE) Special sense (SVA/VA) Somatic sense (GSA/SA) Visceral sense (GVA/VA)	Motor to muscles of facial expression plus others (see Figs. on pp. 230–233) To parasympathetic ganglia (see Figs. on pp. 230–233) Taste from anterior two-thirds of tongue (see Figs. on pp. 202–203, 206–207) Sensation on pinna (see Figs. on pp. 202–203) Visceral sense from salivary glands	Pons–medulla junction (intermediate location)	Internal acoustic meatus and stylomastoid foramen Internal acoustic meatus Internal acoustic meatus and stylomastoid foramen Internal acoustic meatus and stylomastoid foramen Internal acoustic meatus and stylomastoid foramen	Weakness/paralysis of facial muscles and loss of efferent limb corneal reflex (see Figs. on pp. 230–233) Decrease in secretions Loss of taste on anterior two-thirds of tongue (see Figs. on pp. 206–207, 232–233) Loss of ear sensation (see Figs. on pp. 232–233)
Vestibulocochlear (CN VIII)	Special sense (SSA/SA)	Hearing, balance, and equilibrium (see Figs. on pp. 270–273)	Pons–medulla junction (lateral location)	Internal acoustic meatus Associated	Deafness, tinnitus, vertigo, unsteady gait, and nystagmus (see Figs. on pp. 270–273)

Cranial Nerve	Component(s)	Function	Attachment to Brain	Associated Foramen/Foramina	Deficits
Glossopharyngeal (CN IX)	Pharyngeal motor (SVE/SE)	Motor to stylopharyngeus muscle (see Figs. on pp. 230–233)	Postolivary sulcus	Jugular foramen	Difficulty swallowing and loss of gag reflex (see Figs. on pp. 230–233)
	Visceral motor (GVE/VE)	To otic ganglion then parotid (see Figs. on pp. 230–233)			Decrease of secretory function
	Special sense (SVA/VA)	Taste from posterior third of tongue (see Figs. on pp. 206–207, 232–233)	Postolivary sulcus	Jugular foramen	Loss of taste on posterior third of tongue; not tested (see Figs. on pp. 230–233)
	Somatic sense (GSA/SA)	Sensation in external auditory meatus (see Figs. on pp. 202–203, 232–233)			Loss of sensation in external auditory meatus (see Figs. on pp. 230–233)
	Visceral sense (GVA/VA)	From carotid body/sinus, parotid, and pharynx			Possible bradycardia or tachycardia
Vagus (CN X)	Pharyngeal motor (SVE/SE)	Motor to constrictors of pharynx, intrinsic laryngeal muscles, much of palate, upper esophagus, and vocalis (see Figs. on pp. 230–231)	Postolivary sulcus	Jugular foramen	Dysphagia, dysarthria, loss of vocalis function (hoarseness), and loss of gag reflex (see Figs. on pp. 214–217, 230–233)
	Visceral motor (GVE/VE)	To ganglia in/on trachea, bronchi, gut, and heart (see Figs. on pp. 230–231)			Decrease in secretory action and effect on intestinal motility and heart rate (see Figs. on pp. 230–233)
	Special sense (SVA/VA)	From taste buds on epiglottis, base of tongue, and palate (see Figs. on pp. 206–207)			Loss of taste; not tested
	Somatic sense (GSA/SA)	Sensation on eardrum, external auditory meatus, and dura of posterior fossa (see Figs. on pp. 202–203)			Loss of sensation in external auditory meatus and on eardrum (see Figs. on pp. 230–233)
	Visceral sense (GVA/VA)	From larynx, pharynx, heart, trachea and bronchi, esophagus, and gut (see Figs. on pp. 206–207)			Decrease/loss of sensations from viscera; may affect gag reflex
Accessory (CN XI)	Somatic motor (GSE/SE)	Motor to sternocleidomastoid and trapezius muscles (see Figs. on pp. 226–227)	Lateral aspect of spinal cord C1–C4/C5	Enters foramen magnum; exits jugular foramen	Weakness of trapezius and sternocleidomastoid muscles (see Figs. on pp. 214–217)
Hypoglossal (CN XII)	Somatic motor (GSE/SE)	Motor to extrinsic and intrinsic tongue muscles (see Figs. on pp. 226–227)	Preolivary sulcus	Hypoglossal canal	Deviation of the tongue on protrusion (see Figs. on pp. 214–217, 226–229)

*This table is not intended to be all inclusive, but to serve as a brief overview. Details of structures innervated and their functions and of the various deficits seen following root lesions of cranial nerves (or central lesions that influence cranial nerve function) are available in the respective figures indicated in this table and in other portions of this chapter and Chapter 6. The functional component designations used on this table integrate the traditional and contemporary versions that are explained in Figure 6-1 on p. 96.

CN, cranial nerve; TMJ, temporomandibular joint; V₁, ophthalmic nerve; V₂, maxillary nerve; V₃, mandibular nerve.

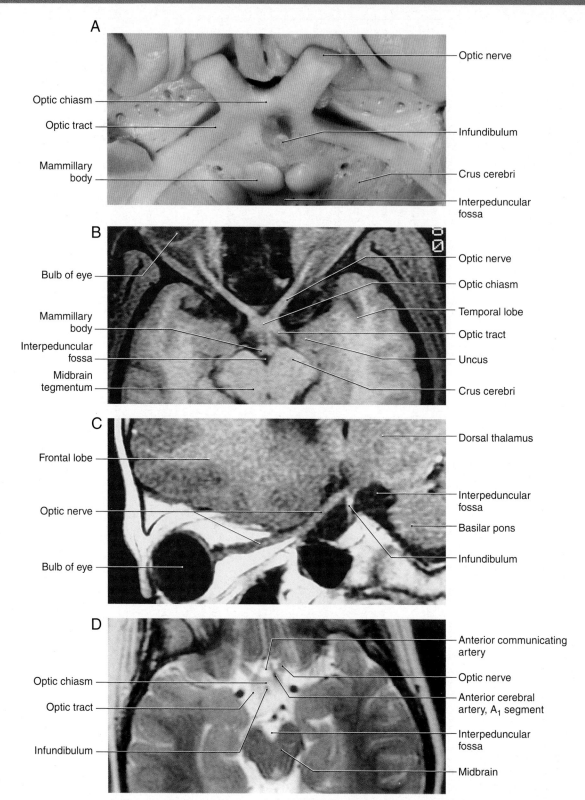

A

Optic chiasm
Optic tract
Mammillary body

Optic nerve
Infundibulum
Crus cerebri
Interpeduncular fossa

B

Bulb of eye
Mammillary body
Interpeduncular fossa
Midbrain tegmentum

Optic nerve
Optic chiasm
Temporal lobe
Optic tract
Uncus
Crus cerebri

C

Frontal lobe
Optic nerve
Bulb of eye

Dorsal thalamus
Interpeduncular fossa
Basilar pons
Infundibulum

D

Optic chiasm
Optic tract
Infundibulum

Anterior communicating artery
Optic nerve
Anterior cerebral artery, A$_1$ segment
Interpeduncular fossa
Midbrain

3-1 Inferior view of the hemisphere showing the optic nerve (II), chiasm, tract, and related structures (**A**). The MRIs of cranial nerve (CN) II are shown in axial (**B**, T1-weighted; **D**, T2-weighted) and in oblique sagittal (**C**, T1-weighted) planes. Note the similarity between the axial planes, especially (**B**), and the gross anatomical specimen. In addition, note the relationship between the anterior cerebral artery, anterior communicating artery, and the structures around the optic chiasm (**D**).

The anterior communicating artery or its junction with the anterior cerebral artery (**D**) is the most common site of supratentorial (carotid system) **aneurysms**. Rupture of aneurysms at this location is one of the more common causes of **spontaneous** (also called **nontraumatic**) sub-arachnoid hemorrhage. The proximity of these vessels to optic structures and the hypothalamus (**D**) explains the variety of visual and hypothalamic disorders that may be experienced by these patients. A lesion of the optic nerve results in **blindness** in that eye and loss of the afferent limb of the **pupillary light reflex**. Lesions caudal to the optic chiasm result in deficits in the visual fields of both eyes (**contralateral [right or left] homonymous hemianopia**).

The anterior choroidal artery serves the optic tract and portions of the internal capsule immediately internal to this structure. This explains the unusual combination of a **homonymous hemianopia** coupled with a contralateral **hemiplegia** and **hemianesthesia** (to all somatosensory modalities) in the **anterior choroidal artery syndrome**.

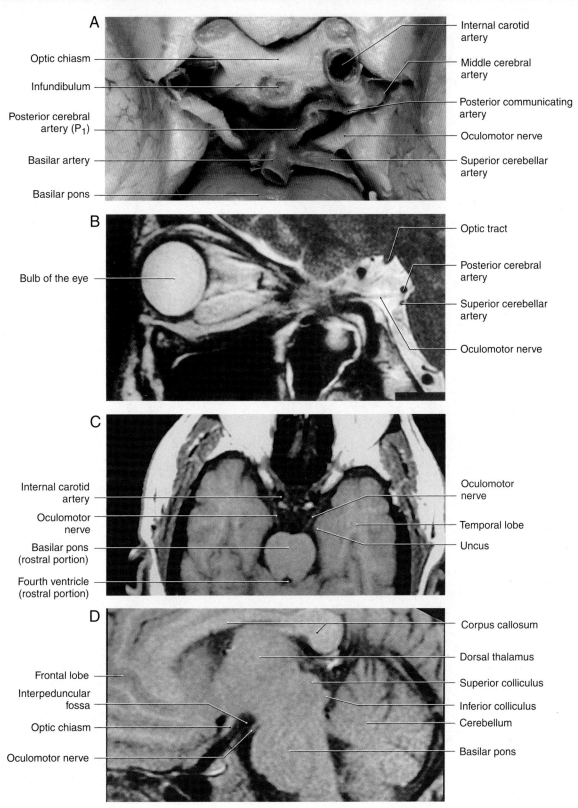

A

- Optic chiasm
- Infundibulum
- Posterior cerebral artery (P₁)
- Basilar artery
- Basilar pons
- Internal carotid artery
- Middle cerebral artery
- Posterior communicating artery
- Oculomotor nerve
- Superior cerebellar artery

B

- Bulb of the eye
- Optic tract
- Posterior cerebral artery
- Superior cerebellar artery
- Oculomotor nerve

C

- Internal carotid artery
- Oculomotor nerve
- Basilar pons (rostral portion)
- Fourth ventricle (rostral portion)
- Oculomotor nerve
- Temporal lobe
- Uncus

D

- Frontal lobe
- Interpeduncular fossa
- Optic chiasm
- Oculomotor nerve
- Corpus callosum
- Dorsal thalamus
- Superior colliculus
- Inferior colliculus
- Cerebellum
- Basilar pons

3-2 Inferior view of the hemisphere showing the exiting fibers of the oculomotor nerve (III), and their relationship to the posterior cerebral and superior cerebellar arteries (**A**). The MRIs of cranial nerve III are shown in sagittal (**B**, T2-weighted; **D**, T1-weighted) and in axial (**C**, T1-weighted) planes. Note the relationship of the exiting fibers of the oculomotor nerve to the posterior cerebral and superior cerebellar arteries (**A, B**) and the characteristic appearance of CN III as it passes through the subarachnoid space toward the superior orbital fissure (**C**). The sagittal section (**D**) is just off the midline and shows the position of the oculomotor nerve in the interpeduncular fossa rostral to the basilar pons and caudal to optic structures.

That portion of the posterior cerebral artery located between the basilar artery and posterior communicating artery (**A**) is the P₁ segment. The most common site of **aneurysms** in the infratentorial area (vertebrobasilar system) is at the bifurcation of the basilar artery, also called the basilar tip. Patients with aneurysms at this location may present with **eye movement disorders, pupillary dilation** caused by damage to the root of the third nerve, and **diplopia.**

Rupture of a **basilar tip aneurysm** may result in the cardinal signs (sudden **severe headache, nausea, vomiting,** and possibly **syncope**) that signal a stroke as broadly defined. In addition, the extravasated blood may dissect its way into the ventricular system through the floor of the third ventricle.

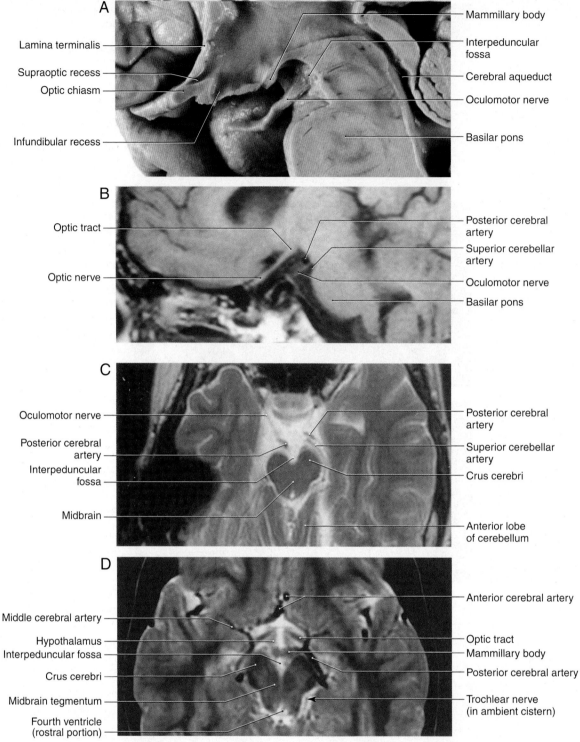

A

Lamina terminalis
Supraoptic recess
Optic chiasm
Infundibular recess

Mammillary body
Interpeduncular fossa
Cerebral aqueduct
Oculomotor nerve
Basilar pons

B

Optic tract
Optic nerve

Posterior cerebral artery
Superior cerebellar artery
Oculomotor nerve
Basilar pons

C

Oculomotor nerve
Posterior cerebral artery
Interpeduncular fossa
Midbrain

Posterior cerebral artery
Superior cerebellar artery
Crus cerebri
Anterior lobe of cerebellum

D

Middle cerebral artery
Hypothalamus
Interpeduncular fossa
Crus cerebri
Midbrain tegmentum
Fourth ventricle (rostral portion)

Anterior cerebral artery
Optic tract
Mammillary body
Posterior cerebral artery
Trochlear nerve (in ambient cistern)

3-3 A median sagittal view of the brainstem and diencephalon (A) reveals the position of the oculomotor nerve (III) in relation to adjacent structures. The MRI in B and C show the position of the oculomotor nerve in sagittal (B, T1-weighted) and in axial (C, T2-weighted) planes. Note the relationship of the oculomotor nerve to the adjacent posterior cerebral and superior cerebellar arteries (B, C). Also compare these images with that of Figure 3-2B on p. 47. In D (T2-weighted), the trochlear nerve is seen passing through the ambient cistern around the lateral aspect of the midbrain (compare with Figures 2-39 on p. 35 and 5-15 on p. 91).

The oculomotor (III) and trochlear (IV) nerves are the cranial nerves of the midbrain. The third nerve exits via the interpeduncular fossa to innervate four major extraocular muscles (see Figure 8-19 on p. 226), and through the ciliary ganglion, the sphincter pupillae muscles. Damage to the oculomotor nerve may result in **paralysis of most eye movement, a dilated pupil**, and loss of the efferent limb of the **pupillary light reflex**, all in the ipsilateral eye. The fourth nerve is unique in that it is the only cranial nerve to exit the posterior (dorsal) aspect of the brainstem and is the only cranial nerve motor nucleus to innervate, exclusively, a muscle on the contralateral side of the midline. Damage to the third and fourth nerves also results in **diplopia**.

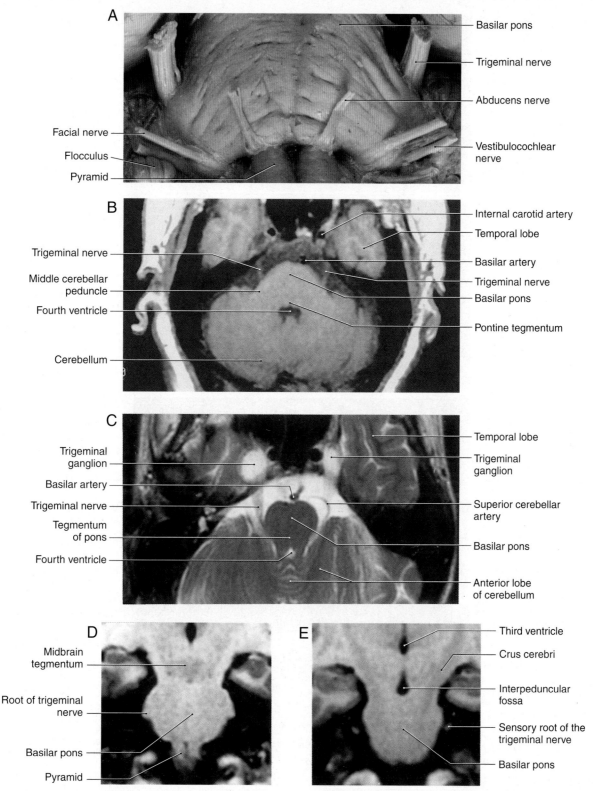

A
— Basilar pons
— Trigeminal nerve
— Abducens nerve
Facial nerve —
Flocculus —
Pyramid —
— Vestibulocochlear nerve

B
Trigeminal nerve —
Middle cerebellar peduncle —
Fourth ventricle —
Cerebellum —
— Internal carotid artery
— Temporal lobe
— Basilar artery
— Trigeminal nerve
— Basilar pons
— Pontine tegmentum

C
Trigeminal ganglion —
Basilar artery —
Trigeminal nerve —
Tegmentum of pons —
Fourth ventricle —
— Temporal lobe
— Trigeminal ganglion
— Superior cerebellar artery
— Basilar pons
— Anterior lobe of cerebellum

D
Midbrain tegmentum —
Root of trigeminal nerve —
Basilar pons —
Pyramid —

E
— Third ventricle
— Crus cerebri
— Interpeduncular fossa
— Sensory root of the trigeminal nerve
— Basilar pons

3-4 The trigeminal nerve (V) is the largest of the cranial nerve roots of the brainstem (**A**). It exits at an intermediate position on the lateral aspect of the pons roughly in line with CNs VII, IX, and X. The fifth nerve and these latter three are mixed nerves in that they have motor and sensory components. The trigeminal nerve is shown in axial MRI (**B**, T1-weighted; **C**, T2-weighted) and coronal planes (**D, E**, both T1-weighted images). Note the characteristic appearance of the root of the trigeminal nerve as it traverses the subarachnoid space (**B, C**), origin of the trigeminal nerve, and position of the sensory root of the nerve at the lateral aspect of the pons in the coronal plane (**D, E**). In addition, the MRI in C clearly illustrates the position of the trigeminal ganglion in the middle cranial fossa.

Trigeminal neuralgia (tic douloureux) is a lancinating paroxysmal pain within the V_2 to V_3 territories frequently triggered by stimuli around the corner of the mouth. The causes probably are multiple and may include neurovascular compression by aberrant branches of the superior cerebellar artery (see the apposition of this vessel to the nerve root in C), **multiple sclerosis, tumors,** and ephaptic transmission within the nerve or ganglion.

There are multiple medical treatments for trigeminal neuralgia; when these fail, surgical therapy may include peripheral nerve section or neurectomy, microvascular decompression, or percutaneous trigeminal rhizotomy.

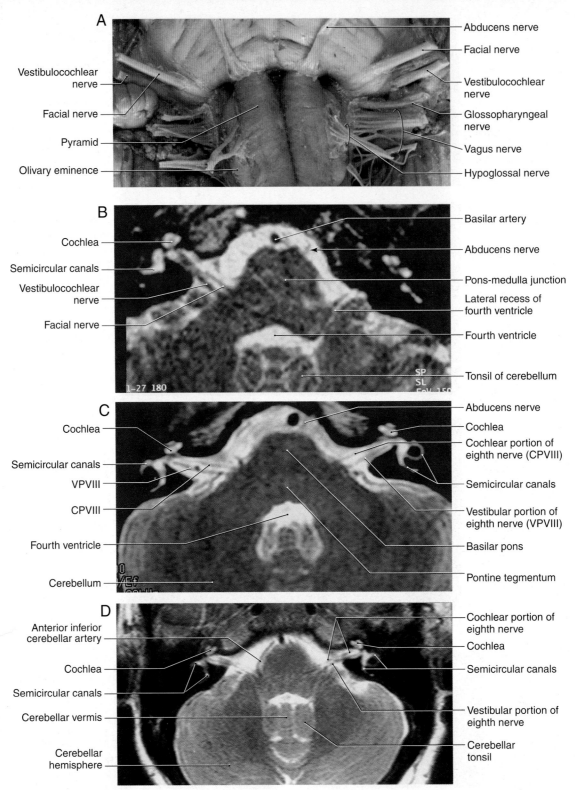

A

Vestibulocochlear nerve
Facial nerve
Pyramid
Olivary eminence

Abducens nerve
Facial nerve
Vestibulocochlear nerve
Glossopharyngeal nerve
Vagus nerve
Hypoglossal nerve

B

Cochlea
Semicircular canals
Vestibulocochlear nerve
Facial nerve

Basilar artery
Abducens nerve
Pons-medulla junction
Lateral recess of fourth ventricle
Fourth ventricle
Tonsil of cerebellum

C

Cochlea
Semicircular canals
VPVIII
CPVIII
Fourth ventricle
Cerebellum

Abducens nerve
Cochlea
Cochlear portion of eighth nerve (CPVIII)
Semicircular canals
Vestibular portion of eighth nerve (VPVIII)
Basilar pons
Pontine tegmentum

D

Anterior inferior cerebellar artery
Cochlea
Semicircular canals
Cerebellar vermis
Cerebellar hemisphere

Cochlear portion of eighth nerve
Cochlea
Semicircular canals
Vestibular portion of eighth nerve
Cerebellar tonsil

3-5 The cranial nerves at the pons–medulla junction are the abducens (VI), the facial (VII), and the vestibulocochlear (VIII) (**A**). The facial and vestibulocochlear nerves both enter the internal acoustic meatus, the facial nerve distributing eventually to the face through the stylomastoid foramen, and the vestibulocochlear nerve to structures of the inner ear. MRIs in the axial plane, **B, C, D** (all T2-weighted images) show the relationships of the vestibulocochlear root and the facial nerve to the internal acoustic meatus. Also notice the characteristic appearance of the cochlea (**B, C**) and the semicircular canals (**B, C**). In addition to these two cranial nerves, the labyrinthine branch of the anterior inferior cerebellar artery also enters the internal acoustic meatus and sends branches to serve the cochlea and semicircular canals and their respective ganglia.

The tumor commonly associated with the eighth nerve is correctly called a **vestibular schwannoma** because it arises from the **neurilemma sheath of the vestibular root**. It is not correct to refer to this as an *acoustic neuroma*; it is neither acoustic (does not arise for the cochlear root) nor a neuroma (does not arise from nerve tissue).

Most patients with this tumor have **hearing loss, tinnitus,** and **equilibrium problems,** or **vertigo.** As the tumor enlarges (to more than about 2 cm) it may cause **facial weakness** (seventh root), numbness (fifth root), or abnormal **corneal reflex** (fifth or seventh root). Treatment is usually by surgery, radiation therapy, or a combination thereof.

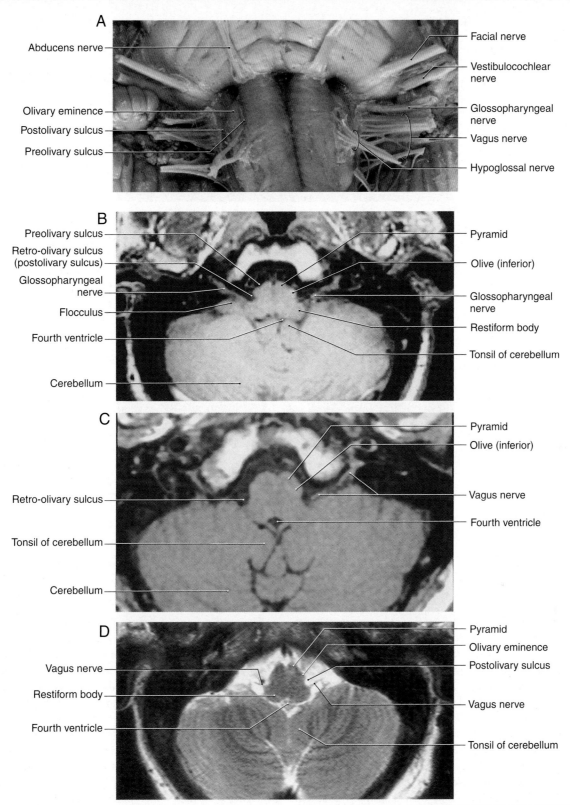

A

Abducens nerve

Olivary eminence
Postolivary sulcus
Preolivary sulcus

Facial nerve
Vestibulocochlear nerve
Glossopharyngeal nerve
Vagus nerve
Hypoglossal nerve

B

Preolivary sulcus
Retro-olivary sulcus (postolivary sulcus)
Glossopharyngeal nerve
Flocculus
Fourth ventricle
Cerebellum

Pyramid
Olive (inferior)
Glossopharyngeal nerve
Restiform body
Tonsil of cerebellum

C

Retro-olivary sulcus
Tonsil of cerebellum
Cerebellum

Pyramid
Olive (inferior)
Vagus nerve
Fourth ventricle

D

Vagus nerve
Restiform body
Fourth ventricle

Pyramid
Olivary eminence
Postolivary sulcus
Vagus nerve
Tonsil of cerebellum

3-6 The glossopharyngeal (IX) and vagus (X) nerves (**A**) exit the lateral aspect of the medulla via the postolivary sulcus; the ninth nerve exits rostral to the row of rootlets comprising the tenth nerve (**A**). These nerves are generally in line with the exits of the facial and trigeminal nerves; all of these are mixed nerves. The exit of the glossopharyngeal nerve (**A, B**) is close to the pons–medulla junction and correlates with the corresponding shape (more rectangular) of the medulla. The vagus nerve exits at a slightly more caudal position (**A, C, D**); the shape of the medulla is more square and the fourth ventricle is smaller. The ninth and tenth cranial nerves and the spinal portion of the accessory nerve (XI) exit the skull via the jugular foramen.

Glossopharyngeal neuralgia is a lancinating pain originating from the territories served by the ninth and tenth nerves at the base of the tongue and throat. Trigger events may include chewing and swallowing. Lesions of nerves passing through the jugular foramen (IX, X, XI) may result in loss of the **gag reflex** (motor limb via ninth nerve), drooping of the ipsilateral shoulder accompanied by an inability to turn the head to the opposite side against resistance (eleventh nerve), and **dysarthria** and **dysphagia** (tenth nerve). **Syndromes of the jugular foramen** may result from lesions/tumors located inside the cranial cavity adjacent to the foramen (as in the **Vernet syndrome**, roots of IX, X, XI), within the foramen itself, or external to the foramen at the skull base. In the latter case, the lesion may encompass the roots of the ninth, tenth, and eleventh nerves as well as the twelfth (the **Collet-Sicard syndrome**).

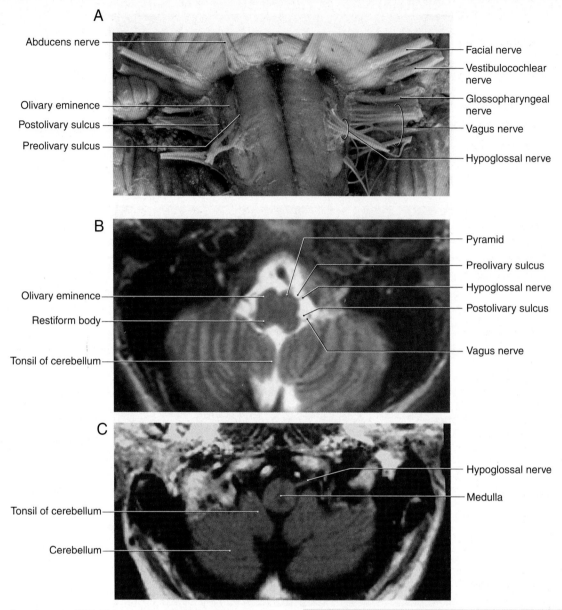

A

Abducens nerve
Olivary eminence
Postolivary sulcus
Preolivary sulcus

Facial nerve
Vestibulocochlear nerve
Glossopharyngeal nerve
Vagus nerve
Hypoglossal nerve

B

Olivary eminence
Restiform body
Tonsil of cerebellum

Pyramid
Preolivary sulcus
Hypoglossal nerve
Postolivary sulcus
Vagus nerve

C

Tonsil of cerebellum
Cerebellum

Hypoglossal nerve
Medulla

3-7 The hypoglossal nerve (XII) (**A**) exits the inferolateral aspect of the medulla via the preolivary sulcus. This cranial nerve exits in line with the abducens nerve found at the pons–medulla junction and in line with the exits of the third and fourth nerves of the midbrain. The twelfth nerve exit is characteristically located laterally adjacent to the pyramid, which contains corticospinal fibers.

In axial MRI (**B**, T2-weighted; **C**, T1-weighted), note the characteristic position of the hypoglossal nerve in the subarachnoid space and its relation to the overall shape of the medulla. This shape is indicative of a cranial nerve exiting at more mid-to-caudal medullary levels. In **B**, note its relationship to the preolivary sulcus and olivary eminence. The hypoglossal exits the base of the skull by traversing the hypoglossal canal. A lesion of the hypoglossal root, or in its peripheral distribution, will result in a deviation of the tongue to the side of the root damage on attempted protrusion; the **genioglossus muscle** on that side is paralyzed. A lesion in the medulla, such as a **medial medullary syndrome (Déjèrine syndrome)**, can result in the same deviation of the tongue (to the side of the lesion on protrusion) plus additional motor (corticospinal) and sensory (medial lemniscus) deficits on the opposite side of the body.

The total picture of deficits seen in medullary lesions that involve the hypoglossal nucleus, or nerve, or in posterior fossa lesions that involve the hypoglossal root and other roots, will depend on what additional structures are recruited into the lesion or are damaged. For example, **syndromes of the jugular foramen** commonly involve roots of cranial nerves (CNs) IX, X, and XI either together or in various combinations.

Recall that the jugular foramen (CNs IX, X, XI) and the hypoglossal canal (CN XII) are closely adjacent to each other, separated only by a small bar of bone on the inner aspect of the skull (see Figure 2-23 on p. 24). This separation may preclude an intracranial lesion from damaging all of these roots simultaneously. However, the roots of CNs IX–XII come into close apposition immediately upon their exit from the skull base and may be collectively damaged by a lesion in this confined area. Deficits in the **Collet-Sicard syndrome** (one of the jugular foramen syndromes) reflect damage to CNs IX, X, XI, and XII.

These roots may be collectively damaged in a basal skull fracture involving both foramina or by a tumor involving these roots in a confined area.

Patient's Right   Patient's Left

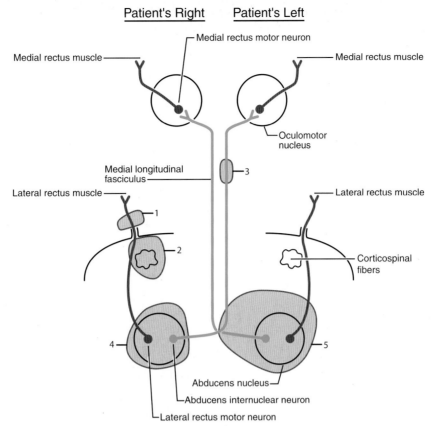

3-8 Lesions (#1 to #5) of the abducens nerve and/or nucleus and of the medial longitudinal fasciculus that result in deficits of eye movements in the horizontal plane.

Lesion of the abducens root (#1): Motor neurons in the abducens nucleus innervate the ipsilateral lateral rectus muscle. Consequently, a patient with a lesion of the abducens root external to the pons (see Figure 3-5 for the position of the sixth root) experiences a loss of voluntary lateral gaze in the eye on the side of the lesion, indicating a paralysis of the lateral rectus muscle. Other movements in the affected eye, and all movements in the contralateral eye, are normal. This patient will experience **diplopia**. When looking straight ahead, the eye on the lesioned side will deviate slightly toward the midline (unopposed action of the medial rectus in the same eye) and the diplopia is made worse when attempting to look toward the lesioned side in a horizontal plane.

Caudal basilar pontine lesion (#2): As axons arising from abducens motor neurons pass through the basilar pons, they are located laterally adjacent to corticospinal fibers (see Figure 6-19 on pp. 130–131). A lesion in this portion of the pons may simultaneously damage the exiting abducens fibers and corticospinal axons. A patient with this lesion experiences an **alternating** (or **crossed**) **hemiplegia**, a paralysis of the lateral rectus muscle on the side of the lesion (loss of voluntary lateral gaze to that side, and **diplopia**), and a paralysis of the upper and lower extremities on the opposite side of the body. Alternating, or crossed, deficits are characteristic of brainstem lesions.

Internuclear ophthalmoplegia (INO) (#3): In addition to abducens motor neurons that innervate the ipsilateral lateral rectus muscle, the abducens nucleus also contains interneurons. The axons of these interneurons cross the midline, enter the medial longitudinal fasciculus (MLF), and ascend to terminate on motor neurons in the oculomotor nucleus that innervate the medial rectus muscle on that side. A lesion in the MLF interrupts these axons and results in a **loss of medial gaze** (medial rectus paralysis) in the eye on the side of the lesion during attempted conjugate eye movements. Other movements in the affected eye and all movements in the contralateral eye are normal. The laterality of the deficit reflects the side of the lesion and of the deficit. For example, a **right internuclear ophthalmoplegia** specifies a lesion in the right MLF and paralysis of the right medial rectus muscle; a **left internuclear ophthalmoplegia** indicates a lesion in the left MLF and left medial rectus weakness.

Lesion of the abducens nucleus (#4): A lesion of the abducens nucleus damages alpha motor neurons innervating the ipsilateral lateral rectus muscle and the interneurons that terminate on medial rectus alpha motor neurons residing in the contralateral oculomotor nucleus. A patient with this lesion experiences a **loss of horizontal gaze** in both eyes during attempted voluntary eye movement toward the side of the lesion; horizontal gaze toward the contralateral side is normal. This is basically an abducens root lesion plus an INO.

The one-and-a-half syndrome (#5): This syndrome is so named because a unilateral pontine lesion may result in **a loss of medial and lateral voluntary eye movement on the side of the lesion** (the "one") and **a loss of medial horizontal eye movement on the contralateral side** (the "one-half"). The lesion resulting in this pattern of deficits involves the abducens nucleus on one side (deficits = lateral rectus paralysis on the side of the lesion, medial rectus paralysis on the contralateral side) and the immediately adjacent MLF conveying the axons of abducens interneurons originating in the opposite abducens nucleus (deficit = medial rectus paralysis on the side of the lesion). These lesions are usually large and involve portions of the paramedian pontine reticular formation, commonly called the horizontal gaze center.

Table 3-2 Summary of Brainstem Lesions that Involve Cranial Nerve Nuclei and/or the Roots of Cranial Nerves and the Correlated Deficits of Cranial Nerve Function

Lesion(s)/Syndrome	Structures Damaged	Deficits
Medulla Medial medullary (Déjérine) syndrome Lateral medullary (PICA or Wallenberg) syndrome	Hypoglossal nerve/nucleus Corticospinal fibers Medial lemniscus	Ipsilateral paralysis of tongue Contralateral hemiplegia Contralateral loss of discriminative touch, vibratory and position sense on UE, trunk, and LE
	Spinal trigeminal tract nucleus Nucleus ambiguus Vestibular nuclei Anterolateral system	Ipsilateral loss of pain and thermal sense on face Dysphagia, hoarseness, deviation of uvula to contralateral side Nystagmus, vertigo, nausea Contralateral loss of pain and thermal sense on UE, trunk, and LE
Pons Raymond syndrome* (Foville syndrome) Gubler syndrome	Corticospinal fibers Abducens fibers in pons Corticospinal fibers Facial nucleus or fibers (Anterolateral system) (Trigeminal nerve)	Contralateral hemiplegia Ipsilateral abducens palsy, diplopia Contralateral hemiplegia Ipsilateral paralysis of facial muscles (Contralateral loss of pain and thermal sensation on UE, trunk, and LE) (Ipsilateral paralysis of masticatory muscles, ipsilateral loss of pain and thermal sensation on face)
	Corticospinal fibers Trigeminal nerve	Contralateral hemiplegia Ipsilateral paralysis of masticatory muscles, ipsilateral loss of pain and thermal sensation on face
Midbrain Weber (cerebral peduncle) syndrome Claude (red nucleus) syndrome	Corticospinal fibers Oculomotor fibers Corticonuclear fibers	Contralateral hemiplegia Ipsilateral oculomotor paralysis, diplopia, dilated pupil Contralateral weakness of facial muscles on lower face; deviation of tongue to contralateral side on protrusion; ipsilateral trapezius + sternocleidomastoid weakness
	Oculomotor nerve Cerebellothalamic fibers	Ipsilateral oculomotor palsy, diplopia, dilated pupil Contralateral ataxia, tremor, + red nucleus hyperkinesias
Benedikt syndrome = Deficits of Weber syndrome + deficits of Claude syndrome.		

*According to Wolf (1971) in his excellent book describing brainstem syndromes from their original sources, Fulgence Raymond described a female patient, with several medical complications, with right hemiparesis and left abducens palsy. Raymond localized the probable lesion (he acknowledged more than one potential cause) to the basilar pons involving corticospinal fibers and the abducens root. This is also commonly called the Foville syndrome, although Foville is also described as recruiting adjacent structures with their corresponding deficits. Both eponyms are acceptable.

LE, lower extremity; UE, upper extremity.

Cranial Nerves in Their Larger Functional/Clinical Context (Figures 3-9 to 3-15)

Cranial nerves are usually an integral part of any neurological examination; this is certainly the case in injuries and/or diseases that involve the head and neck. This chapter details their exit points (or, one could argue, the entrance points in the case of sensory nerves), their corresponding appearance in MRI, and examples of lesions causing deficits of eye movements in the horizontal plane and of brainstem lesions that include cranial nerve deficits.

This is, however, only part of a much larger picture that places cranial nerves in a functional context and views their connections in the periphery as well as within the central nervous system. Although these more comprehensive cranial nerve connections, and their corresponding functions, are illustrated in Chapter 8 in their appropriate *systems context*, they are briefly listed here to facilitate cross reference for those users wishing to consider cranial nerves in a more integrated format at this point.

Functional Components of Spinal and Cranial Nerves (see also Figures 6-1 and 6-2 on pp. 96–97)

3-9 The columns of cells within the spinal cord are rostrally continuous with comparable cell columns in the brainstem that have similar functions. For example, general motor cell columns of the spinal cord are continuous with the groups of motor nuclei that innervate the tongue and the extraocular muscles; both cell columns innervate skeletal muscles. The same is the case for general sensation. Nuclei conveying special senses are found only in the brainstem and are associated with only certain cranial nerves.

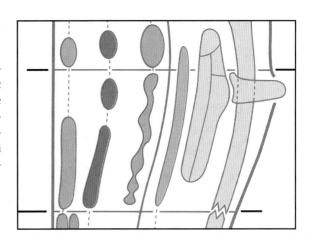

Trigeminal Pathways and Deficits (see also Figures 8-7 and 8-8A, B on pp. 202–205)

3-10 The trigeminal nerve conveys sensory input from the face and oral cavity and provides motor innervation to the muscles of mastication. The spinal trigeminal tract and nucleus also receive general sensation via CNs VII, IX, and X. In this respect, the *spinal trigeminal tract is the center for all general sensory sensations entering the brainstem on all cranial nerves.* In the same sense, the solitary tract and nucleus (Figure 8-9 on pp. 206–207) *is the brainstem center for all visceral sensation that enters the brainstem on CNs VII, IX, and X.* Both of these cranial nerve brainstem nuclei convey information to the thalamus and eventually to the cerebral cortex.

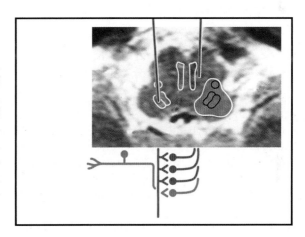

Corticonuclear Pathways and Deficits (see also Figures 8-13 and 8-14A, B on pp. 214–217)

3-11 The cerebral cortex influences cranial nerve nuclei via corticonuclear fibers. In the neurological examination, this is most evident when testing motor functions of CNs VII, IX, X, XI, and XII. In many situations, the deficit is seen by the inability of the patient to perform a movement "against resistance." Comparing the deficit(s) of a lesion of these fibers to damage of cranial nerves within the brainstem, or the periphery, is essential to localizing the lesion within the central nervous system.

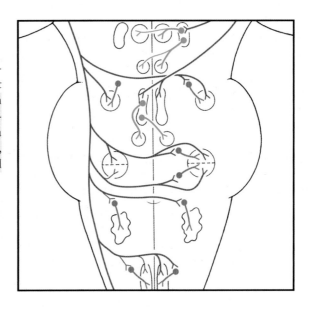

Cranial Nerve Efferents (III–VII and IX–XII) and Deficits (see also Figures 8-19 to 8-22B on pp. 226–233)

3-12 Cranial nerve nuclei are either motor to skeletal muscle or visceromotor to ganglia in the periphery. Lesions involving the nuclei, or roots, of motor nuclei result in paralysis of the muscles served, with the predictable deficits, such as weakness of the facial muscles or deviation of the tongue on protrusion. Lesions that damage the visceromotor fibers of a cranial nerve result in an expected visceromotor response, such as dilation of the pupil, or a decrease in secretory function or smooth muscle motility.

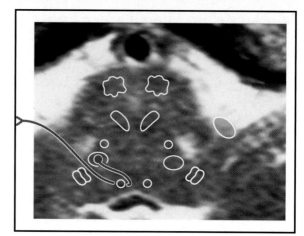

Cranial Nerve Reflex Pathways and Deficits (see also Figures 8-23 to 8-32 on pp. 234–240)

3-13 Testing cranial nerve reflexes is a routine part of any complete neurological examination. This part of the neurological exam tests the integrity of the afferent and efferent limbs of the reflex. Sometimes both of these are on the same cranial nerve; sometimes they are on different cranial nerves. In addition, deficits may be seen that reflect damage **affecting** cranial nerve function, but this damage is not in the afferent or efferent limbs of the reflex; this suggests a broader problem within the central nervous system.

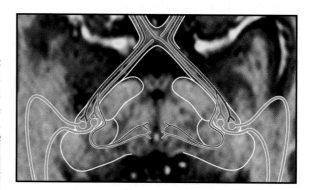

Pupillary and Visual Pathways and Deficits (see also Figures 8-44 to 8-47B on pp. 262–267)

3-14 The pupillary reflex (commonly called the **pupillary light reflex**) has its afferent limb via the second cranial nerve and its efferent limb via the third cranial nerve. The reaction of the pupil when light is shined in one eye is a clear hint as to the location of the lesion. The optic nerve, chiasm, tract, and radiations and the visual cortex have a retinotopic representation throughout. Lesions of any of these structures result in visual deficits, such as a **hemianopia** or **quadrantanopia**, that reflect the particular portion of the visual system that is damaged. Because visual pathways are widespread within the brain, lesions at various different locations may result in visual deficits.

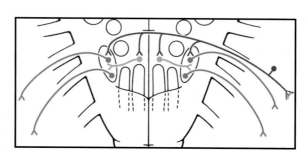

Auditory and Vestibular Pathways and Deficits (see also Figures 8-49 to 8-50 on pp. 270–273).

3-15 The auditory portion of the eighth cranial nerve is concerned with the perception of sound. Damage to the cochlea itself, or the cochlear root, may profoundly alter one's perception of sound or may result in deafness. The vestibular portion of the eighth cranial nerve functions in the arena of balance, equilibrium, and maintenance of posture. Damage to the semicircular canals, to the vestibular root, or to central structures that receive vestibular input, may result in **vertigo**, **ataxia**, difficulty walking or maintaining balance, and/or a variety of eye movement problems.

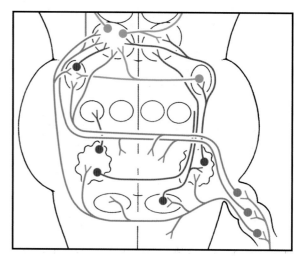

Q&A for this chapter is available online on thePoint

Meninges, Cisterns, Ventricles, and Related Hemorrhages

4

Table 4-1 Comparison of Cerebral Versus Spinal Meninges

CEREBRAL	SPINAL
Dura	*Dura*
• Adherent to inner table of skull (no epidural space) • Composed of two fused layers (periosteal and meningeal), which split to form sinuses	• Separated from vertebrae by epidural space • Composed of one layer (spinal dura only; vertebrae have their own periosteum)
Arachnoid (outer part of leptomeninges)	*Arachnoid (outer part of leptomeninges)*
• Attached to dura in living condition (no subdural space) • Arachnoid villi (in superior sagittal sinus) • Arachnoid trabeculae • Subarachnoid space with many cisterns	• Attached to dura in living condition (no subdural space) • No arachnoid villi • Few or no arachnoid trabeculae but larger arachnoid septae • Subarachnoid space with one cistern
Pia (inner part of leptomeninges)	*Pia (inner part of leptomeninges)*
• Intimately adherent to surface of brain • No pial specializations • Follows vessels as they pierce the cerebral cortex	• Intimately adherent to surface of cord • Specializations in the form of denticulate ligaments, filum terminale, and linea splendens • Follows vessels as they pierce the cord

Meningitis, Meningeal Hemorrhages, and Meningiomas

A wide variety of disease processes and lesions may involve the meninges; only a few examples are mentioned here.

Infections of the meninges (**bacterial meningitis**) may be called **leptomeningitis** because the causative organisms localize to the subarachnoid space and involve the pia and arachnoid. Extension into the dura is called **pachymeningitis**. A variety of organisms cause **bacterial meningitis**; those most commonly associated with certain groups are as follows: neonate = *Streptococcus agalactiae, Escherichia coli, Listeria monocytogenes*; neonate to about 24 months = *S. agalactiae, E. coli, Haemophilus influenzae*; about 2 to 50 years = *Streptococcus pneumoniae, Neisseria meningitidis*; about 50 years + = *S. pneumoniae, N. meningitidis, L. monocytogenes*; basal skull fracture = *S. pneumoniae, H. influenzae*; head trauma = **Staphylococcus**. The patient becomes acutely ill (i.e., headache, confusion, fever, stiff neck [**meningismus**], stupor), may have generalized or focal signs/symptoms, and, if not rapidly treated (with appropriate antibiotics), will likely die. Patients with **viral meningitis** may become ill over a period of several days, experience headache, confusion, and fever, but, with supportive care, will usually recover after an acute phase of about 1 to 2 weeks with no permanent deficits.

The most common cause of an **epidural (extradural) hematoma** is a skull fracture that results in a laceration of a major dural vessel, such as the middle meningeal artery. In approximately 15% of cases, bleeding may come from a venous sinus. The extravasated blood dissects the dura mater off the inner table of the skull; there is no pre-existing cerebral extradural space for the blood to enter. These lesions are frequently large, lens (lenticular) shaped, may appear loculated, and are "short and thick" compared with subdural hematomas (see Figure 4-4 on p. 62). The fact that epidural hematomas do not cross suture lines correlates with their characteristic shape. The patient may lapse into a coma and, if the lesion is left untreated, death may result. In some cases, the patient may be unconscious initially, followed by a lucid interval (the patient is wide awake), then subsequently deteriorate rapidly and die; this is called "talk and die." Treatment of choice for large lesions is surgical removal of the clot and coagulation of the damaged vessel.

Tearing of bridging veins (veins passing from the brain outward through the arachnoid and dura), usually the result of trauma, is a common cause of **subdural hematoma**. This designation is somewhat a misnomer because the extravasated blood actually dissects through a specialized, yet structurally weak, cell layer at the dura–arachnoid interface; this is the **dural border cell layer.** There is no pre-existing "subdural space" in the normal brain. Acute subdural hematomas, more commonly seen in younger patients, usually are detected immediately or within a few hours after the precipitating incident. Chronic subdural hematomas, usually seen in the elderly, or in patients on anticoagulation therapy, are frequently of unknown origin. They may take days or weeks to become symptomatic and, in the process, cause a progressive change in the mental status of the patient. This lesion appears "long and thin" compared with an epidural hematoma, follows the surface of the brain, and may extend for considerable distances (see Figures 4-4 on p. 62 and 4-5 on p. 63). Treatment is surgical evacuation (for larger or acute lesions) or close monitoring for small, asymptomatic, or chronic lesions.

The most common cause of **subarachnoid hemorrhage** is trauma. In approximately 75% to 80% of patients with **spontaneous (nontraumatic) subarachnoid hemorrhage**, the precipitating event is rupture of an intracranial aneurysm. Symptomatic bleeding from an arteriovenous malformation occurs in approximately 5% of cases. Blood collects in and percolates through the subarachnoid space and cisterns (see Figure 4-7 on p. 65). Sometimes, the deficits seen (assuming the patient is not in a coma) may be a clue as to location, especially if cranial nerves are nearby. Onset is sudden; the patient complains of a sudden and excruciatingly painful headache ("the worst of my life," "thunderclap," "felt like my head exploded") and may remain conscious, become lethargic and disoriented, or may be comatose. Treatment of an aneurysm is to surgically separate the sac of the aneurysm from the parent vessel (by clip or coil), if possible, and protect against the development of vasospasm. During surgery, some blood in the subarachnoid space and cisterns may be removed.

Tumors of the meninges (**meningiomas**) are classified in different ways, but usually they arise from arachnoid cap/stem cells (a small number are dural in origin) around the villi or at places where vessels or cranial nerves penetrate the dura–arachnoid. These tumors may present with seizure, grow slowly (symptoms may develop almost imperceptibly over years), are histologically benign, may result in hyperostosis of the overlying skull, and frequently contain calcifications. In decreasing order, meningiomas are found in the following locations: parasagittal area + falx cerebri (together 29%), convexity 15%, sella 13%, sphenoid ridge 12%, and olfactory groove 10%. Treatment is primarily by surgical removal, although some meningiomas are treated by radiotherapy.

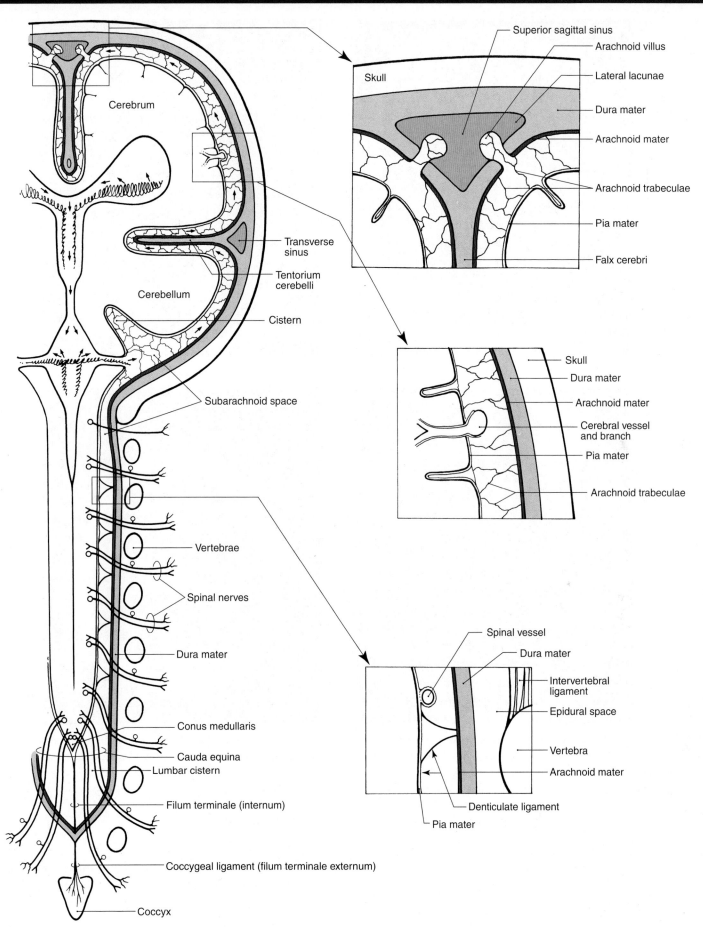

4-1 Semi-diagrammatic representation of the central nervous system and its associated meninges. The details show the relationships of the meninges in the area of the superior sagittal sinus, on the lateral aspect of the cerebral hemisphere, and around the spinal cord. Cerebrospinal fluid is produced by the choroid plexuses of the lateral, third, and fourth ventricles. It circulates through the ventricular system (**small arrows**) and enters the subarachnoid space via the medial foramen of Magendie and the two lateral foramina of Luschka. In the living situation, the arachnoid is attached to the inner surface of the dura. There is no **actual** or **potential** subdural space. This space is created resultant to a traumatic, infectious, or pathologic process.

A

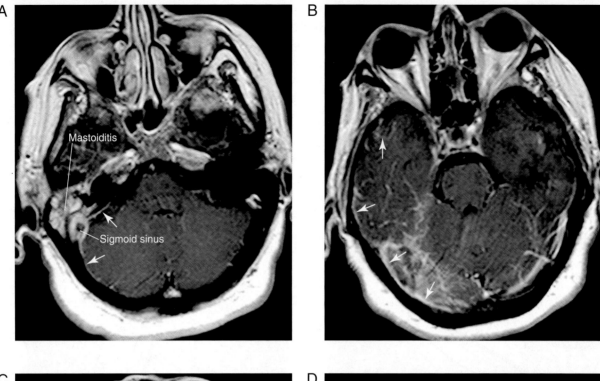

B

C

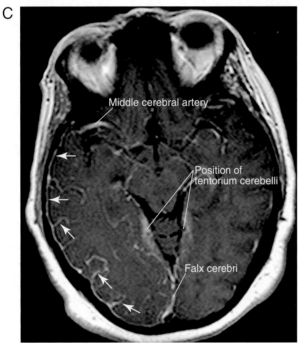

D

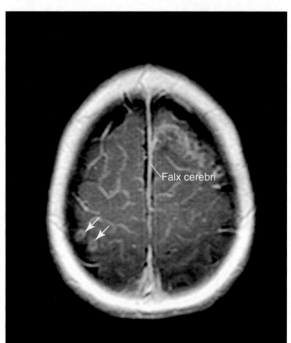

4-2 Examples of **meningitis** (A–D, all axial) in the adult. Meningitis is a disease that generally involves the subarachnoid space (SAS) and the membranes bordering on this space, namely the **arachnoid mater** and the **pia mater**. Consequently, it is commonly called **leptomeningitis** (or **arachnoiditis**, or **pia-arachnitis**). Meningitis may preferentially affect one side more that the other in some cases.

Sources of infections that may lead to meningitis are those involving the paranasal sinuses or the mastoid air cells (**mastoiditis, A**). Mastoiditis is almost always accompanied by other disease processes, most notably acute or chronic **otitis media**. The close association of mastoid air cells to the sigmoid sinus represents one comparatively direct route into the central nervous system.

Once an infection of the mastoid accesses the central nervous system, it may involve the venous sinuses (**A**), which appear bright when enhanced. The infection will layer out over the surface of brain within the SAS, enter the sulci, and occupy the SAS immediately above and below the tentorium cerebelli (see arrows in **A, B, C**). The SAS and the sulci enhance when the patient is treated with IV gadolinium (**C, D**) and appear bright in the image. In addition to these features, small enhancements may appear within the SAS (**D,** arrows) that indicate the formation of small abscesses. This inflammation may also extend to involve the dura mater in which case it is called **pachymeningitis**.

A

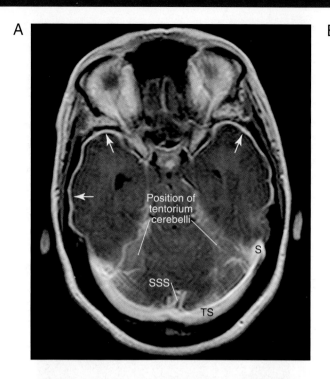

B

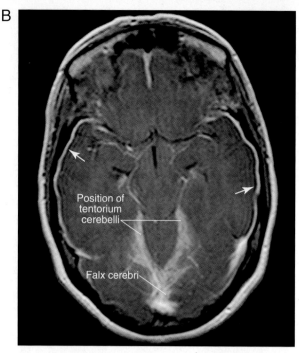

C

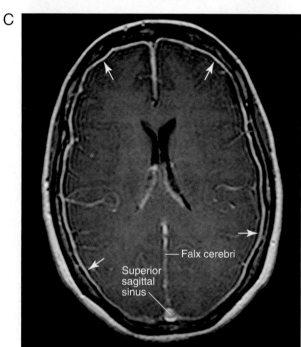

D

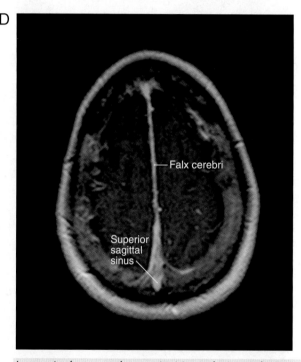

4-3 Examples of **meningitis** (**leptomeningitis**) that extensively involves both sides of the central nervous system (**A–D**, all axial) in the adult. In **A**, note the enhancement of the meninges over the temporal lobe, at the location of the tentorium cerebelli, and of the venous sinuses (SSS = superior sagittal; S = sigmoid; TS = transverse). At different axial levels, enhancement is clearly visible on the brain surface (**B, C, arrows**), along the dural reflections (tentorium cerebelli and falx cerebri, **B–D**), and within the sulci (**C**). In addition, enhancements over the curvature of the hemisphere are suggestive of focal collections of inflammation.

As seen in these samples, meningitis can be imaged using gadolinium and to a reasonable level its degree and extent visualized. However, it is also apparent that the lesion, the inflamed meninges, and SAS, are more subtle than lesions such as meningioma, hemorrhage, or brain tumor. Vessels located within the subarachnoid space may also enhance as they most likely contain infectious material and the organisms may infiltrate the vessel walls. As noted in Figure 4-2, the inflammation may also extend to involve the dura mater (**pachymeningitis**). The more common causative agents for meningitis, and the age groups with which they are more frequently associated, are discussed on p. 58.

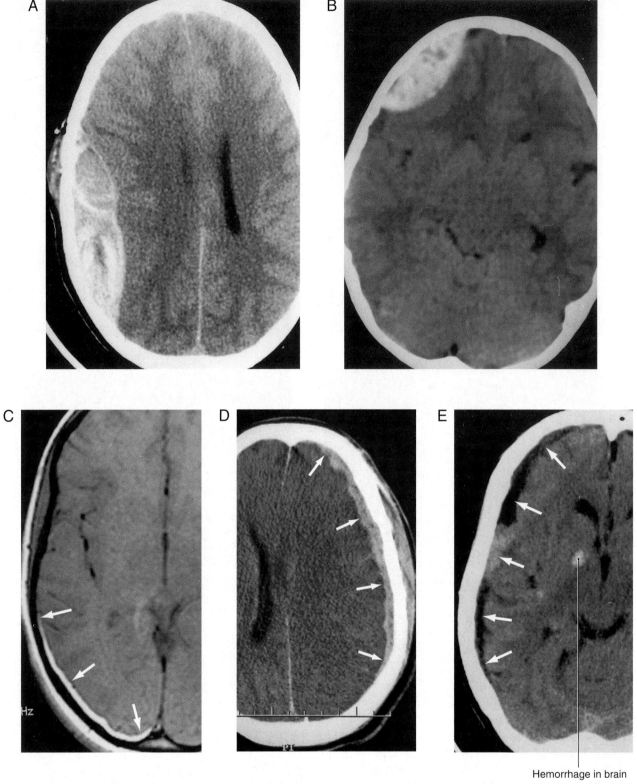

Hemorrhage in brain

4-4 Examples of **epidural (extradural) hemorrhage/hematoma (A, B)** and of acute **(C, D)** and subacute **(E)** **subdural hematoma/ hemorrhage**. Note the lenticular shape of the epidural lesions (they do not cross suture lines—**A, B**), their loculated appearance, and their location external to the substance of the brain (see also Figure 4-5, facing page). In contrast, the acute subdural lesions (**C, D, arrows**) are quite thin and extend over a longer distance on the cortex; they are not constrained by suture lines. Note the midline shift in patients (**A, D**).

In **E**, the subdural hematoma has both **chronic** and **subacute** phases. The chronic phase is indicated by the upper two and lower two arrows where the blood is replaced by fluid, and the subacute phase by the middle arrow, where fresher blood has entered the lesion. Note the extent of this lesion on the surface of the cortex and its narrowness compared

with epidural lesions. The patient in **E** also has small hemorrhages into the substance of the brain in the region of the genu of the internal capsule. Images **A–E** are CT. For additional comments on epidural and subdural hemorrhages, see p. 58.

The treatment of choice for **epidural hematoma**, especially if the patient is symptomatic, or if the patient is asymptomatic but the acute lesion is greater than 1 cm thick at its widest point and has a volume of greater than 30 cm³, is surgical removal and hemostasis of bleeders. In **subdural hematoma**, surgical evacuation is the preferred treatment in symptomatic patients with acute lesions that are 1 cm thick (0.5 in pediatric patients) and a midline shift of greater than 5 mm. On the other hand, asymptomatic patients with thin subdural lesions may be followed medically and may not require surgery.

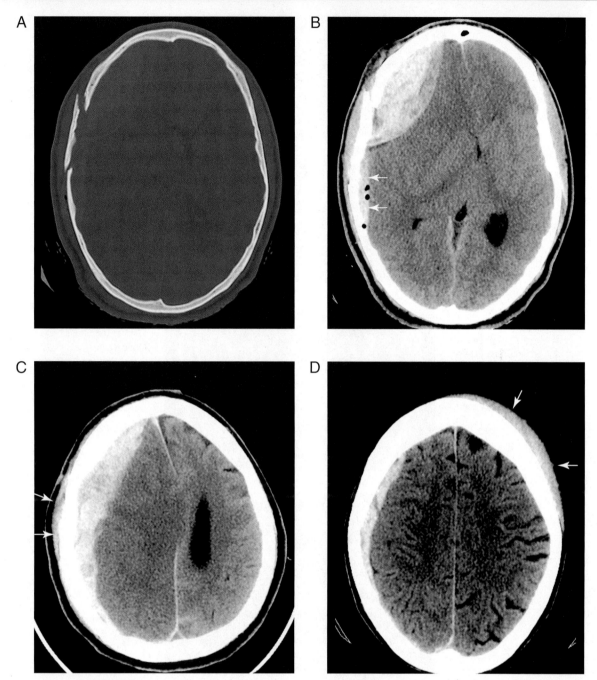

4-5 Examples of **epidural (extradural) hemorrhage/hematoma (A, B)** and **subdural hematoma/hemorrhage (C, D)** resultant to trauma to the head; all are CT and all are in the axial plane.

Epidural hematoma may occur in cases of skull fracture (**A**, on the right side) in which the middle meningeal artery (or its larger branches) is lacerated. The resulting hematoma is formed between the inner table of the skull and the outer aspect of the dura (**epidural, B**, on the right). In this significant trauma, there is a large epidural, a small lesion, probably also an epidural (small arrows), and small amounts or air within the cranial cavity (**B**, black dots).

The mechanism of epidural hematoma formation is most likely twofold. First, the dura is stripped from the inner table of the skull during the traumatic event creating an artifactual space. Second, the sharp edges of bone lacerate arteries, which bleed into this space, and, it is believed, may further dissect the dura from the skull. Epidural hematomas do not cross suture lines.

Trauma to the head, without skull fracture, may result in subdural hemorrhage/hematoma; in such cases, it is called **acute subdural hematoma**

(**C, D**). Subdural hematomas may also be **subacute** or **chronic** and do occur in cases where trauma is not involved. In these examples, trauma on the right side of the head (**C**, soft tissue damage at **arrows**) resulted in a large **acute subdural hematoma** on the patient's right side, and trauma on the left side of the head (**D**, soft tissue damage at **arrows**) resulted in a subdural lesion on the patient's right. This latter lesion is a type of **contrecoup injury** in which the lesion is on the side opposite the initial impact. Note that the larger subdural lesion (**C**) has caused considerable midline shift. Subdural hematomas are not restrained by suture lines.

As seen in **B** and **C** in this figure, and in Figure 4-4A and **D** on the facing page, epidural and subdural lesions may be sufficiently large to result in effacement of the midline as indicated by a shift in the position of the falx cerebri. This appearance, plus the frequent loss of sulci and sometimes cisterns on the side of the lesion, foretells the very real possibility of brain herniation. This may present as a **subfalcine herniation**, which may impinge on both hemispheres, or morph into a **transtentorial herniation**; all result in characteristic deficits (see Chapter 9 for further information of herniation syndromes).

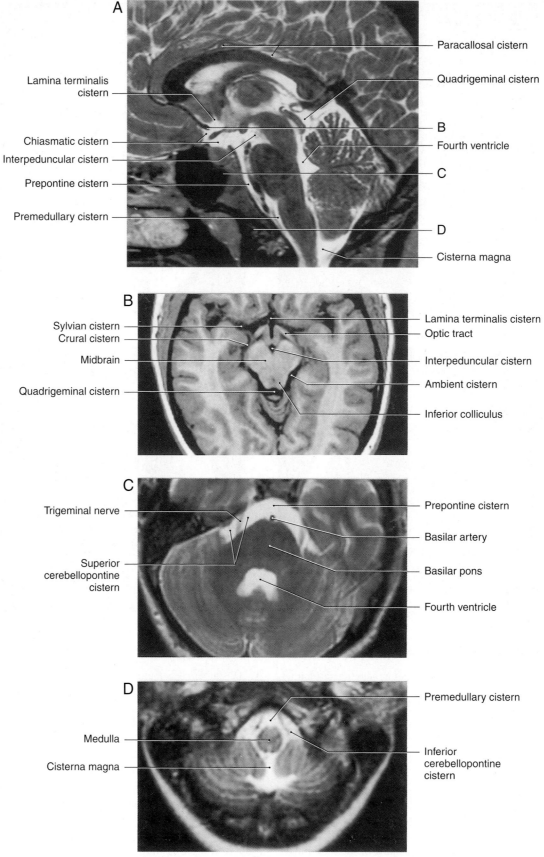

A

Paracallosal cistern

Lamina terminalis cistern

Quadrigeminal cistern

B

Chiasmatic cistern

Fourth ventricle

Interpeduncular cistern

C

Prepontine cistern

Premedullary cistern

D

Cisterna magna

B

Sylvian cistern

Lamina terminalis cistern

Crural cistern

Optic tract

Midbrain

Interpeduncular cistern

Ambient cistern

Quadrigeminal cistern

Inferior colliculus

C

Trigeminal nerve

Prepontine cistern

Basilar artery

Superior cerebellopontine cistern

Basilar pons

Fourth ventricle

D

Premedullary cistern

Medulla

Cisterna magna

Inferior cerebellopontine cistern

4-6 A median sagittal MRI (**A**, T2-weighted) of the brain showing the positions of the major cisterns associated with midline structures. Axial views of the midbrain (**B**, T1-weighted), pons (**C**, T2-weighted), and medulla (**D**, T2-weighted) represent the corresponding planes indicated in the sagittal view (**A**).

Cisterns are the enlarged portions of the subarachnoid space that contain arteries and veins, roots of cranial nerves, and, of course,

cerebrospinal fluid. Consequently, the subarachnoid space and cisterns are continuous one with the other. In addition, the subarachnoid space around the brain is continuous with that around the spinal cord. Compare the locations and shapes of these cisterns with the blood-filled parts of the subarachnoid space and contiguous cisterns shown in Figure 4-7 on the facing page.

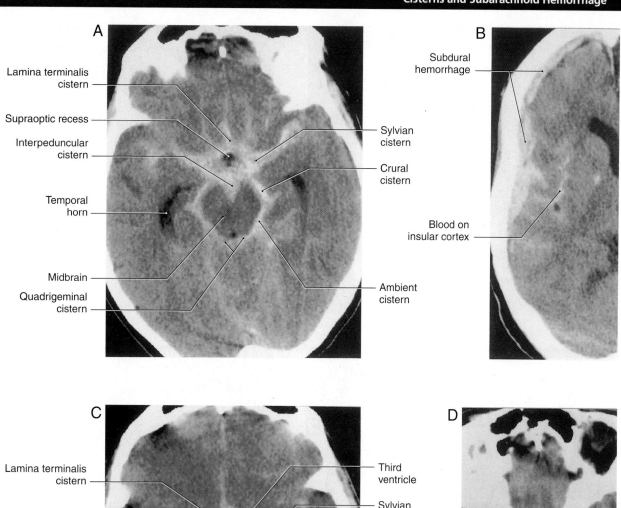

A

Lamina terminalis cistern

Supraoptic recess

Interpeduncular cistern

Temporal horn

Midbrain

Quadrigeminal cistern

Sylvian cistern

Crural cistern

Ambient cistern

B

Subdural hemorrhage

Blood on insular cortex

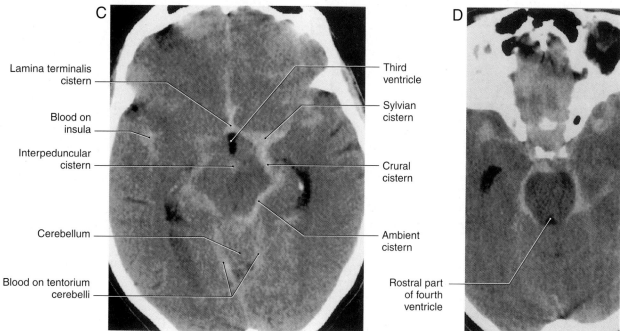

C

Lamina terminalis cistern

Blood on insula

Interpeduncular cistern

Cerebellum

Blood on tentorium cerebelli

Third ventricle

Sylvian cistern

Crural cistern

Ambient cistern

D

Rostral part of fourth ventricle

4-7 Blood in the **subarachnoid space** and **cisterns** (**subarachnoid hemorrhage**). In these CT examples, blood occupies the subarachnoid space and cisterns, outlining these areas in white. Consequently, the shape of the cisterns is indicated by the configuration of the white area, the white area representing blood.

Around the base of the brain (**A**), it is easy to identify the cisterns related to the midbrain, the supraoptic recess, which is devoid of blood, and blood extending laterally into the Sylvian cistern. In some cases (**B**), subdural hemorrhage may penetrate the arachnoid membrane and result in blood infiltrating between gyri, such as this example with blood on the cortex of the insula. In **C**, the blood is located around the midbrain (crural and ambient cisterns), extends into the Sylvian cistern, and into the cistern of the lamina terminalis. The sharp interface between the lamina terminalis cistern (containing blood) and the third ventricle (devoid of blood) represents the position of the lamina terminalis. In **D**, blood is located in cisterns around the pons, but avoids the rostral part of the fourth ventricle. Also note the clearly enlarged temporal horn of the lateral ventricle in **D**; enlargement of this particular part of the ventricle is indicative of increased pressure within the ventricular system.

Subarachnoid hemorrhage (SAH) is always a serious medical event. In the case of SAH resulting from aneurysm rupture (about 75% to 80% of all spontaneous cases), 10% to 15% die prior to receiving medical attention and about 20% after hospital admission; about 30% have permanent disability; and approximately 30% who survive may have moderate to severe deficits, particularly depression and cognitive compromise. Other comparable statistics indicate that about 45% to 50% die within the first 2 to 4 weeks, and about 30% have moderate to severe deficits.

About 65% of patients who have the aneurysms successfully clipped have a diminished quality of life. Compare these images with the locations of some of the comparable cisterns as seen in Figure 4-6 on the facing page. Images A–D are CT.

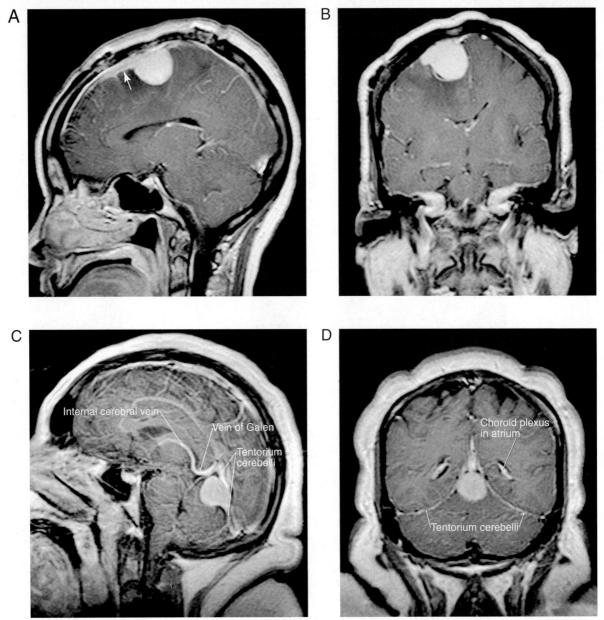

A

B

C

Internal cerebral vein

Vein of Galen

Tentorium cerebelli

D

Choroid plexus in atrium

Tentorium cerebelli

4-8 Examples of a right-sided **convexity meningioma** (**A, B**) and a **meningioma of the tentorium cerebelli** (**C, D**). Meningiomas are slow growing, usually benign extra-axial tumors that are curable assuming they can be completely removed (91%+, 5-year survival). They may present with headache or seizure, but many are asymptomatic and some are discovered as an incidental finding. The **convexity meningioma** (**A**, sagittal; **B**, coronal) is located in the medial aspect of the superior frontal gyrus rostral to the paracentral gyri. It is slightly off the midline; meningiomas that are directly adjacent to the midline and involve the superior sagittal sinus are called **parasagittal meningiomas**. Note its attachment to the dura (**A, arrow**); this attachment, seen in many meningiomas, is commonly called the **dural tail**. Convexity meningiomas are seen in about 15% of cases, and parasagittal meningiomas are found in about 21% of patients.

The **tentorial meningioma** (**C**, sagittal; **D**, coronal) is located on the midline, close to the rostral edge of the tentorium, and on its inferior surface. The tumor significantly impinges on the cerebellum (**C, D**), but does not involve the occipital lobes. This patient has motor deficits of the cerebellar type due to the involvement of the cerebellum. Due to its location, this tumor presents a greater surgical challenge than does the convexity meningioma and may contribute to eventual occlusion of the cerebral aqueduct. Tentorial meningiomas are seen in 3% to 4% of cases.

A

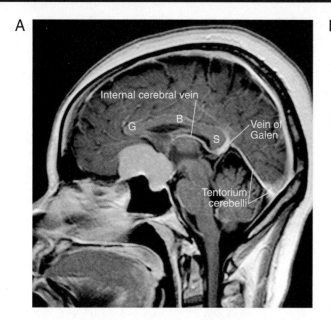

B

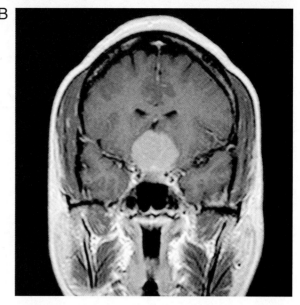

C

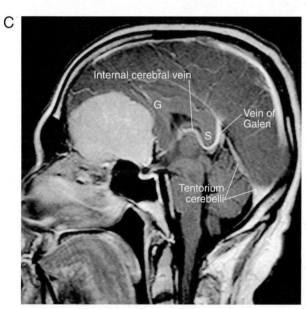

D

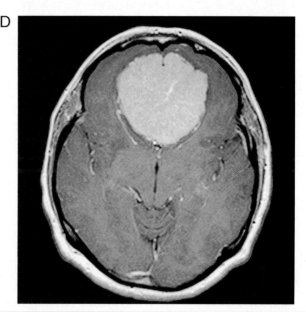

4-9 Examples of meningiomas that are located on the midline. The **sellar meningioma** (**A**, sagittal; **B**, coronal, also called **tuberculum sellae meningioma**), arises from the sella turcica and, due to its position, may impinge on optic structures and/or cause deficits indicative of involvement of the hypothalamus. Note that, although the tumor has reached significant size, major structures in the central region of the hemisphere, such as large veins and the corpus callosum (G = genu, B = body, S = splenium), are in their normal positions. Tumors are seen in this area in about 10% to 12% of cases and may require special surgical approaches.

The large meningioma in **C** and **D** was diagnosed as a **falcine meningioma,** a tumor that arises from the falx cerebri. Such tumors may arise at any point along the course of the falx cerebri, are frequently bilateral, and may impinge on the medial aspects of both hemispheres. Note that the central portions of the hemisphere have been pushed caudally

as seen by the foreshortened internal cerebral vein and the change in shape and position of the corpus callosum(G = genu, S = splenium). At the same time, **olfactory groove meningiomas** are also seen in this location and have a similar appearance. These arise from the area of the cribriform plate and enlarge upward to impinge on the frontal lobes. Falcine meningiomas constitute about 8% and olfactory groove meningiomas about 10% of all tumors of this type.

The general appearance of these examples, and those in Figure 4-8 (facing page), illustrate that these lesions, in many cases, grow so slowly that a significant portion of the brain can be displaced without untoward effects. The presenting deficits may be **persistent headache** and **seizure.** The sulci and midline may not be effaced and brain structures may not be displaced from their normal position. However, meningiomas that may block the egress of cerebrospinal fluid will likely result in deficits that reflect the point of the blockage.

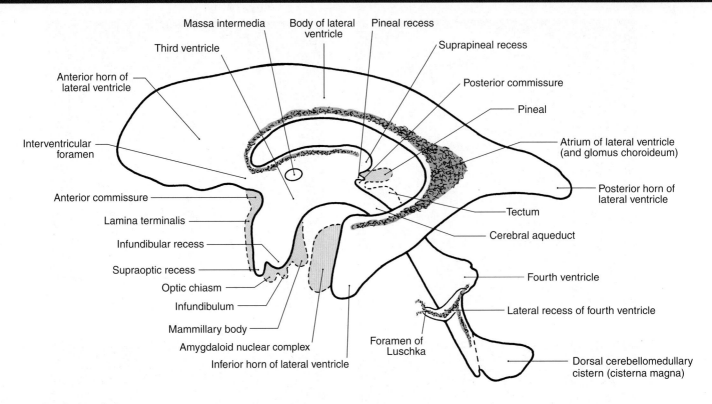

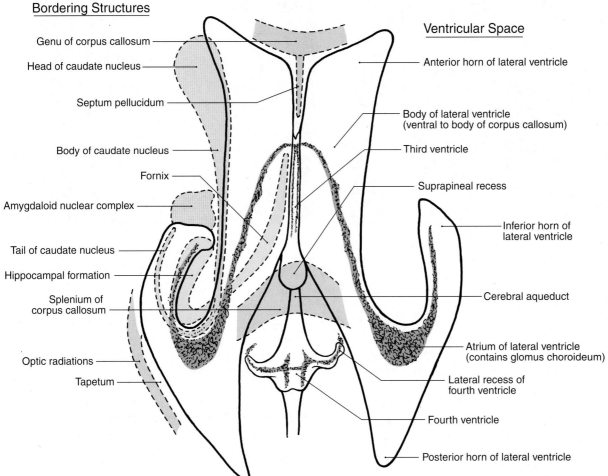

4-10 Lateral (**above**) and dorsal (**below**) views of the ventricles and the choroid plexus. The **dashed lines** show the approximate positions of some of the important structures that border on the ventricular space. The **choroid plexus** is shown in **red**, and structures bordering on the various portions of the ventricular spaces are color coded; these colors are continued in Figure 4-11 on the facing page. Note the relationships between the choroid plexus and various parts of the ventricular system. The large expanded portion of the choroid plexus found in the area of the atrium is the glomus (**glomus choroideum**).

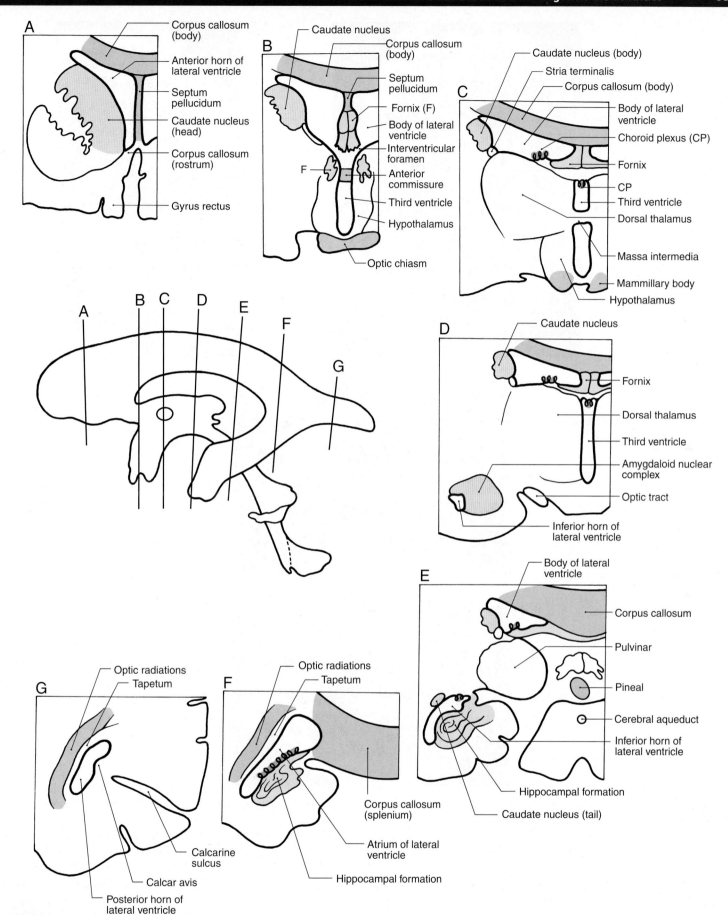

4-11 Lateral view of the ventricular system and corresponding semi-diagrammatic cross-sectional representations from rostral (**A**) to caudal (**G**) identifying specific structures that border on the ventricular space. In the cross-sections, the ventricle is outlined by a heavy line, and the majority of structures labeled have some direct relevance to the ventricular space at that particular level. The color coding corresponds to that shown in Figure 4-10 on the facing page.

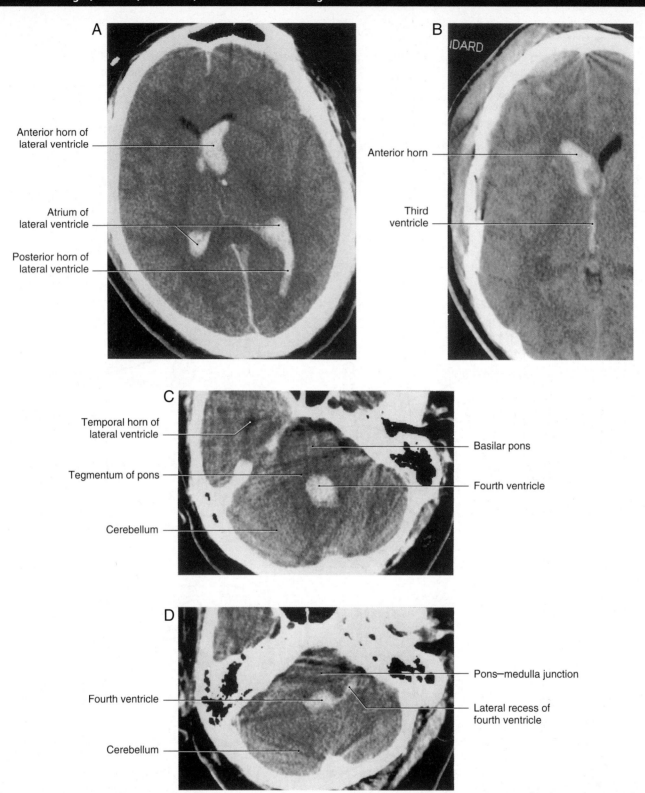

4-12 Examples of hemorrhage occupying portions of the ventricular system (**intraventricular hemorrhage**). In these CT images, blood appears white within the ventricles. Consequently, the shape of the ventricular system is outlined by the white area, and the specific portion of the ventricular system is correspondingly labeled.

Note blood in the anterior horn, atrium, and posterior horn of the lateral ventricles (**A, B**), and blood clearly outlining the shape of the third ventricle (**B**). Blood also clearly outlines central portions of the fourth ventricle (**C**) and caudal portions of the fourth ventricle (**D**), including an extension of blood into the left lateral recess of the fourth ventricle. In addition to these images, Figure 4-13C on the facing page

shows blood in the most inferior portions of the third ventricle. Images A–D are CT.

The presence of blood within the ventricular system occurs in about 25% of cases with ruptured aneurysm. The most common aneurysm sites, and point at which blood may enter the ventricular system upon rupture, are as follows: the distal posterior inferior cerebellar artery, through the roof of the fourth ventricle or foramen of Luschka (fourth ventricle); the basilar tip, through the floor of the third ventricle (third ventricle); at the junction of the anterior communicating and anterior cerebral arteries, through the lamina terminalis (third ventricle); from this same location into the anterior horn of the lateral ventricle.

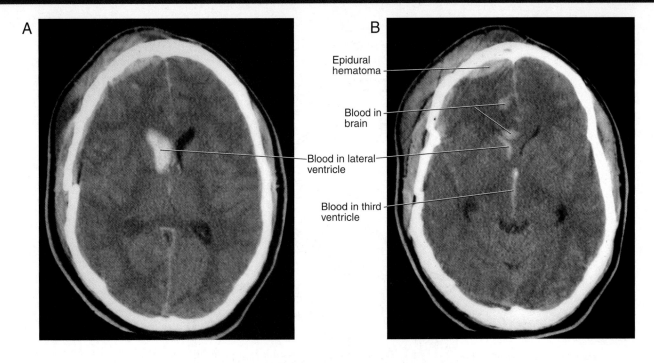

A

B

Epidural
hematoma

Blood in
brain

Blood in lateral
ventricle

Blood in third
ventricle

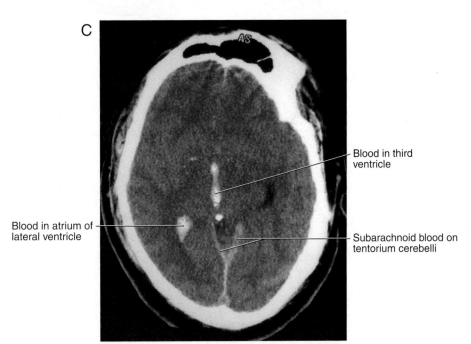

C

AS

Blood in third
ventricle

Blood in atrium of
lateral ventricle

Subarachnoid blood on
tentorium cerebelli

4-13 Examples of blood in the ventricles resulting from head trauma and traumatic brain injuries. Note the soft tissue damage and skull fractures (especially in patients **A** and **B**). In patient **A**, there is blood in the right anterior horn of the lateral ventricle. Patient **B** has blood in the right anterior horn, in the third ventricle, in the substance of the brain in the right frontal lobe as well as a small epidural at the right frontal pole. Patient **C** has blood in the third ventricle and in the atrium of the lateral ventricle on the right side. In addition to trauma, as illustrated here, **intraventricular hemorrhage** (also called **intraventricular blood**) may occur in a variety of situations. **Intracerebral hemorrhage**, a bleed into the substance of the brain (also called **parenchymatous hemorrhage**), may extend into a ventricular space, bleeding from a brain tumor, arteriovenous malformation, or from a

tumor of the choroid plexus. In addition, blood from a ruptured aneurysm may preferentially dissect into adjacent ventricular spaces as described in Figure 4-12. Intraventricular blood may also occur in newborns who have bleeding internal to the ependymal lining of the ventricle (**subependymal hemorrhage**) that extends into the ventricle, in a patient of any age who may bleed from an arteriovenous malformation, or from a highly vascular tumor of the choroid plexus within the ventricular space. As a general principle, the larger the ventricles become, in cases of intraventricular blood, the worse the prognosis for the patient.

These images illustrate the important fact that, especially in patients with head trauma, blood may be found at different locations (meningeal, intraventricular, within the substance of the brain [**parenchymatous**]) in the same patient. All images are axial CTs.

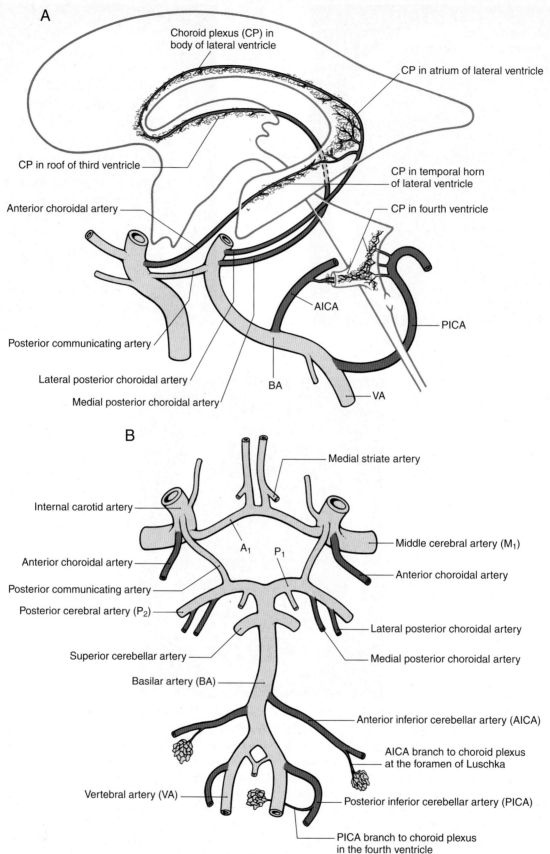

A

Choroid plexus (CP) in
body of lateral ventricle

CP in atrium of lateral ventricle

CP in roof of third ventricle

CP in temporal horn
of lateral ventricle

Anterior choroidal artery

CP in fourth ventricle

AICA

PICA

Posterior communicating artery

Lateral posterior choroidal artery

BA

Medial posterior choroidal artery

VA

B

Medial striate artery

Internal carotid artery

A₁   P₁

Middle cerebral artery (M₁)

Anterior choroidal artery

Anterior choroidal artery

Posterior communicating artery

Posterior cerebral artery (P₂)

Lateral posterior choroidal artery

Superior cerebellar artery

Medial posterior choroidal artery

Basilar artery (BA)

Anterior inferior cerebellar artery (AICA)

AICA branch to choroid plexus
at the foramen of Luschka

Vertebral artery (VA)

Posterior inferior cerebellar artery (PICA)

PICA branch to choroid plexus
in the fourth ventricle

4-14 Blood supply to the choroid plexus of the lateral, third, and fourth ventricles. Those branches of the vertebrobasilar system and of the internal carotid artery and P₂ segment of the posterior cerebral artery that supply the choroid plexus are accentuated by appearing in a darker red shade. In **A,** a representation of these vessels (origin, course, termination) is shown from the lateral aspect. Anterior, medial posterior, and lateral posterior choroidal arteries serve the plexuses of the lateral and third ventricles. The choroid plexus in the fourth ventricle and the clump of choroid plexus protruding out of the foramen of Luschka are served by posterior inferior and anterior inferior cerebellar arteries, respectively. In **B,** the origins of these branches from their main arterial trunks are shown. See also Figures 2-24 (p. 25), 2-32 (p. 31), and 2-35 (p. 33).

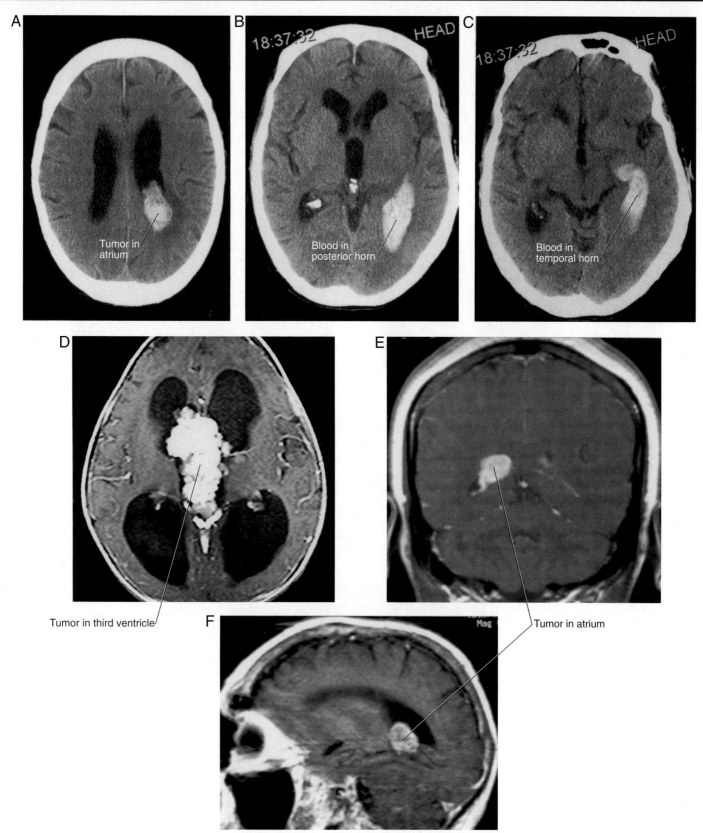

A — Tumor in atrium

B — Blood in posterior horn

C — Blood in temporal horn

D — Tumor in third ventricle

E — Tumor in atrium

F

4-15 Tumors of the choroid plexus (CP) constitute about 1% of all intracranial tumors and are generally classified as **choroid plexus papilloma** (benign, most common of CP tumors) or **choroid plexus carcinoma** (malignant, rare). These tumors are most commonly seen in children younger than 2 years and may present with **symptoms/ signs of increased intracranial pressure** (nausea/vomiting, lethargy, headache, enlarged ventricles, craniomegaly). The CP is highly vascularized; consequently, tumors of this structure may bleed into the ventricular space (**intraventricular hemorrhage**) and create a cast outlining its shape. Examples of tumors of the choroid plexus in axial (**A–D**), coronal (**E**), and sagittal (**F**) planes. The tumor in **A–C** is from the same patient and shows the lesion in the area of the atrium of the lateral ventricle on the left (**A**) with bleeding from the tumor into the posterior and temporal horns of the lateral ventricle on the same side (**B, C**). Note the enlarged ventricles (**A–C**). The image in **D** shows a large tumor originating from the choroid plexus in the roof of the third ventricle. This tumor has partially obstructed the interventricular foramina, with consequent enlargement of the lateral ventricles. Images **E** and **F** are of patients with tumors in the glomus choroideum of the choroid plexus of the lateral ventricle. Images **A–C** are CT, and **D–F** are MRI with enhancement of the tumor.

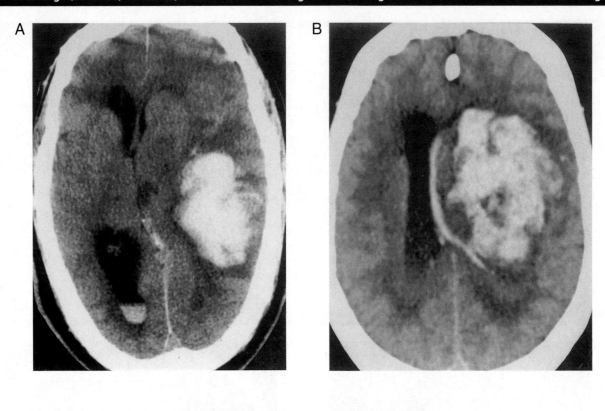

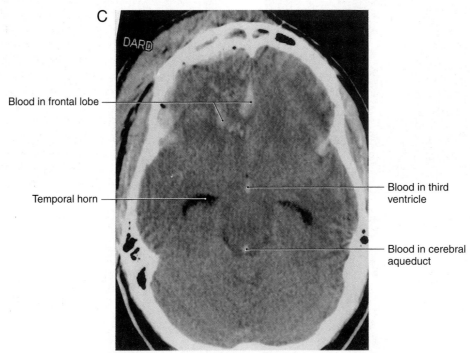

Blood in frontal lobe

Temporal horn

Blood in third ventricle

Blood in cerebral aqueduct

4-16 The presence of blood within the substance of the brain may be called **parenchymatous hemorrhage** (a more general and global term), or **cerebral hemorrhage** (hemorrhage into the cerebral hemisphere), **brainstem hemorrhage** (hemorrhage into the brainstem), **pontine hemorrhage** (hemorrhage into the pons), or by any of a number of other terms that indicate a more specific location and size (**Duret hemorrhage**), shape (**splinter hemorrhage**), or extent of the extravasated blood. The large hemorrhages into the hemisphere (**A, B**) have resulted in enlargement of the ventricles, a **midline shift** (with the real possibility of brain herniation), and, in the case of **A**, a small amount of blood in the posterior horn of the lateral ventricle. In these examples, the lesion is most likely a result of hemorrhage from lenticulostriate branches of the M_1 segment.

Blood in the substance of the brain and in the ventricular system may also result from trauma (**C**). In this example (**C**), blood is seen in the frontal lobe and in the third ventricle and cerebral aqueduct. The enlarged temporal horns (**C**) of the lateral ventricles are consistent with the interruption of CSF flow through the cerebral aqueduct (noncommunicating *hydrocephalus*). Images **A–C** are CT.

Other causes of blood within the brain include bleeding from a variety of tumors, more commonly from malignant tumors and metastatic tumors and less so from benign tumors. Traumatic injury, commonly referred to as **traumatic brain injury** (**TBI**), may be a source of blood within the brain as well as the transformation of an **ischemic stroke** into a **hemorrhagic stroke**.

Q&A for this chapter is available online on thePoint

Internal Morphology of the Brain in Unstained Slices and MRI

5

Part I

Brain Slices in the Coronal Plane Correlated with MRI

Orientation to Coronal MRIs: When looking at a coronal MRI, you are viewing the image as if you are looking at the face of the patient. *Consequently, the observer's right is the left side of the brain in the MRI and the left side of the patient's brain. Conversely, the observer's left is the right side of the brain in the MRI and the right side of the patient's brain.* Obviously, the concept of what is the left side versus what is the right side of the patient's brain is enormously important when using MRI (or CT) to diagnose a neurologically impaired individual.

To reinforce this concept, the rostral surface of each coronal brain slice appears in each photograph. So, when looking at the slice, the observer's right field of view is the left side of the brain slice, and the observer's left field of view is the right side of the brain slice. This view of the slice correlates exactly with the orientation of the brain as seen in the accompanying coronal MRIs.

Orientation to Axial MRIs: When looking at an axial MRI, you are viewing the image as if standing at the patient's feet and looking toward his or her head while the patient is lying on his or her back. *Consequently, and as is the case in coronal images, the observer's right is the left side of the brain in the MRI and the left side of the patient's brain.* It is absolutely essential to have a clear understanding of this right-versus-left concept when using MRI (or CT) in the diagnosis of the neurologically impaired patient.

To reinforce this concept, the ventral surface of each axial slice was photographed. So, when looking at the slice, the observer's right is the left side of the brain slice. This view of the slice correlates exactly with the orientation of the brain as seen in the accompanying axial MRIs.

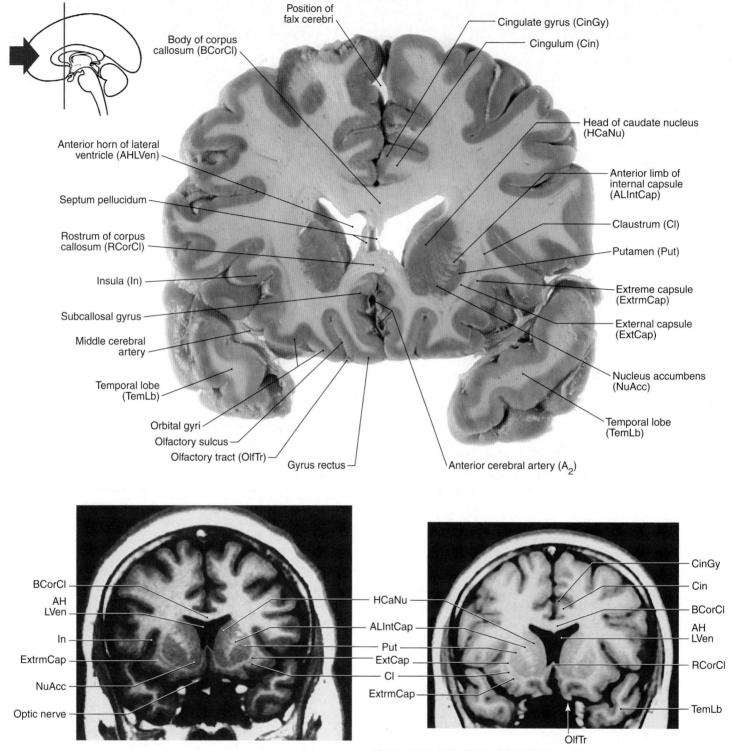

5-1 The rostral surface of a coronal section of brain through the **anterior limb of the internal capsule** and the **head of the caudate nucleus**. The head of the **caudate nucleus** is especially prominent at this coronal plane. In patients with **Huntington disease** (an inherited neurodegenerative disease), the head of the caudate has largely, or completely, disappeared, and the anterior horn of the lateral ventricle would be noticeably large at this level. The two MRIs (both are inversion recovery) are at the same plane and show many of the structures identified in the brain slice.

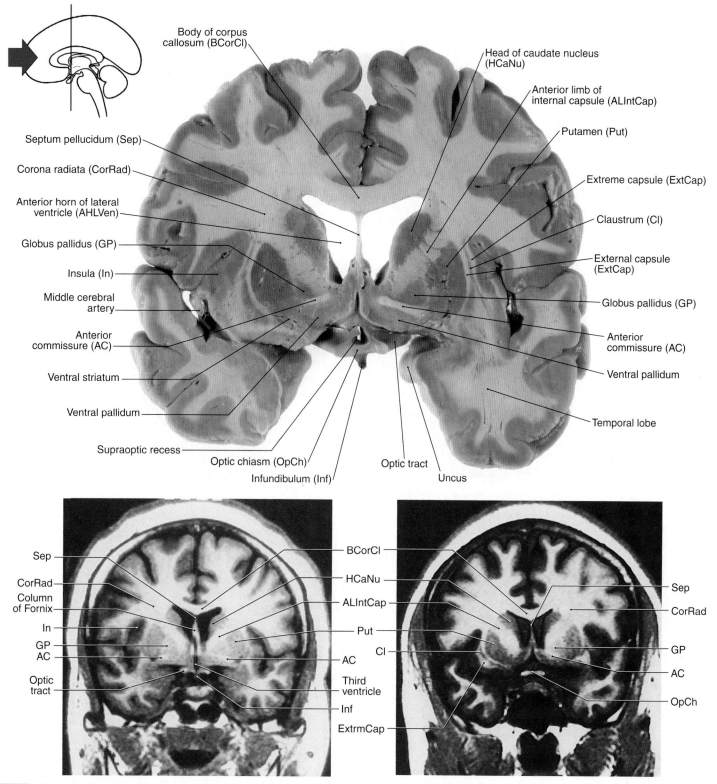

Body of corpus callosum (BCorCl)

Head of caudate nucleus (HCaNu)

Anterior limb of internal capsule (ALIntCap)

Putamen (Put)

Septum pellucidum (Sep)

Extreme capsule (ExtCap)

Corona radiata (CorRad)

Claustrum (Cl)

Anterior horn of lateral ventricle (AHLVen)

External capsule (ExtCap)

Globus pallidus (GP)

Globus pallidus (GP)

Insula (In)

Middle cerebral artery

Anterior commissure (AC)

Anterior commissure (AC)

Ventral striatum

Ventral pallidum

Ventral pallidum

Temporal lobe

Supraoptic recess

Optic chiasm (OpCh)

Optic tract

Infundibulum (Inf)

Uncus

Sep

BCorCl

CorRad

HCaNu

Column of Fornix

ALIntCap

Sep

In

Put

CorRad

GP

Cl

AC

GP

Optic tract

AC

AC

Third ventricle

OpCh

Inf

ExtrmCap

5-2 The rostral surface of a coronal section of brain through the level of the **anterior commissure** and just rostral to the level of the column of the fornix and genu of the internal capsule. The **caudate nucleus** is smaller in size (when compared to the more rostral plane in Figure 5-1) and the **globus pallidus** is obvious in its position medially adjacent to the **putamen.** The two MRIs (both are inversion recovery) are at the same plane and show many of the structures identified in the brain slice.

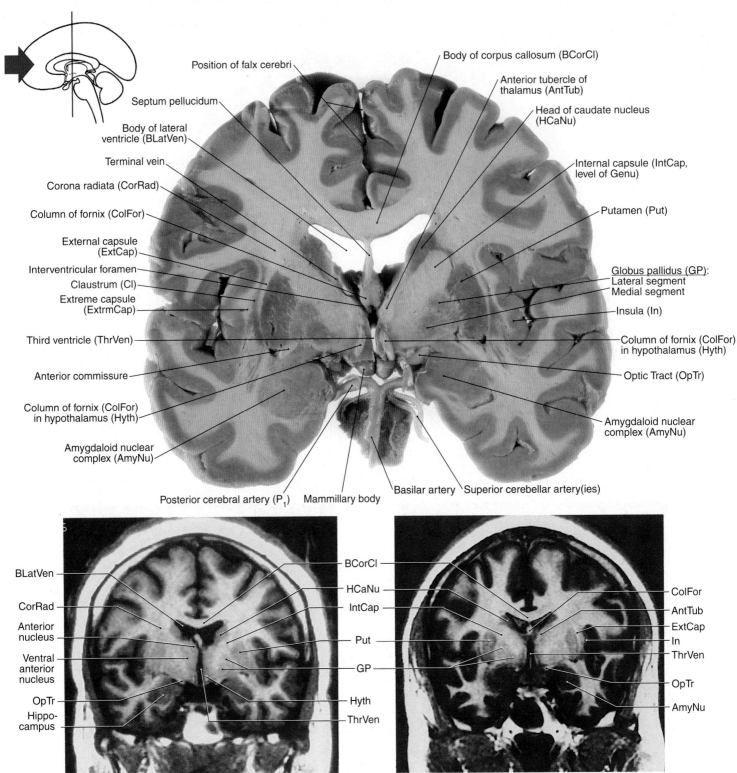

Position of falx cerebri

Body of corpus callosum (BCorCl)

Septum pellucidum

Anterior tubercle of thalamus (AntTub)

Body of lateral ventricle (BLatVen)

Head of caudate nucleus (HCaNu)

Terminal vein

Internal capsule (IntCap, level of Genu)

Corona radiata (CorRad)

Column of fornix (ColFor)

Putamen (Put)

External capsule (ExtCap)

Interventricular foramen

Globus pallidus (GP):
Lateral segment
Medial segment

Claustrum (Cl)

Extreme capsule (ExtrmCap)

Insula (In)

Third ventricle (ThrVen)

Column of fornix (ColFor) in hypothalamus (Hyth)

Anterior commissure

Optic Tract (OpTr)

Column of fornix (ColFor) in hypothalamus (Hyth)

Amygdaloid nuclear complex (AmyNu)

Amygdaloid nuclear complex (AmyNu)

Posterior cerebral artery (P$_1$)   Mammillary body   Basilar artery   Superior cerebellar artery(ies)

BLatVen

BCorCl

HCaNu

ColFor

CorRad

IntCap

AntTub

Anterior nucleus

Put

ExtCap

In

Ventral anterior nucleus

GP

ThrVen

OpTr

Hyth

OpTr

Hippo-campus

ThrVen

AmyNu

5-3 The rostral surface of a coronal section of brain through the level of the **anterior tubercle of the thalamus** and the **column of the fornix** just caudal to the anterior commissure. A level that includes these structures also passes through the **genu of the internal capsule.** This section also includes the two portions of the globus pallidus: a **medial** or **internal segment** and a **lateral** or **external segment.** The terminal vein is also called the superior thalamostriate vein. The two MRIs (both are inversion recovery) are at the same plane and show many of the structures identified in the brain slice.

The **hippocampus** is located in the ventromedial aspect of the temporal horn of the lateral ventricle and appears to have texture in MRI representing its alternating layers of cell bodies and fibers (see Figure 5-4 on the facing page). On the other hand, the **amygdaloid nucleus** is located in the rostral end of the temporal horn and appears very homogenous in MRI (see above). An easy way to recall these relationships is: ventricular space + texture = hippocampus, whereas no ventricular space + homogenous appearance = amygdala. Based on the coronal plane, the transition from one to the other may take place quickly.

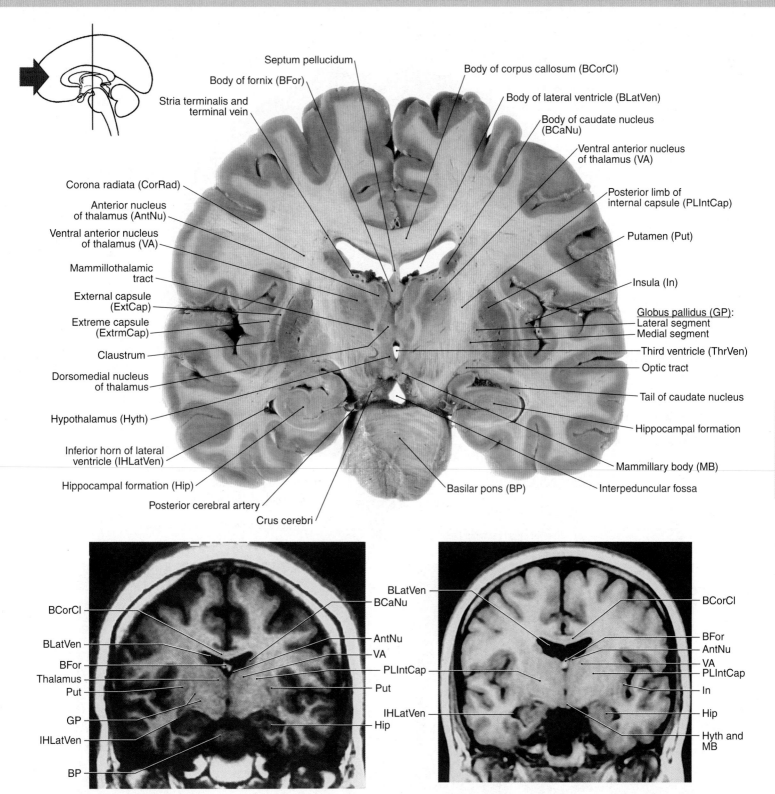

Septum pellucidum
Body of fornix (BFor)
Stria terminalis and terminal vein
Body of corpus callosum (BCorCl)
Body of lateral ventricle (BLatVen)
Body of caudate nucleus (BCaNu)
Ventral anterior nucleus of thalamus (VA)
Posterior limb of internal capsule (PLIntCap)
Putamen (Put)
Insula (In)
Globus pallidus (GP):
Lateral segment
Medial segment
Third ventricle (ThrVen)
Optic tract
Tail of caudate nucleus
Hippocampal formation
Mammillary body (MB)
Interpeduncular fossa

Corona radiata (CorRad)
Anterior nucleus of thalamus (AntNu)
Ventral anterior nucleus of thalamus (VA)
Mammillothalamic tract
External capsule (ExtCap)
Extreme capsule (ExtrmCap)
Claustrum
Dorsomedial nucleus of thalamus
Hypothalamus (Hyth)
Inferior horn of lateral ventricle (IHLatVen)
Hippocampal formation (Hip)
Posterior cerebral artery
Crus cerebri
Basilar pons (BP)

BCorCl
BLatVen
BFor
Thalamus
Put
GP
IHLatVen
BP

BLatVen
BCaNu
AntNu
VA
PLIntCap
Put
IHLatVen
Hip

BCorCl
BFor
AntNu
VA
PLIntCap
In
Hip
Hyth and MB

5-4 The rostral surface of a section of brain through the **anterior nucleus of the thalamus, mammillothalamic tract,** and **mammillary bodies.** This plane also includes the basilar pons (seen in the slice and MRI) and structures associated with the **interpeduncular fossa** (seen in the slice). The two MRIs (both are inversion recovery) are at the same plane and show many of the structures identified in the brain slice. The **globus pallidus** is clearly divided into its **lateral** and **medial segments** in the brain slice. In addition, the terminal vein is also called the superior thalamostriate vein.

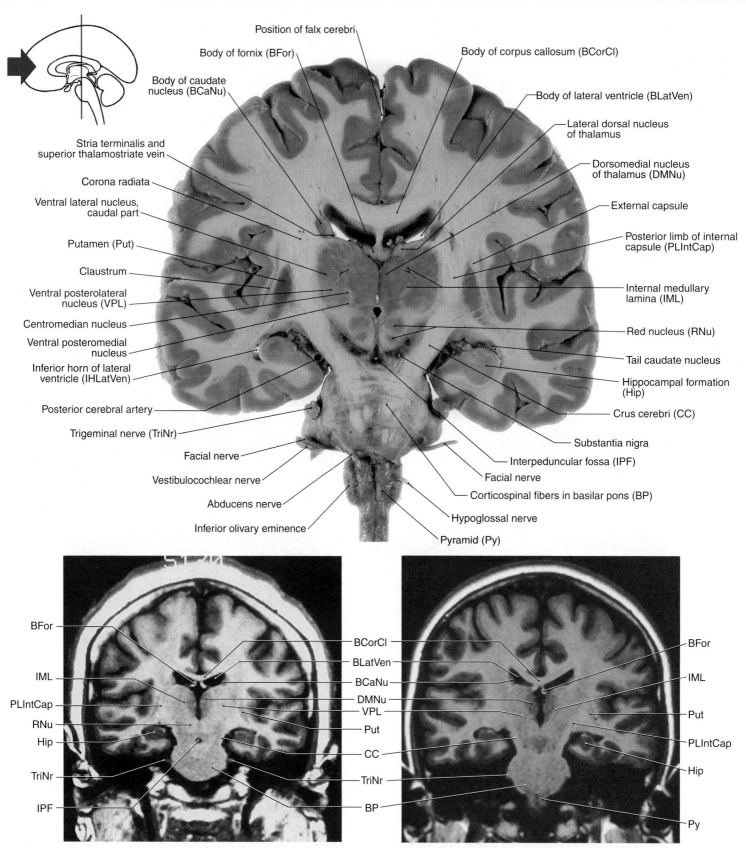

Position of falx cerebri

Body of fornix (BFor)

Body of caudate nucleus (BCaNu)

Stria terminalis and superior thalamostriate vein

Corona radiata

Ventral lateral nucleus, caudal part

Putamen (Put)

Claustrum

Ventral posterolateral nucleus (VPL)

Centromedian nucleus

Ventral posteromedial nucleus

Inferior horn of lateral ventricle (IHLatVen)

Posterior cerebral artery

Trigeminal nerve (TriNr)

Facial nerve

Vestibulocochlear nerve

Abducens nerve

Inferior olivary eminence

Body of corpus callosum (BCorCl)

Body of lateral ventricle (BLatVen)

Lateral dorsal nucleus of thalamus

Dorsomedial nucleus of thalamus (DMNu)

External capsule

Posterior limb of internal capsule (PLIntCap)

Internal medullary lamina (IML)

Red nucleus (RNu)

Tail caudate nucleus

Hippocampal formation (Hip)

Crus cerebri (CC)

Substantia nigra

Interpeduncular fossa (IPF)

Facial nerve

Corticospinal fibers in basilar pons (BP)

Hypoglossal nerve

Pyramid (Py)

BFor

IML

PLIntCap

RNu

Hip

TriNr

IPF

BCorCl

BLatVen

BCaNu

DMNu

VPL

Put

CC

TriNr

BP

BFor

IML

Put

PLIntCap

Hip

Py

5-5 The rostral surface of a coronal section of brain through caudal parts of the **ventral lateral nucleus, massa intermedia, ventral posterolateral nucleus, red nucleus, substantia nigra,** and **basilar pons.** This slice beautifully illustrates that fibers within the internal capsule (posterior limb in this slice) traverse the crus cerebri and enter the basilar pons (MRI and brain slice); these within the crus are the **corticospinal, corticopontine (parieto-, occipito-, temporo-,** and **frontopontine),** and the **corticonuclear fibers.** The two MRIs (both are inversion recovery) are at the same plane and show many of the structures identified in the brain slice.

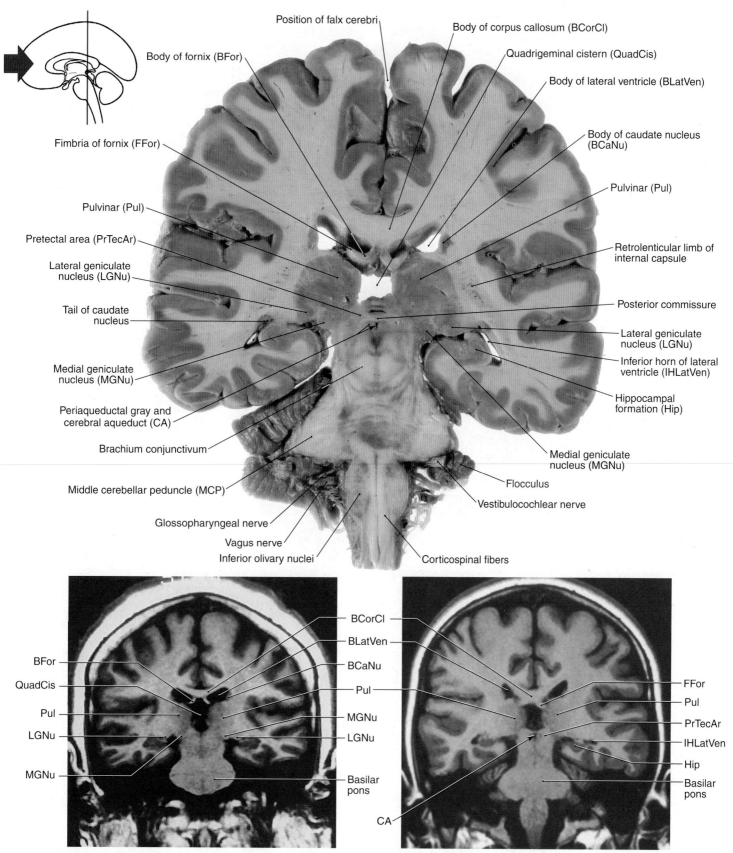

Position of falx cerebri

Body of corpus callosum (BCorCl)

Quadrigeminal cistern (QuadCis)

Body of fornix (BFor)

Body of lateral ventricle (BLatVen)

Fimbria of fornix (FFor)

Body of caudate nucleus (BCaNu)

Pulvinar (Pul)

Pulvinar (Pul)

Pretectal area (PrTecAr)

Retrolenticular limb of internal capsule

Lateral geniculate nucleus (LGNu)

Posterior commissure

Tail of caudate nucleus

Lateral geniculate nucleus (LGNu)

Inferior horn of lateral ventricle (IHLatVen)

Medial geniculate nucleus (MGNu)

Hippocampal formation (Hip)

Periaqueductal gray and cerebral aqueduct (CA)

Medial geniculate nucleus (MGNu)

Brachium conjunctivum

Flocculus

Middle cerebellar peduncle (MCP)

Vestibulocochlear nerve

Glossopharyngeal nerve

Vagus nerve

Inferior olivary nuclei

Corticospinal fibers

BFor

BCorCl

BLatVen

QuadCis

BCaNu

FFor

Pul

Pul

Pul

MGNu

PrTecAr

LGNu

LGNu

IHLatVen

MGNu

Basilar pons

Hip

Basilar pons

CA

5-6 The rostral surface of a coronal section of brain through the **pulvinar nucleus, medial** and **lateral geniculate nuclei,** the **tegmentum of the midbrain and pons,** and the ventral medulla. The corticospinal fibers that had traversed the posterior limb, crus cerebri, and basilar pons are now located in the pyramid of the medulla as **corticospinal fibers.** Note the position and relations of the **quadrigeminal cistern** and that it is clearly different from the position of the third ventricle. The **geniculate bodies** are characteristically located inferior to the overlying **pulvinar** in both the brain slice and MRI. The MRIs (T1) are at the same plane and show many of the structures identified in the brain slice.

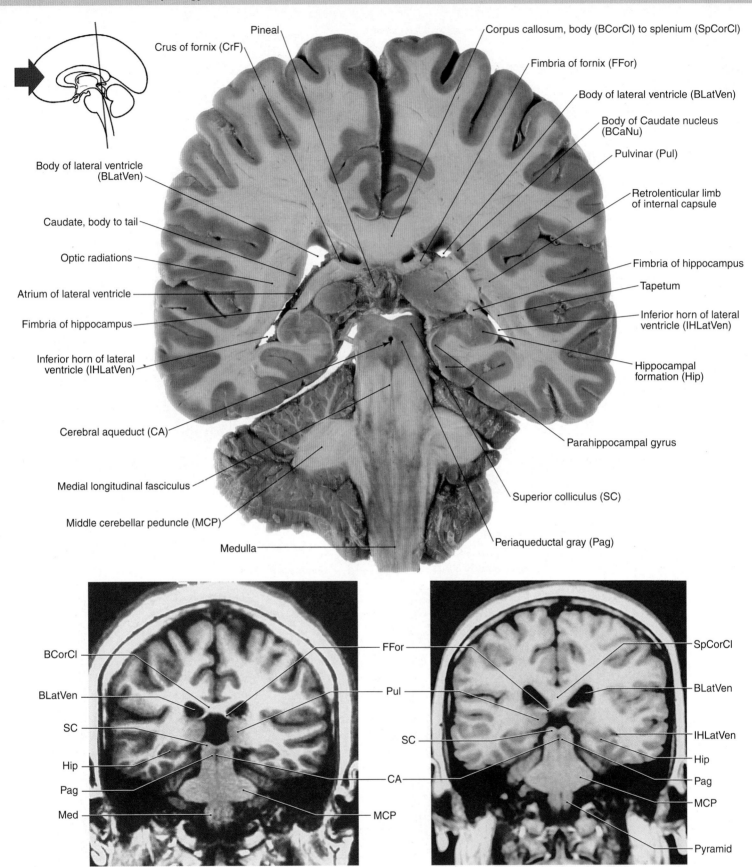

Pineal

Crus of fornix (CrF)

Corpus callosum, body (BCorCl) to splenium (SpCorCl)

Fimbria of fornix (FFor)

Body of lateral ventricle (BLatVen)

Body of Caudate nucleus (BCaNu)

Pulvinar (Pul)

Retrolenticular limb of internal capsule

Body of lateral ventricle (BLatVen)

Caudate, body to tail

Optic radiations

Atrium of lateral ventricle

Fimbria of hippocampus

Inferior horn of lateral ventricle (IHLatVen)

Cerebral aqueduct (CA)

Medial longitudinal fasciculus

Middle cerebellar peduncle (MCP)

Medulla

Fimbria of hippocampus

Tapetum

Inferior horn of lateral ventricle (IHLatVen)

Hippocampal formation (Hip)

Parahippocampal gyrus

Superior colliculus (SC)

Periaqueductal gray (Pag)

BCorCl

BLatVen

SC

Hip

Pag

Med

FFor

Pul

SC

CA

MCP

SpCorCl

BLatVen

IHLatVen

Hip

Pag

MCP

Pyramid

5-7 The rostral surface of a coronal section of brain through the **pineal,** caudal aspects of the **pulvinar, superior colliculi, brainstem tegmentum,** and the **middle cerebellar peduncle.** Note the characteristics and relationships of the middle cerebellar peduncle. The two MRIs (both are inversion recovery) are at the same plane and show many of the structures identified in the brain slice. For details of the cerebellum, see Figures 2-37 and 2-38 (pp. 34–35).

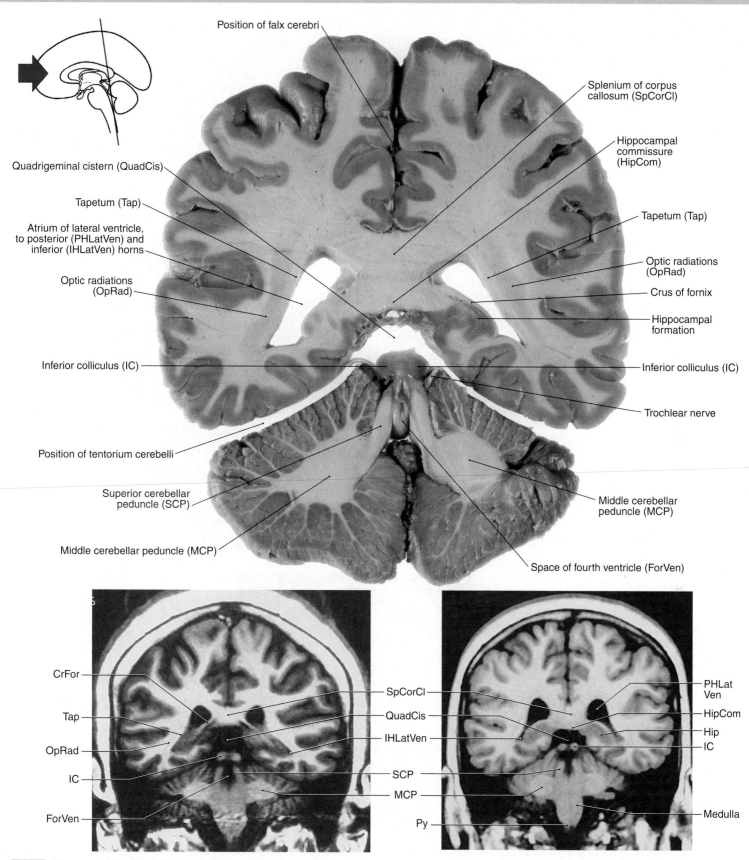

Position of falx cerebri

Splenium of corpus callosum (SpCorCl)

Hippocampal commissure (HipCom)

Quadrigeminal cistern (QuadCis)

Tapetum (Tap)

Atrium of lateral ventricle, to posterior (PHLatVen) and inferior (IHLatVen) horns

Tapetum (Tap)

Optic radiations (OpRad)

Optic radiations (OpRad)

Crus of fornix

Hippocampal formation

Inferior colliculus (IC)

Inferior colliculus (IC)

Trochlear nerve

Position of tentorium cerebelli

Superior cerebellar peduncle (SCP)

Middle cerebellar peduncle (MCP)

Middle cerebellar peduncle (MCP)

Space of fourth ventricle (ForVen)

CrFor

Tap

OpRad

IC

ForVen

SpCorCl

QuadCis

IHLatVen

SCP

MCP

Py

PHLat Ven

HipCom

Hip

IC

Medulla

5-8 The rostral surface of a coronal section of brain through the **splenium of the corpus callosum,** caudal portions on the **quadrigeminal cistern, atrium of the lateral ventricle,** the **superior** and **middle cerebellar peduncles,** and the medially adjacent **fourth ventricle.**

Note the relationship of the **inferior colliculi** to the space of the quadrigeminal cistern. The two MRIs (T1) are at the same plane and show many of the structures identified in the brain slice. For details of the cerebellum, see Figures 2-37 and 2-38 (pp. 34–35).

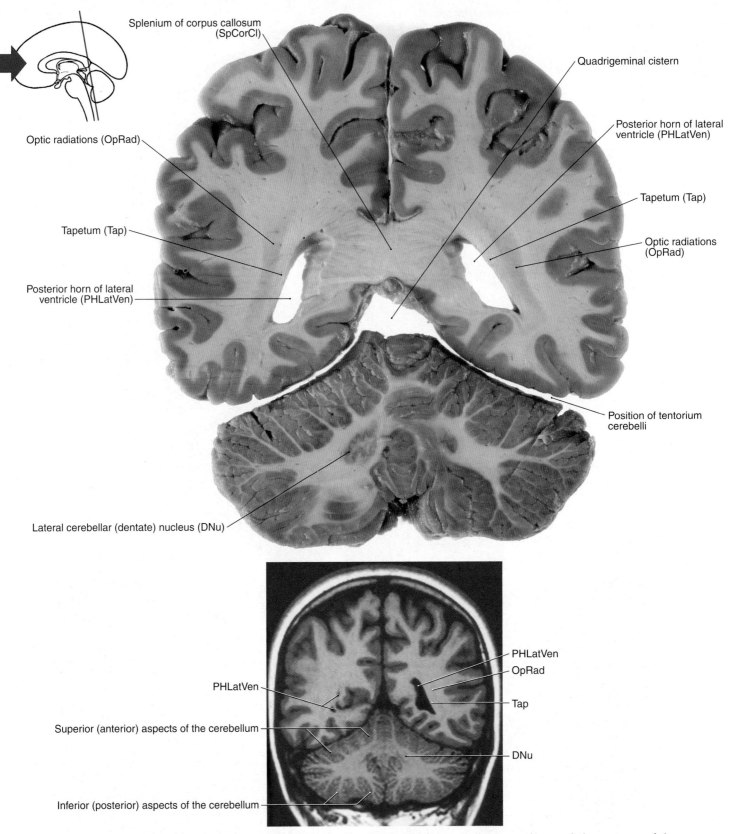

Splenium of corpus callosum (SpCorCl)

Quadrigeminal cistern

Optic radiations (OpRad)

Posterior horn of lateral ventricle (PHLatVen)

Tapetum (Tap)

Optic radiations (OpRad)

Tapetum (Tap)

Posterior horn of lateral ventricle (PHLatVen)

Position of tentorium cerebelli

Lateral cerebellar (dentate) nucleus (DNu)

PHLatVen

PHLatVen
OpRad

Tap

Superior (anterior) aspects of the cerebellum

DNu

Inferior (posterior) aspects of the cerebellum

5-9 The rostral surface of a coronal section of brain through the **splenium of the corpus callosum, posterior horn of the lateral ventricle,** and the cerebellum including a portion of the **dentate nucleus.** The MRI (T1) is at the same plane and shows many of the structures identified in the brain slice. For details of the cerebellum, see Figures 2-37 and 2-38 (pp. 34–35).

Internal Morphology of the Brain in Unstained Slices and MRI

Part II

Brain Slices in the Axial Plane Correlated with MRI

Orientation to Axial MRIs: When looking at an axial MRI, you are viewing the image as if standing at the patient's feet and looking toward his or her head while the patient is lying on his or her back. *Consequently, and as is the case in coronal images, the observer's right is the left side of the brain in the MRI and the left side of the patient's brain, and the observer's left is the right side of the brain in MRI and the right side of the patient's brain.* It is absolutely essential to have a clear understanding of this right-versus-left concept when using MRI or CT in the diagnosis of the neurologically impaired patient.

To reinforce this concept, the ventral surface of each axial slice was photographed. So, when looking at the slice, the observer's right is the left side of the brain slice, and the observer's left is the right side of the brain slice. This view of the slice correlates exactly with the orientation of the brain as seen in the accompanying axial MRIs.

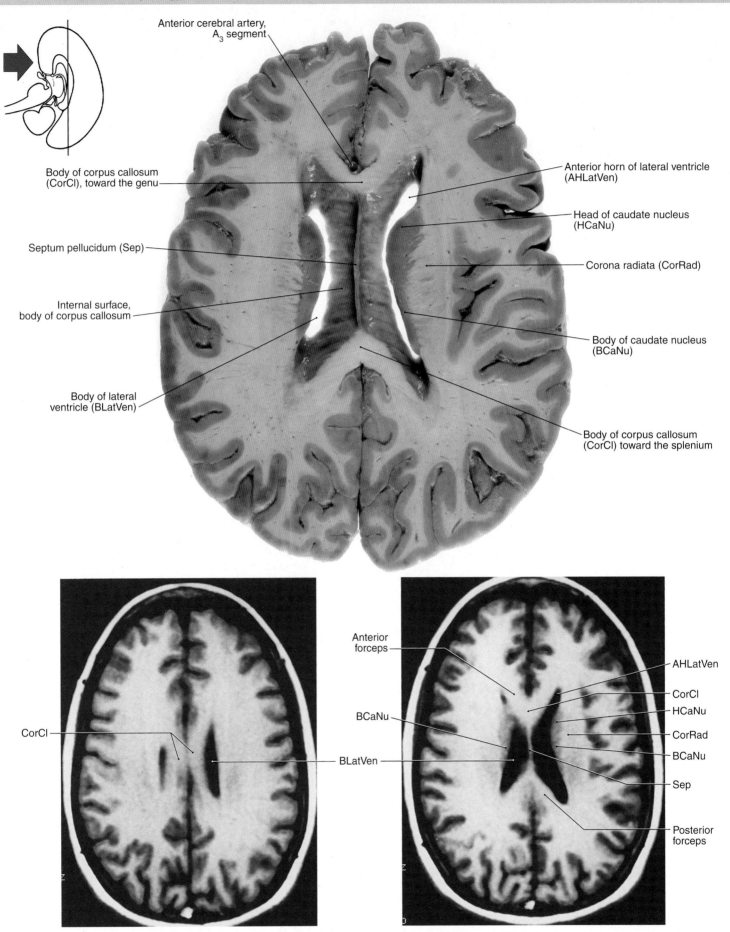

5-10 The ventral surface of an axial section of brain through portions of the **corpus callosum,** the rostrocaudal extent of more superior parts of the lateral **ventricle,** and the head and **body of the** **caudate nucleus.** The two MRIs (both are inversion recovery) are at a similar plane and show some of the structures identified in the brain slice.

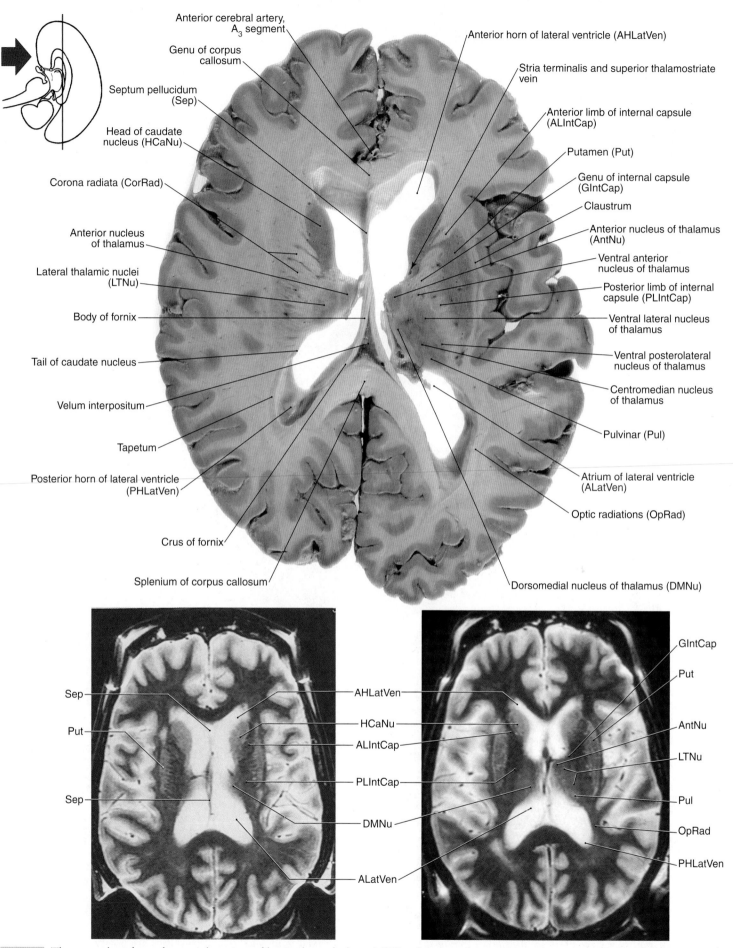

Anterior cerebral artery, A₃ segment

Genu of corpus callosum

Septum pellucidum (Sep)

Head of caudate nucleus (HCaNu)

Corona radiata (CorRad)

Anterior nucleus of thalamus

Lateral thalamic nuclei (LTNu)

Body of fornix

Tail of caudate nucleus

Velum interpositum

Tapetum

Posterior horn of lateral ventricle (PHLatVen)

Crus of fornix

Splenium of corpus callosum

Anterior horn of lateral ventricle (AHLatVen)

Stria terminalis and superior thalamostriate vein

Anterior limb of internal capsule (ALIntCap)

Putamen (Put)

Genu of internal capsule (GIntCap)

Claustrum

Anterior nucleus of thalamus (AntNu)

Ventral anterior nucleus of thalamus

Posterior limb of internal capsule (PLIntCap)

Ventral lateral nucleus of thalamus

Ventral posterolateral nucleus of thalamus

Centromedian nucleus of thalamus

Pulvinar (Pul)

Atrium of lateral ventricle (ALatVen)

Optic radiations (OpRad)

Dorsomedial nucleus of thalamus (DMNu)

Sep

Put

Sep

AHLatVen

HCaNu

ALIntCap

PLIntCap

DMNu

ALatVen

GIntCap

Put

AntNu

LTNu

Pul

OpRad

PHLatVen

5-11 The ventral surface of an axial section of brain through the **splenium of the corpus callosum** and the **head of the caudate nucleus.** *Note that the sides (right/left) of the brain slice are considered the same as the sides (right/left) in the MRIs (see comments on pp. 75 and 85).* This plane is slightly tilted (sometimes seen in MRI), showing the superior most part of the thalamus on the patient's right and a slightly lower axial plane on the patient's left. The two MRIs, both are T2-weighted, are at a comparable plane and show some of the structures identified in the brain slice.

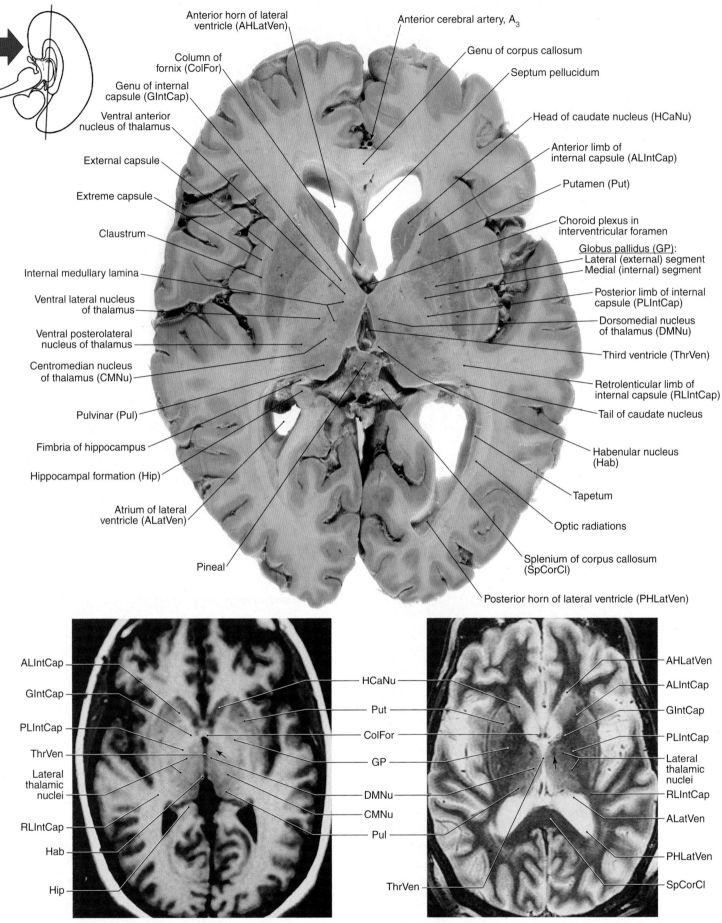

The ventral surface of an axial section of brain through the **lenticular nucleus,** four limbs of the **internal capsule,** the main **thalamic nuclei, third ventricle,** and the **pineal.** The **medial and lateral segments of the globus pallidus** are clearly visible on the left side of the axial brain slice. The arrowheads are pointing to the mammillothalamic tract in both MRIs. The two MRIs (T1, **left;** T2, **right**) are at the same plane and show many of the structures identified in the brain slice.

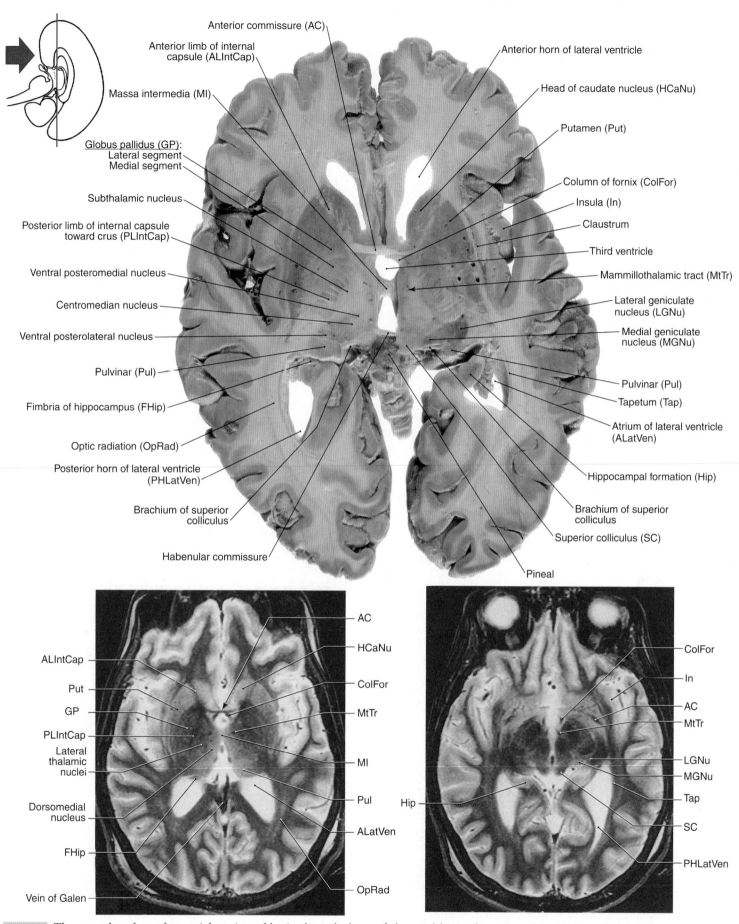

Anterior commissure (AC)

Anterior limb of internal
capsule (ALIntCap)

Massa intermedia (MI)

Globus pallidus (GP):
Lateral segment
Medial segment

Subthalamic nucleus

Posterior limb of internal capsule
toward crus (PLIntCap)

Ventral posteromedial nucleus

Centromedian nucleus

Ventral posterolateral nucleus

Pulvinar (Pul)

Fimbria of hippocampus (FHip)

Optic radiation (OpRad)

Posterior horn of lateral ventricle
(PHLatVen)

Brachium of superior
colliculus

Habenular commissure

Anterior horn of lateral ventricle

Head of caudate nucleus (HCaNu)

Putamen (Put)

Column of fornix (ColFor)

Insula (In)

Claustrum

Third ventricle

Mammillothalamic tract (MtTr)

Lateral geniculate
nucleus (LGNu)

Medial geniculate
nucleus (MGNu)

Pulvinar (Pul)

Tapetum (Tap)

Atrium of lateral ventricle
(ALatVen)

Hippocampal formation (Hip)

Brachium of superior
colliculus

Superior colliculus (SC)

Pineal

ALIntCap

Put

GP

PLIntCap

Lateral
thalamic
nuclei

Dorsomedial
nucleus

FHip

Vein of Galen

AC

HCaNu

ColFor

MtTr

MI

Pul

ALatVen

OpRad

Hip

ColFor

In

AC

MtTr

LGNu

MGNu

Tap

SC

PHLatVen

5-13 The ventral surface of an axial section of brain through the **anterior commissure, column of the fornix**, portions of the **medial** and **lateral geniculate nuclei**, and **superior colliculus**. The **medial** and **lateral segments** of the **globus pallidus** are visible on the right side

of the axial brain slice. Note the position of the **subthalamic nucleus** and its position adjacent to the posterior limb as it condenses to form the crus cerebri. The MRIs (both T2-weighted) are at approximately the same plane and show many of the structures identified in the brain slice.

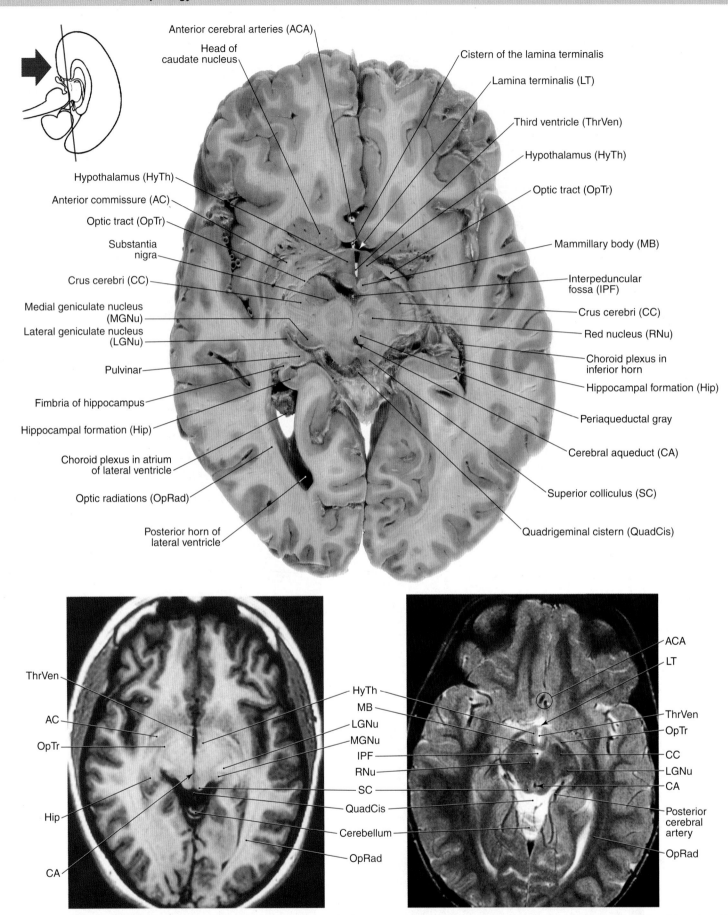

Anterior cerebral arteries (ACA)

Head of caudate nucleus

Cistern of the lamina terminalis

Lamina terminalis (LT)

Third ventricle (ThrVen)

Hypothalamus (HyTh)

Optic tract (OpTr)

Hypothalamus (HyTh)

Anterior commissure (AC)

Optic tract (OpTr)

Substantia nigra

Crus cerebri (CC)

Medial geniculate nucleus (MGNu)

Lateral geniculate nucleus (LGNu)

Pulvinar

Fimbria of hippocampus

Hippocampal formation (Hip)

Choroid plexus in atrium of lateral ventricle

Optic radiations (OpRad)

Posterior horn of lateral ventricle

Mammillary body (MB)

Interpeduncular fossa (IPF)

Crus cerebri (CC)

Red nucleus (RNu)

Choroid plexus in inferior horn

Hippocampal formation (Hip)

Periaqueductal gray

Cerebral aqueduct (CA)

Superior colliculus (SC)

Quadrigeminal cistern (QuadCis)

ThrVen
AC
OpTr
Hip
CA

HyTh
MB
LGNu
MGNu
IPF
RNu
SC
QuadCis
Cerebellum
OpRad

ACA
LT
ThrVen
OpTr
CC
LGNu
CA
Posterior cerebral artery
OpRad

5-14 The ventral surface of an axial section of brain through the **optic tract, hypothalamus, mammillary body, red nucleus, superior colliculi,** and the **medial and lateral geniculate nuclei.** Note that the anterior commissure and the optic tract (brain slice, MRI) may appear similar but have important spatial relationships that differentiate one from the other. The two MRIs (T1, **left;** T2, **right**) are at similar planes and show many of the structures identified in the brain slice.

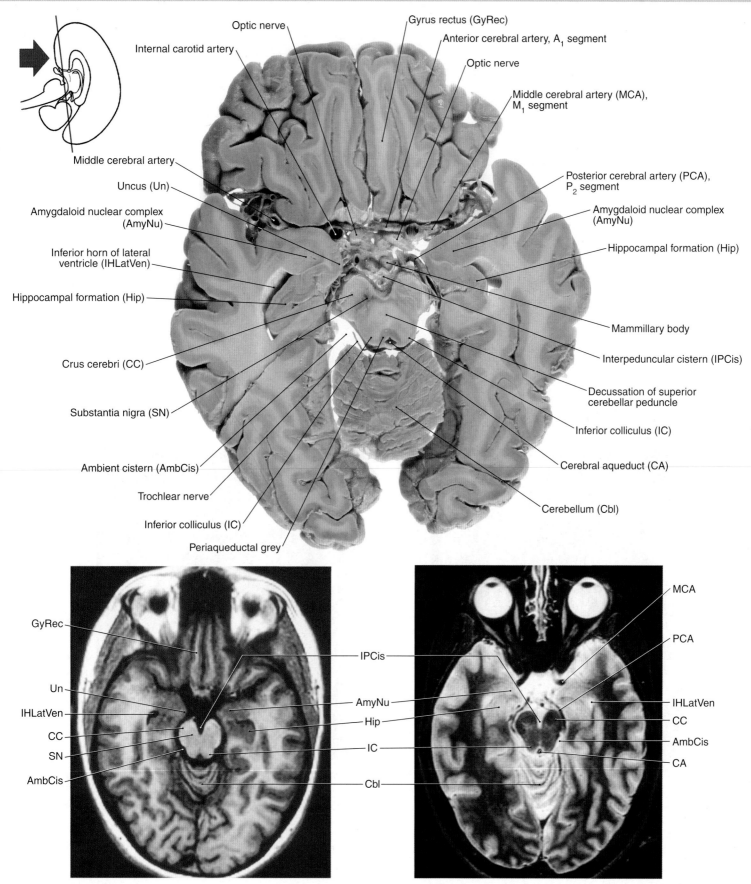

Optic nerve

Gyrus rectus (GyRec)

Internal carotid artery

Anterior cerebral artery, A$_1$ segment

Optic nerve

Middle cerebral artery (MCA), M$_1$ segment

Middle cerebral artery

Posterior cerebral artery (PCA), P$_2$ segment

Uncus (Un)

Amygdaloid nuclear complex (AmyNu)

Amygdaloid nuclear complex (AmyNu)

Inferior horn of lateral ventricle (IHLatVen)

Hippocampal formation (Hip)

Hippocampal formation (Hip)

Mammillary body

Crus cerebri (CC)

Interpeduncular cistern (IPCis)

Substantia nigra (SN)

Decussation of superior cerebellar peduncle

Ambient cistern (AmbCis)

Inferior colliculus (IC)

Trochlear nerve

Cerebral aqueduct (CA)

Inferior colliculus (IC)

Cerebellum (Cbl)

Periaqueductal grey

GyRec

IPCis

MCA

Un

PCA

IHLatVen

AmyNu

IHLatVen

CC

Hip

CC

SN

IC

AmbCis

AmbCis

CA

Cbl

5-15 The ventral surface of an axial section of brain through the **amygdaloid nucleus, hippocampus,** and mid to caudal levels of the **midbrain.** At this midbrain level, note the **decussation of the superior cerebellar peduncle, inferior colliculus,** and the **trochlear nerve** in the ambient cistern. **Mammillary bodies** are also seen in relation to the interpeduncular cistern. The two MRIs (T1, **left;** T2, **right**) are at the same plane and show many of the structures identified in the brain slice. For details of the cerebellum, see Figures 2-37 and 2-38 (pp. 34–35).

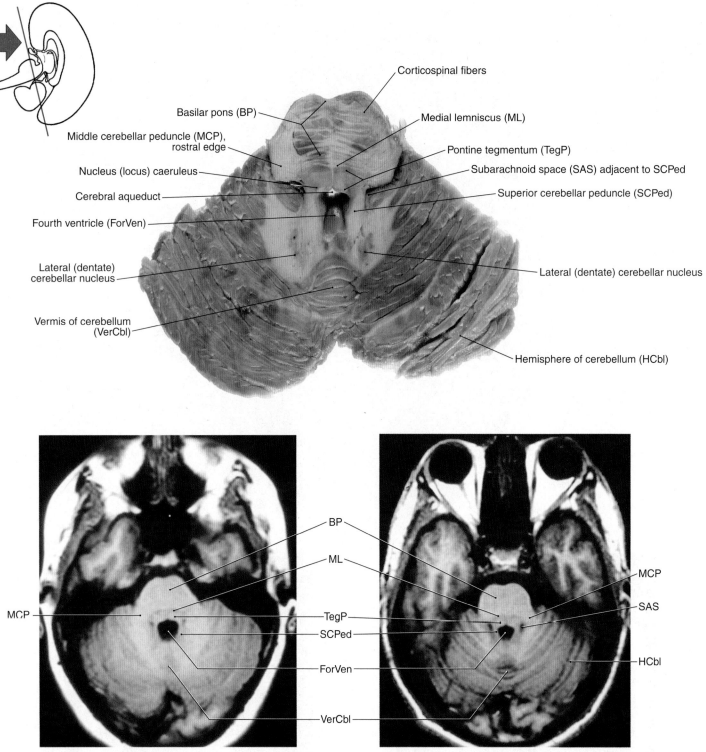

Corticospinal fibers

Basilar pons (BP)

Medial lemniscus (ML)

Middle cerebellar peduncle (MCP), rostral edge

Pontine tegmentum (TegP)

Nucleus (locus) caeruleus

Subarachnoid space (SAS) adjacent to SCPed

Cerebral aqueduct

Superior cerebellar peduncle (SCPed)

Fourth ventricle (ForVen)

Lateral (dentate) cerebellar nucleus

Lateral (dentate) cerebellar nucleus

Lateral (dentate) cerebellar nucleus

Vermis of cerebellum (VerCbl)

Hemisphere of cerebellum (HCbl)

MCP

BP

ML

MCP

MCP

SAS

TegP

SCPed

ForVen

HCbl

VerCbl

5-16   The ventral surface of an axial section of brain through the rostral portions of the **basilar pons,** rostral parts of the **fourth ventricle** and the adjacent **superior cerebellar peduncle,** and the **dentate nucleus** in the white matter core of the cerebellar hemisphere. Note the very characteristic appearance of the small part of the subarachnoid space laterally adjacent to the superior cerebellar peduncle. The two MRIs (both T1-weighted) are at the same plane and show many of the structures identified in the brain slice. For details of the cerebellum, see Figures 2-37 and 2-38 (pp. 34–35).

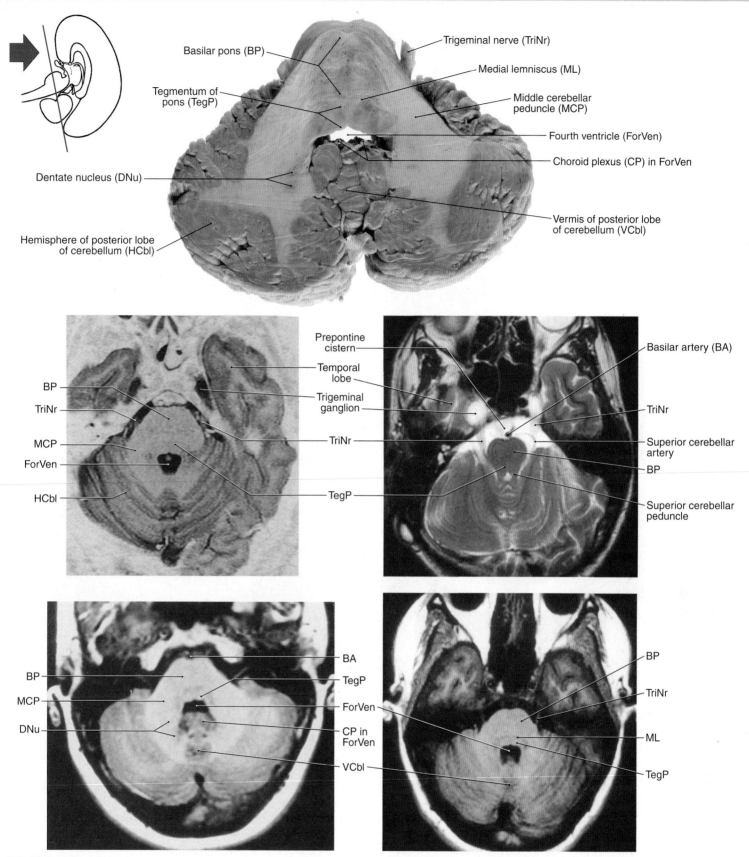

The ventral surface of an axial section of brain through the **basilar pons** at the level of the **trigeminal nerve,** and through the large part of the **middle cerebellar** peduncle. This also correlates with the widest parts of the basilar pons and with the **pontine tegmentum.** The four MRIs (inverted inversion recovery, **upper left;** T2, **upper right;** T1, **both lower**) are at the same general plane and show many of the structures identified in the brain slice. For details of the cerebellum, see Figures 2-37 and 2-38 (pp. 34–35).

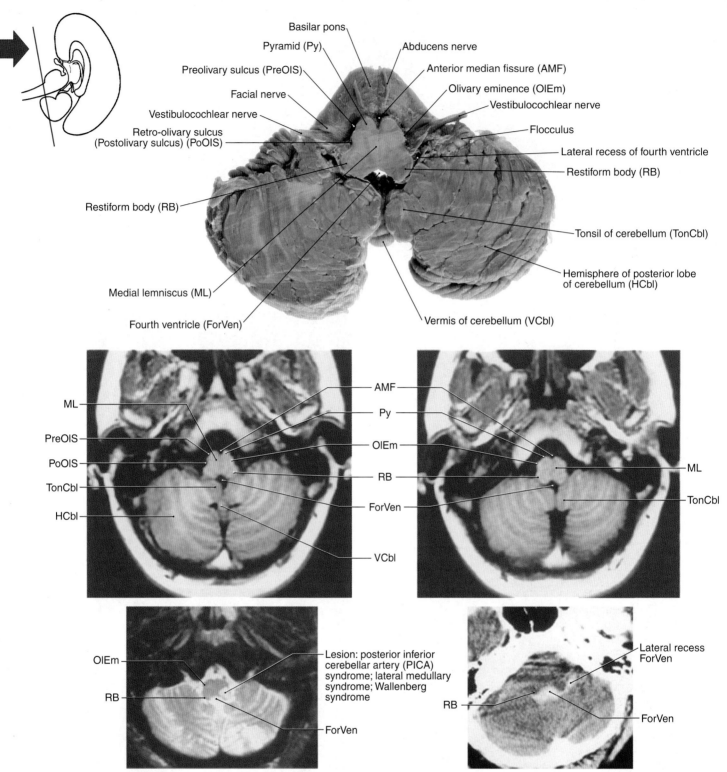

5-18 The ventral surface of an axial section of brain through the medullary surface at the general level of the pons–medulla junction. This level is characterized by the **restiform body, pyramid, olivary eminence** and related **sulci,** and the **fourth ventricle** and the **lateral recess of the fourth ventricle.** Note the close apposition of the cerebellar tonsil to the medulla. The four images (T1 MRI, **both upper;** T2 MRI, **lower left;** CT, **lower right**) are at the same general plane and show many of the structures identified in the brain slice. Note the blood in the fourth ventricle and extending into the lateral recess of the fourth ventricle (compare brain slice with the CT). For details of the cerebellum, see Figures 2-37 and 2-38 (pp. 34–35).

Q&A for this chapter is available online on thePoint

Internal Morphology of the Spinal Cord and Brain: Functional Components, MRI, Stained Sections

6

asic concepts that are essential when one is *initially learning* how to diagnose the neurologically impaired patient include: 1) an understanding of cranial nerve nuclei and 2) how these structures relate to long tracts. The importance of these relationships is clearly seen in the combinations of deficits that generally characterize lesions at different levels of the neuraxis. *First*, deficits of the body only, excluding the head, that may present as motor or sensory losses (long tracts) on the same side, or opposite sides, are indicative of spinal cord lesions (e.g., Brown-Séquard syndrome). Spinal cord injuries characteristically have **motor and sensory levels**; these are the **lowest functional levels** remaining in the compromised patient. *Second*, cranial nerve deficits (on one side of the head) in combination with long tract signs (on the opposite side of the body) characterize lesions in the brainstem (e.g., lateral medullary and Weber syndromes). These patterns of loss are frequently called **alternating** or **crossed deficits**. In these examples, cranial nerve signs are better **localizing signs** than are long tract signs. A **localizing sign** can be defined as an objective neurologic abnormality that correlates with a lesion (or lesions) at a specific neuroanatomical location (or locations). *Third*, motor and sensory deficits on the same side of the head and body are usually indicative of a lesion in the forebrain.

Color-Coded Spinal and Cranial Nerve Nuclei and Long Tracts

Spinal and cranial nerve motor nuclei are coded by their function; those innervating skeletal muscle (**somatic efferent**) are salmon/dark pink, and preganglionic **visceral motor** nuclei are rust. Similarly, the primary sensory nuclei of the spinal cord and brainstem that receive **somatic afferent** sensation are light pink, and those receiving **visceral afferents** are purple. For example, one can easily correlate damage to the hypoglossal nerve root and the corticospinal fibers on one side, while comparing this pattern to a lateral medullary syndrome on the other side.

Long tracts are color coded beginning at the most caudal spinal cord levels (e.g., see Figures 6-3 and 6-4), with these colors extending into the dorsal thalamus (see Figure 6-33) and the posterior limb of the internal capsule (see Figures 6-34 and 6-35). The colorized spinal tracts are the **fasciculus gracilis** (dark blue), the **fasciculus cuneatus** (light blue),* the **anterolateral system** (dark green), and the **lateral corticospinal tract** (gray). In the brainstem, these spinal tracts are joined by the **spinal trigeminal tract** and **ventral trigeminothalamic fibers** (both are light green). The long tracts are color coded on one side only, to emphasize: 1)

laterality of function and dysfunction; 2) points at which fibers in these tracts may decussate; and 3) the relationship of these tracts to cranial nerves.

Each set of facing pages (line drawing/stained section) through spinal and brainstem parts of this chapter feature a version of the overview of motor and sensory nuclei (or cell columns) next to the stained section. The line on this view, and the few labels, specifically identify the sensory and motor nuclei at that particular level, and the color code matches that on the line drawing. This allows the user to easily identify the relationships and continuity of functionally related cell columns at any level.

A color key appears on each page. This key identifies the various tracts and nuclei by their color and specifies the function of each structure on each page.

Correlation of MRI and CT with Internal Spinal Cord and Brainstem Anatomy

As one is learning basic anatomical concepts, it is absolutely essential to understand how this information is used in the clinical environment. To show the relationship between basic anatomy and how MRI (T1- and T2-weighted) and CT (myelogram/cisternogram) are viewed, a series of self-explanatory illustrations is provided on each set of facing pages in the spinal cord and brainstem sections of this chapter. This continuum of visual information consists of: 1) a small version of the colorized line drawing in an **Anatomical Orientation**; 2) a top-to-bottom flip that brings the same image into a **Clinical Orientation**; and 3) a CT (spinal cord) or MRI and CT (brainstem) that follows this clinically oriented image. To further enhance the seamless application of basic neuroscience to clinical images (and to do so in their proper context), especially important anatomical structures are outlined, in white, on CT (spinal cord) and on the T1-weighted MRI (brainstem) images. This allows the user to understand where these anatomical structures are located in clinical images as viewed in the **Clinical Orientation**. One essential aspect of diagnosis is developing the ability to visualize what structures are involved in brainstem lesions and how the patient's deficits correlate with the location and extent of the lesion. In addition, the "flip symbol" at the lower left of each page indicates which anatomical images may be flipped to a clinical orientation (labels on or off) using online resources available with the atlas.

Every effort is made to identify and use MRI and CT that correlate, as closely as possible, with their corresponding line drawing and stained section. This approach recognizes and retains the strength of the anatomical approach and introduces essential clinical concepts while at the same time allowing the user to customize the material to suit a range of educational applications.

---

*The dark and light blue colors represent information originating from lower and upper portions of the body, respectively.

Function Components in the Neural Tube, Spinal Cord, and Brainstem (Figures 6-1 and 6-2)

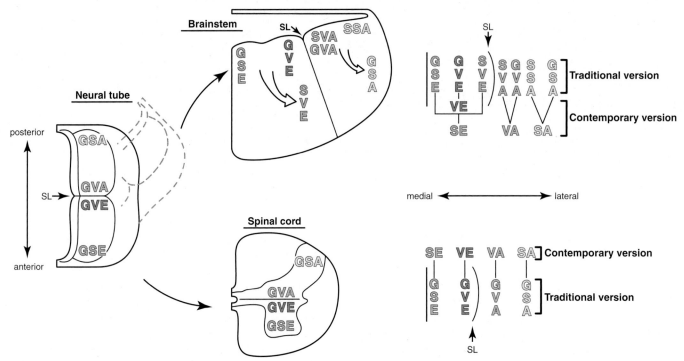

6-1 The concept of **functional components** (of both spinal and cranial nerves) recognizes that primary afferent fibers entering, and the efferent fibers leaving, the spinal cord or brainstem convey **specific types of information**. There are two versions of **functional components**: 1) a **traditional version** that originated early in the 20th century and was the standard for many decades and 2) a **contemporary version** that reflects recent discoveries in head, neck, and brain development. Either of these plans can be used as they are complementary, one to the other.

Traditional version: In this version (Figures 6-1 and 6-2), the components seen in the developing neural tube (**left**), that are associated with the alar plate (GSA, GVA), are located posterior to the sulcus limitans (SL); those associated with the basal plate (GVE, GSE) are located anterior to the SL (Figure 6-1, **left**). These are general features also seen in the contemporary version. In the adult spinal cord, this general posterior/anterior relationship is maintained (Figure 6-1, **lower center**).

At the spinal cord–brainstem transition, two important changes occur. *First*, as the central canal enlarges into the fourth ventricle, and the cerebellum develops, the alar portion of the neural tube is rotated laterally. The SL is present in the adult brainstem and separates the medially located basal plate derivatives (motor nuclei) from the laterally located alar plate derivatives (sensory nuclei). *Second*, in the brainstem, special functional components, as traditionally identified (SVE to muscles of the pharyngeal arches; SVA to taste; SSA to vestibular and auditory), form cell columns that are restricted to the brainstem and not represented in the spinal cord.

Within the brainstem, there are transpositions of the SVE and GSA components. Early in development, cells associated with the SVE component (nucleus ambiguus, facial and trigeminal motor nuclei) appear in the floor of the ventricle, but then migrate ventrolaterally to their adult locations. In like manner, cells with the GSA component (spinal trigeminal, principal sensory) that appear in the ventricular floor in the alar area also migrate ventrolaterally to their adult locations. Cells of the mesencephalic nucleus arise from the neural crest and migrate into the brainstem to become part of the GSA cell column. The border between motor and sensory areas of the brainstem is represented by an oblique line beginning at the SL. The relative positions, and color coding, of the various components shown in the above image (right) is directly translatable to Figure 6-2 on the facing page.

Contemporary version: This version (Figure 6-1, right), as was the traditional version, is based on development, but incorporates more detailed data concerning neuron and muscle origin and their respective migration patterns. For example, striated muscles innervated by cranial nerves (CNs) III, IV, V, VI, VII, IX, X, and XII all arise from the epimere (paraxial mesoderm), which segments into somitomeres. Consequently, the cells of all of these motor nuclei are designated as an SE (Somatic Efferent) functional component. The neurons of CN III that influence orbital smooth muscles, the cells of CNs VII and IX which influence vascular smooth muscle and glandular epithelium in the head, and cells of CN X that influence the same tissues in the thorax and abdomen, are all designated as VE (Visceral Efferent). All visceral afferent information (traditionally divided into General and Special) is associated with the solitary tract and nuclei and is designated VA (Visceral Afferent). The components traditionally associated with the vestibulocochlear nuclei (SSA) and with the trigeminal sensory nuclei (GSA) are consolidated into an SA (Somatic Afferent) category. The correlation between the traditional and contemporary versions is shown in Figure 6-1, far right.

ABBREVIATIONS			
GSA	General Somatic Afferent	**SVE**	Special Visceral Efferent
GSE	General Somatic Efferent	**SL**	Sulcus Limitans
GVA	General Visceral Afferent	**SA**	Somatic Afferent
GVE	General Visceral Efferent	**SE**	Somatic Efferent
SSA	Special Somatic Afferent	**VA**	Visceral Afferent
SVA	Special Visceral Afferent	**VE**	Visceral Efferent

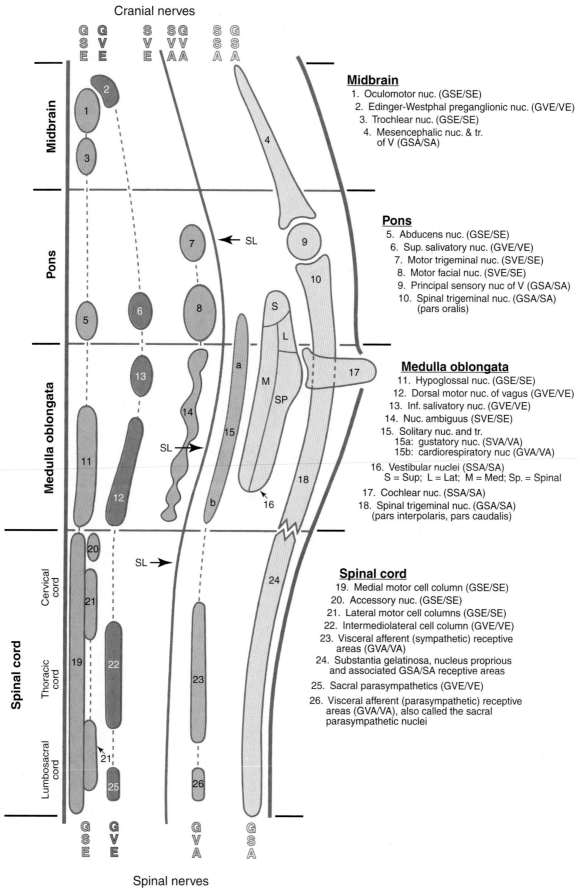

Cranial nerves

Midbrain
1. Oculomotor nuc. (GSE/SE)
2. Edinger-Westphal preganglionic nuc. (GVE/VE)
3. Trochlear nuc. (GSE/SE)
4. Mesencephalic nuc. & tr. of V (GSA/SA)

Pons
5. Abducens nuc. (GSE/SE)
6. Sup. salivatory nuc. (GVE/VE)
7. Motor trigeminal nuc. (SVE/SE)
8. Motor facial nuc. (SVE/SE)
9. Principal sensory nuc of V (GSA/SA)
10. Spinal trigeminal nuc. (GSA/SA) (pars oralis)

Medulla oblongata
11. Hypoglossal nuc. (GSE/SE)
12. Dorsal motor nuc. of vagus (GVE/VE)
13. Inf. salivatory nuc. (GVE/VE)
14. Nuc. ambiguus (SVE/SE)
15. Solitary nuc. and tr.
    15a: gustatory nuc. (SVA/VA)
    15b: cardiorespiratory nuc (GVA/VA)
16. Vestibular nuclei (SSA/SA)
    S = Sup; L = Lat; M = Med; Sp. = Spinal
17. Cochlear nuc. (SSA/SA)
18. Spinal trigeminal nuc. (GSA/SA) (pars interpolaris, pars caudalis)

Spinal cord
19. Medial motor cell column (GSE/SE)
20. Accessory nuc. (GSE/SE)
21. Lateral motor cell columns (GSE/SE)
22. Intermediolateral cell column (GVE/VE)
23. Visceral afferent (sympathetic) receptive areas (GVA/VA)
24. Substantia gelatinosa, nucleus proprious and associated GSA/SA receptive areas
25. Sacral parasympathetics (GVE/VE)
26. Visceral afferent (parasympathetic) receptive areas (GVA/VA), also called the sacral parasympathetic nuclei

Spinal nerves

6-2 The medial-to-lateral positions of brainstem cranial nerve and spinal cord nuclei as shown here are the same as in Figure 6-1. This diagrammatic posterior (dorsal) view shows: 1) the relative positions and names of specific cell groups and their associated functional components; 2) the approximate location of particular nuclei in their specific division of brainstem and/or spinal cord; and 3) the rostrocaudal continuity of cell columns (either as continuous or discontinuous cell groups) from one division of the brainstem to the next or from brainstem to spinal cord. The nucleus ambiguus is a column of cells composed of distinct cell clusters interspersed with more diffusely arranged cells, much like a string of beads. Nuclei associated with CNs I and II are not shown. The color coding used on this figure correlates with that on Figure 6-1 (facing page).

6-3A   Transverse section of the spinal cord showing the characteristics of a sacral level. The gray matter occupies most of the cross-section; its H-shaped appearance is not especially obvious at sacral–coccygeal levels. The white matter is a comparatively thin mantle. The sacral cord, although small, appears round in the CT myelogram. Note the appearance of the sacral spinal cord surrounded by the upper portion of the **cauda equina (left)** and the cauda equina as it appears caudal to the conus medullaris in the **lumbar cistern (right)**. Compare with Figure 2-4 on p. 10.

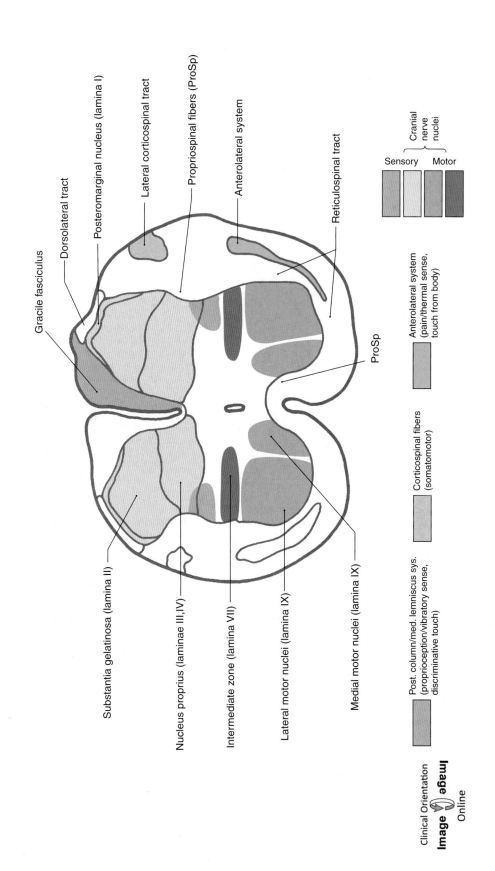

Gracile fasciculus

Dorsolateral tract

Posteromarginal nucleus (lamina I)

Lateral corticospinal tract

Propriospinal fibers (ProSp)

Anterolateral system

Reticulospinal tract

ProSp

Substantia gelatinosa (lamina II)

Nucleus proprius (laminae III,IV)

Intermediate zone (lamina VII)

Lateral motor nuclei (lamina IX)

Medial motor nuclei (lamina IX)

Sensory   Motor

Cranial nerve nuclei

Post. column/med. lemniscus sys. (proprioception/vibratory sense, discriminative touch)

Corticospinal fibers (somatomotor)

Anterolateral system (pain/thermal sense, touch from body)

Clinical Orientation

Image Online

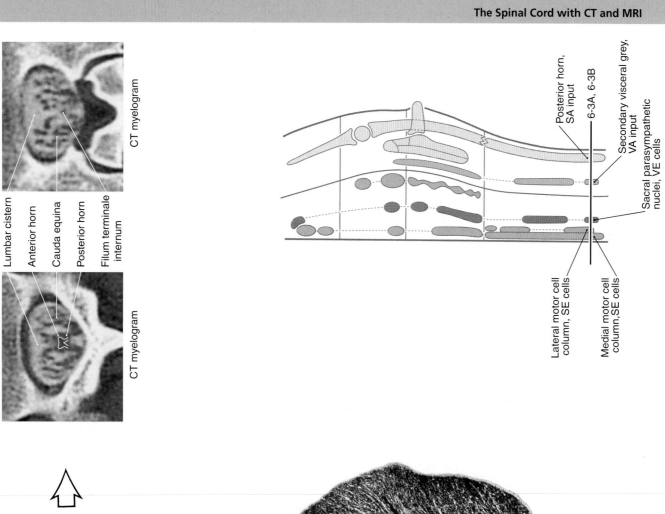

Lumbar cistern
Anterior horn
Cauda equina
Posterior horn
Filum terminale internum

CT myelogram

CT myelogram

Posterior horn, SA input

6-3A, 6-3B

Secondary visceral grey, VA input

Sacral parasympathetic nuclei, VE cells

Lateral motor cell column, SE cells

Medial motor cell column, SE cells

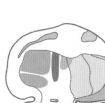

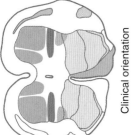

Clinical orientation

Anatomical orientation

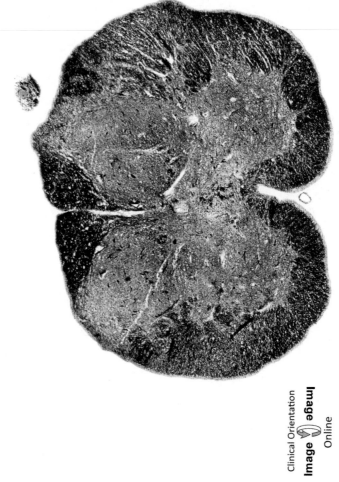

Clinical Orientation
Image
Image
Online

6-3B

6-4A Transverse section of the spinal cord showing its characteristic appearance at lumbar levels (L4). Posterior and anterior horns are large in relation to a modest amount of white matter, and the general shape of the cord is round. Fibers of the **medial division of the posterior root** directly enter the gracile fasciculus. The lumbar spinal cord appears round in the CT myelogram. The roots of upper portions of the cauda equina surround the lower levels of the lumbar spinal cord (**right**), see also Figure 2-4 on p. 10.

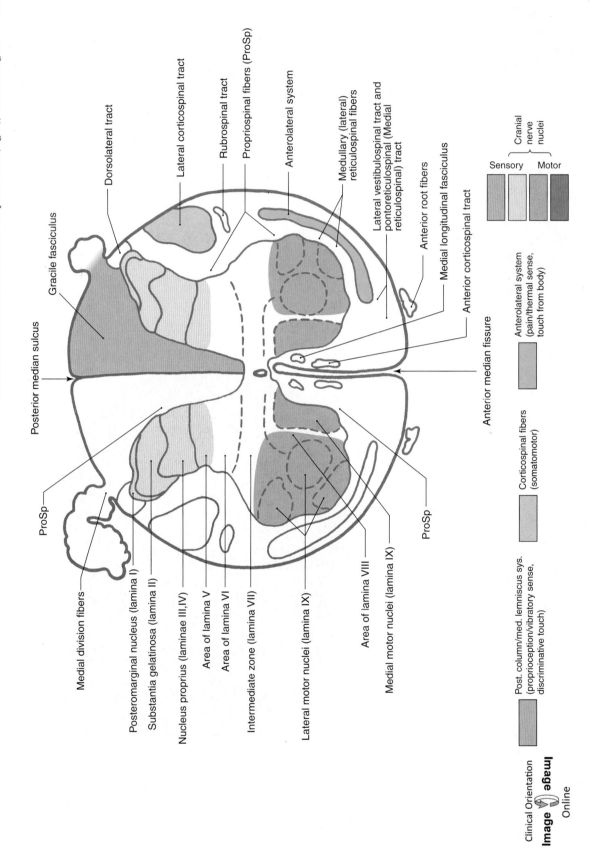

Dorsolateral tract

Lateral corticospinal tract

Rubrospinal tract

Propriospinal fibers (ProSp)

Anterolateral system

Medullary (lateral) reticulospinal fibers

Lateral vestibulospinal tract and pontoreticulospinal (Medial reticulospinal) tract

Anterior root fibers

Medial longitudinal fasciculus

Anterior corticospinal tract

Anterior median fissure

Gracile fasciculus

Posterior median sulcus

ProSp

Medial division fibers

Posteromarginal nucleus (lamina I)

Substantia gelatinosa (lamina II)

Nucleus proprius (laminae III,IV)

Area of lamina V

Area of lamina VI

Intermediate zone (lamina VII)

Lateral motor nuclei (lamina IX)

Area of lamina VIII

Medial motor nuclei (lamina IX)

ProSp

Sensory

Cranial nerve nuclei

Motor

Post. column/med. lemniscus sys. (proprioception/vibratory sense, discriminative touch)

Anterolateral system (pain/thermal sense, touch from body)

Corticospinal fibers (somatomotor)

Clinical Orientation

Image 🔄 **Image**

Online

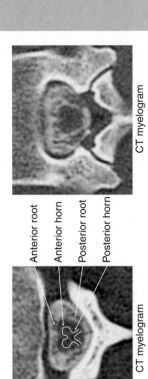

Anterior root
Anterior horn
Posterior root
Posterior horn

CT myelogram

CT myelogram

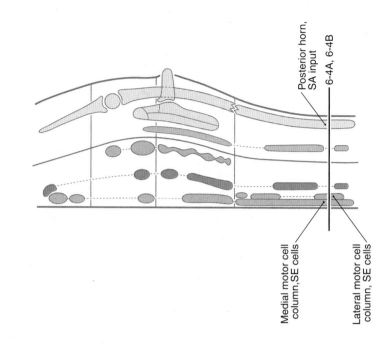

Posterior horn, SA input

6-4A, 6-4B

Medial motor cell column, SE cells

Lateral motor cell column, SE cells

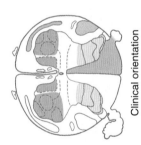

Clinical orientation

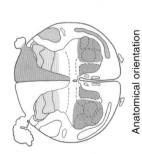

Anatomical orientation

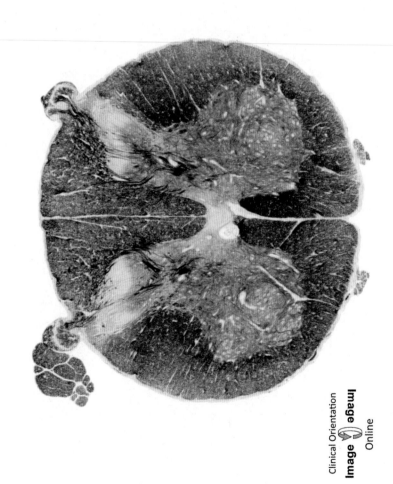

Clinical Orientation
Image Online

6-4B

6-5A Transverse section of the spinal cord showing its characteristic appearance at thoracic levels (T4). The white matter appears large in relation to the rather diminutive amount of gray matter. Posterior and anterior horns are small, especially when compared to low cervical levels and to lumbar levels. The overall shape of the cord is round. The thoracic spinal cord appears round in CT myelogram.

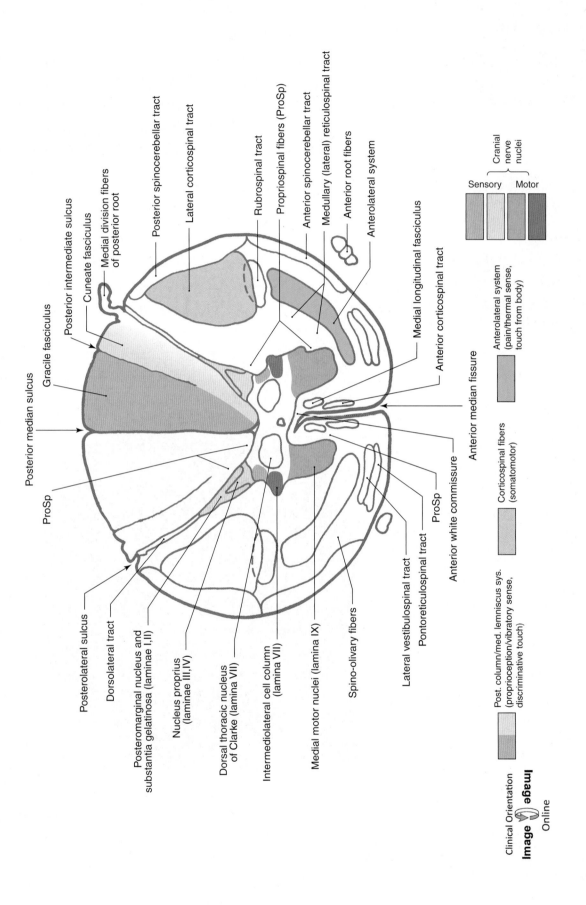

Medial division fibers of posterior root

Cuneate fasciculus

Posterior intermediate sulcus

Gracile fasciculus

Posterior median sulcus

Posterior spinocerebellar tract

Lateral corticospinal tract

Rubrospinal tract

Propriospinal fibers (ProSp)

Anterior spinocerebellar tract

Medullary (lateral) reticulospinal tract

Anterior root fibers

Anterolateral system

Medial longitudinal fasciculus

Anterior corticospinal tract

Anterior median fissure

ProSp

Posterolateral sulcus

Dorsolateral tract

Posteromarginal nucleus and substantia gelatinosa (laminae I,II)

Nucleus proprius (laminae III,IV)

Dorsal thoracic nucleus of Clarke (lamina VII)

Intermediolateral cell column (lamina VII)

Medial motor nuclei (lamina IX)

Spino-olivary fibers

Lateral vestibulospinal tract

Pontoreticulospinal tract

ProSp

Anterior white commissure

Sensory

Cranial nerve nuclei

Motor

Anterolateral system (pain/thermal sense, touch from body)

Corticospinal fibers (somatomotor)

Post. column/med. lemniscus sys. (proprioception/vibratory sense, discriminative touch)

Clinical Orientation

Image Online

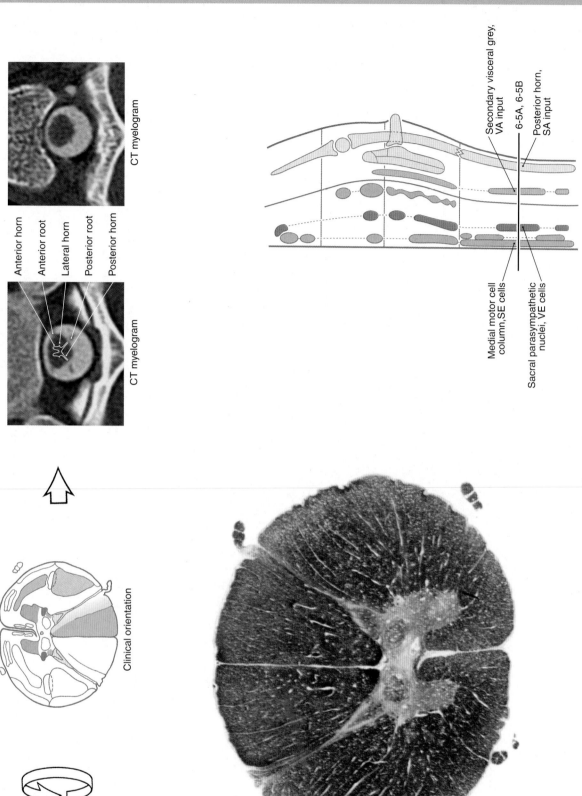

CT myelogram

Anterior horn
Anterior root
Lateral horn
Posterior root
Posterior horn

CT myelogram

Secondary visceral grey,
VA input

6-5A, 6-5B

Posterior horn,
SA input

Medial motor cell
column, SE cells

Sacral parasympathetic
nuclei, VE cells

Clinical orientation

Anatomical orientation

Clinical Orientation
Image Image
Online

6-5B

6-6A Transverse section of the spinal cord showing its characteristic appearance at lower cervical levels (C7). The anterior horn is large, and there is—proportionally and absolutely—a large amount of white matter. The overall shape of the cord is oval. The lower portions of the cervical spinal cord (beginning at about C4 and extending through C8) appear oval in MRI (**left**) and in CT myelogram (**center and right**). Although frequently called lamina X, Rexed (1954) clearly describes nine laminae (I–IX) and an "area X," the central gray substance." This original designation is used here.

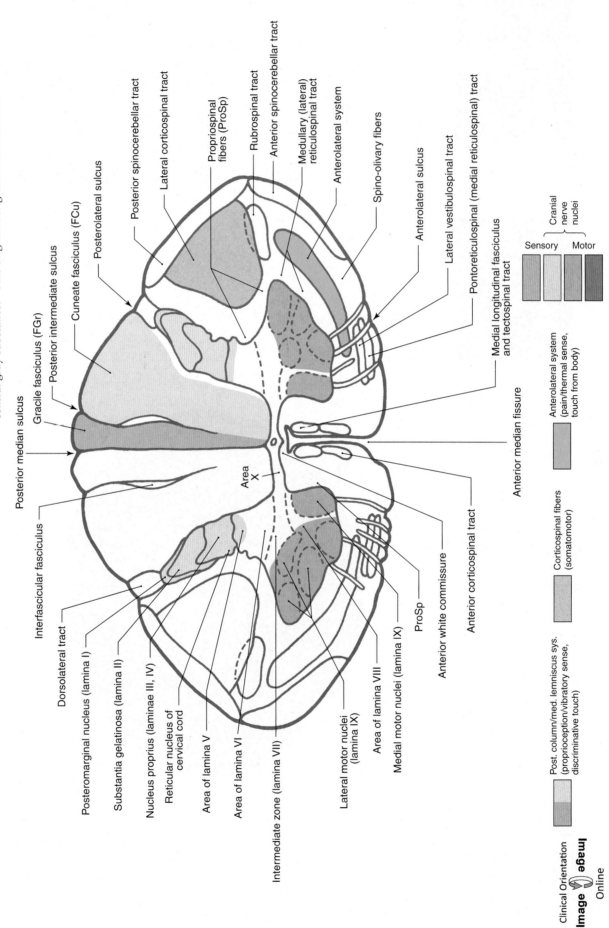

Posterior spinocerebellar tract

Lateral corticospinal tract

Propriospinal fibers (ProSp)

Rubrospinal tract

Anterior spinocerebellar tract

Medullary (lateral) reticulospinal tract

Anterolateral system

Spino-olivary fibers

Cuneate fasciculus (FCu)

Posterolateral sulcus

Posterior intermediate sulcus

Gracile fasciculus (FGr)

Posterior median sulcus

Anterolateral sulcus

Lateral vestibulospinal tract

Pontoreticulospinal (medial reticulospinal) tract

Medial longitudinal fasciculus and tectospinal tract

Interfascicular fasciculus

Dorsolateral tract

Posteromarginal nucleus (lamina I)

Substantia gelatinosa (lamina II)

Nucleus proprius (laminae III, IV)

Reticular nucleus of cervical cord

Area of lamina V

Area of lamina VI

Intermediate zone (lamina VII)

Lateral motor nuclei (lamina IX)

Area of lamina VIII

Medial motor nuclei (lamina IX)

ProSp

Anterior white commissure

Anterior corticospinal tract

Anterior median fissure

Area X

Clinical Orientation

Sensory   Motor

Cranial nerve nuclei

Post. column/med. lemniscus sys. (proprioception/vibratory sense, discriminative touch)

Anterolateral system (pain/thermal sense, touch from body)

Corticospinal fibers (somatomotor)

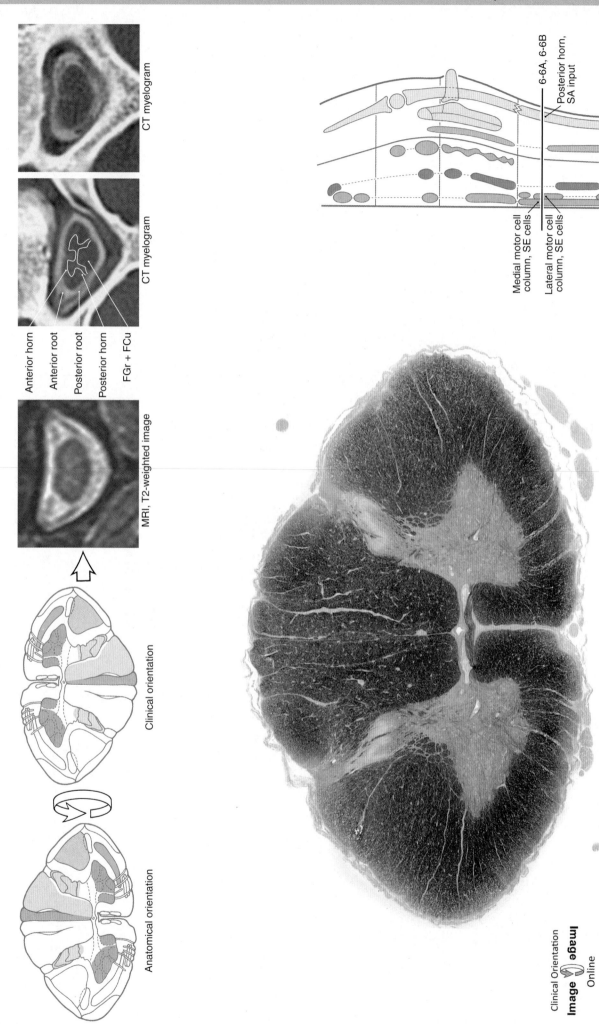

CT myelogram

CT myelogram

Anterior horn
Anterior root
Posterior root
Posterior horn
FGr + FCu

MRI, T2-weighted image

Clinical orientation

Anatomical orientation

6-6A, 6-6B
Posterior horn,
SA input

Medial motor cell
column, SE cells

Lateral motor cell
column, SE cells

Clinical Orientation
Image
Online

6-6B

6-7A Transverse section of the spinal cord at the C1 level. Lateral corticospinal fibers are now located medially toward the decussation of the corticospinal fibers, also called the motor decussation or pyramidal decussation (see also Figure 6-10, p. 112). At this level, fibers of the spinal trigeminal tract are interdigitated with those of the dorsolateral tract. The spinal cord at C1 and C2 levels appears round in CT myelogram when compared to low cervical levels (see Figure 6-6).

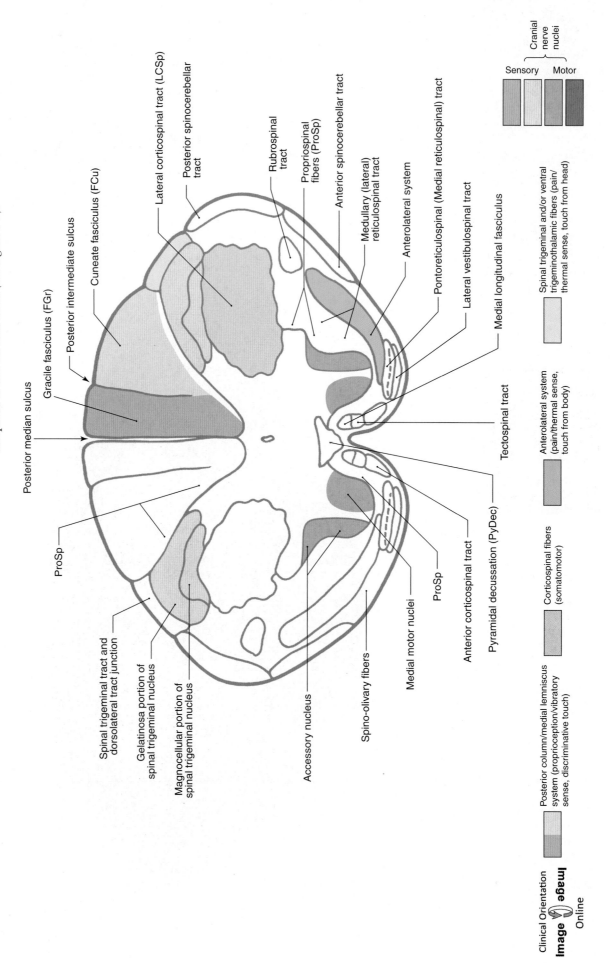

Posterior median sulcus

Gracile fasciculus (FGr)

Posterior intermediate sulcus

Cuneate fasciculus (FCu)

Lateral corticospinal tract (LCSp)

Posterior spinocerebellar tract

Rubrospinal tract

Propriospinal fibers (ProSp)

Anterior spinocerebellar tract

Medullary (lateral) reticulospinal tract

Anterolateral system

Pontoreticulospinal (Medial reticulospinal) tract

Lateral vestibulospinal tract

Medial longitudinal fasciculus

Tectospinal tract

ProSp

Spinal trigeminal tract and dorsolateral tract junction

Gelatinosa portion of spinal trigeminal nucleus

Magnocellular portion of spinal trigeminal nucleus

Accessory nucleus

Spino-olivary fibers

Medial motor nuclei

ProSp

Anterior corticospinal tract

Pyramidal decussation (PyDec)

Cranial nerve nuclei

Sensory   Motor

Posterior column/medial lemniscus system (proprioception/vibratory sense, discriminative touch)

Corticospinal fibers (somatomotor)

Anterolateral system (pain/thermal sense, touch from body)

Spinal trigeminal and/or ventral trigeminothalamic fibers (pain/thermal sense, touch from head)

Clinical Orientation
Image Online

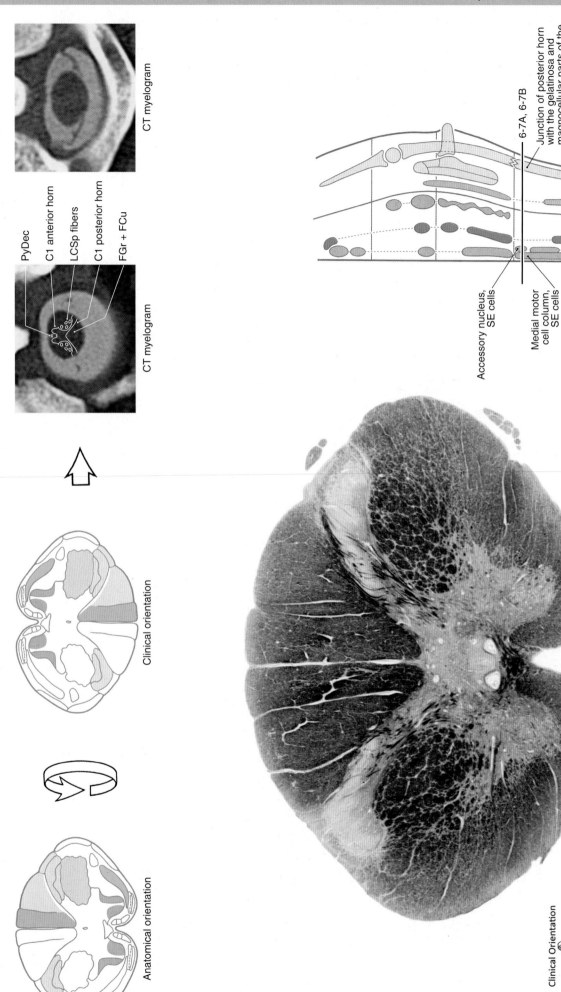

CT myelogram

PyDec
C1 anterior horn
LCSp fibers
C1 posterior horn
FGr + FCu

CT myelogram

Clinical orientation

Anatomical orientation

6-7A, 6-7B

Junction of posterior horn
with the gelatinosa and
magnocellular parts of the
spinal trigeminal nucleus

Accessory nucleus,
SE cells

Medial motor
cell column,
SE cells

Clinical Orientation
Image
Online

6-7B

6-8 Semi-diagrammatic representation of the internal blood supply to the spinal cord. This is a tracing of a C4 level, with the positions of principal tracts shown on the **left**, the general pattern of blood vessels on the **right**, and the color-coded pathways correlate with those on Figure 6-7.

ABBREVIATIONS

AH	Anterior (ventral) horn	N	Representation of neck fibers
AWCom	Anterior white commissure	PH	Posterior (dorsal) horn
CenC	Central canal	S	Representation of sacral fibers
IZ	Intermediate zone	T	Representation of truck fibers
LE	Representation of lower extremity	UE	Representation of upper extremity

Vascular Syndromes or Lesions of the Spinal Cord

Acute Central Cervical Spinal Cord Syndrome

This results from occlusion of the anterior spinal artery.

Deficit	Structure Damage
• Bilateral paresis or flaccid paralysis of upper extremities	• Medial portions of both lateral corticospinal tracts; ventral gray horns at cervical levels
• Irregular loss of pain and temperature sensations bilaterally over body below lesion	• Anterolateral system fibers (partial involvement bilaterally)

Hyperextension of the neck may cause damage to the vertebral arteries (origin of the anterior spinal artery), or it may directly damage the anterior spinal artery, causing a spasm. This vascular damage leads to a temporary or permanent interruption of blood supply. Deficits may resolve within a few hours or may be permanent, depending on the extent of vascular complication. Sparing of the posterior columns (proprioception, vibratory sense) is a hallmark; approximately the anterior two-thirds of the spinal cord is ischemic.

Thrombosis of Anterior Spinal Artery

This may occur in a **hypotensive crisis**, as a result of **trauma resulting from a dissecting aortic aneurysm**, or in patients with **atherosclerosis**. It may occur at all spinal levels, but is more frequently seen in thoracic and lumbosacral levels unless trauma is the primary cause. Results are **bilateral flaccid paraplegia** (if the lesion is below cervical levels) or **quadriplegia** (if the lesion is in cervical levels), **urinary retention**, and **loss of pain and temperature sensation**. Flaccid muscles may become spastic over a period of a day to weeks, with **hyperactive muscle stretch reflexes and extensor plantar (Babinski) reflexes**. In addition, lesions at high cervical levels may also result in **paralysis of respiratory muscles**. The artery of Adamkiewicz (a large spinal medullary artery) is usually located at spinal levels T12–L1 and more frequently arises on the left side. Occlusion of this vessel may infarct lumbosacral levels of the spinal cord.

Hemorrhage in the Spinal Cord

This is *rarely* seen, but may result from trauma or bleeding from congenital vascular lesions. Symptoms may develop rapidly or gradually in stepwise fashion, and blood is usually present in the cerebrospinal fluid.

Arteriovenous Malformation in the Spinal Cord

More frequently found in lower cord levels. Symptoms of a spinal AVM (**micturition problems**, **motor deficits**, **lower back pain**) may appear over time and may seem to resolve then recur (get better, then worse). These lesions are usually found external to the cord (extramedullary) and can be surgically treated, especially when the major feeding vessels are few in number and easily identified. **Foix-Alajouanine syndrome** is an inflammation of spinal veins, with subsequent occlusion that results in infarct of the spinal cord and a **necrotic myelitis**. The symptoms are **ascending pain and a flaccid paralysis**.

Brown-Séquard Syndrome

This syndrome is a hemisection (functional hemisection) of the spinal cord that may result from trauma, compression of the spinal cord by tumors or hematomas, or significant protrusion of an intervertebral disc. The deficits depend on the level of the causative lesion. The classic signs are: 1) a **loss of pain and thermal sensation** on the contralateral side of the body beginning about one to two segments below the level of the lesion (**damage to anterolateral system fibers**); 2) a **loss of discriminative touch and proprioception** on the ipsilateral side of the body below the lesion (**interruption of posterior column fibers**); and 3) a **paralysis on the ipsilateral side of the body below the lesion** (**damage to lateral corticospinal fibers**). This syndrome is classified as an **incomplete spinal cord injury**, and patients with this lesion may regain some degree of motor and sensory function. Compression of the spinal cord may result in some, but not all, of the signs and symptoms of the syndrome.

Syringomyelia

Syringomyelia is a cavitation within the central region of the spinal cord. A cavitation of the central canal with an **ependymal cell lining** is **hydromyelia**. A syrinx may originate in central portions of the spinal cord, may communicate with the central canal, and is most commonly seen in cervical levels of the spinal cord. The most common deficits are a **bilateral loss of pain and thermal sensation due to damage to the anterior white commissure**: the loss reflects the levels of the spinal cord damaged (e.g., a cape distribution over the shoulder and upper extremities). The other commonly seen deficit results from extension of the cavity into the anterior horn(s). The result is **unilateral or bilateral paralysis of the upper extremities** (cervical levels) or **lower extremities** (lumbosacral levels) due to damage to spinal motor neurons. This paralysis is characteristically a **lower motor neuron deficit**. A syrinx in the spinal cord, particularly in cervical levels, may be associated with a variety of other developmental defects in the nervous system.

Spinal Cord Lesions

General Concepts

A **complete spinal cord lesion** is characterized by a bilateral and complete loss of motor and sensory function below the level of the lesion persisting for more than 24 hours. The vast majority of the patients with complete lesions (95%+) will suffer some permanent deficits. **Incomplete spinal cord lesions** are those with preservation of sacral cord function at presentation. The above described cases are examples of incomplete spinal cord lesions.

High Cervical

The **phrenic nucleus** is located in central areas of the anterior horn at levels C3–C7 and receives descending input from nuclei of the medulla (mainly in the reticular formation) that influence respiration, particularly inspiration. The **phrenic nerve** originates primarily from level C4 with some contributions from C3 and C5 and innervates the diaphragm. A **complete spinal cord lesion** between C1 and C3 interrupts medullary input to the phrenic nucleus and may result in immediate respiratory (and potentially cardiac) arrest. This constitutes a medical emergency necessitating intervention within minutes, or the patient will die.

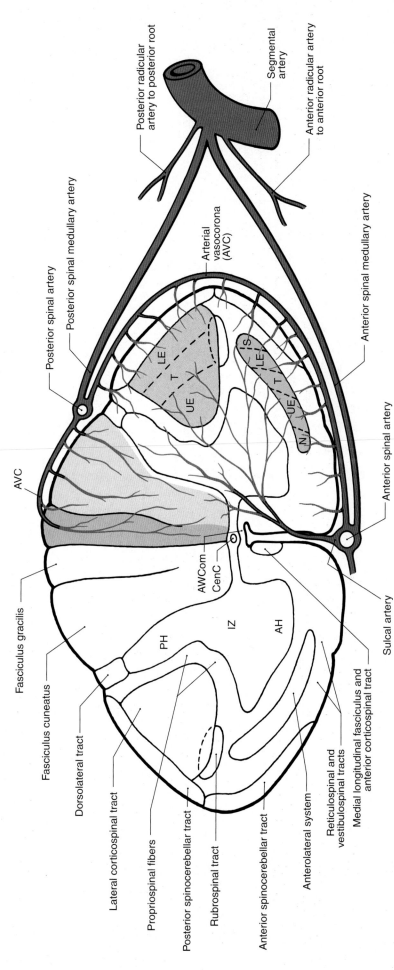

6-8

6-9 All of the brainstem sections used in Figures 6-11 through 6-15 (medulla), 6-19 through 6-22 (pons), and 6-24 through 6-29 (midbrain, except 6-25) are from an individual who had an infarct (green in drawing) in the posterior limb of the internal capsule. This lesion damaged corticospinal fibers (gray in drawing), resulting in a contralateral hemiplegia of the arm and leg, and damaged sensory radiations that travel from thalamic nuclei to the somatosensory cortex through the posterior limb of the internal capsule. Although the patient survived the initial episode, corticospinal fibers (gray) distal to the lesion (green) underwent degenerative changes and largely disappeared. This Wallerian (anterograde) degeneration takes place because the capsular infarct effectively separates the descending corticospinal fibers from their cell bodies in the cerebral cortex. Consequently, the location of corticospinal fibers in the middle one-third of the crus cerebri of the midbrain, in the basilar pons, and in the pyramid of the medulla is characterized by the obvious lack of myelinated axons in these structures when compared to the opposite side. In the brainstem, these degenerated fibers are ipsilateral to their cells of origin, but are contralateral to their destination in the spinal cord—hence, the **contralateral motor deficit** when these fibers are damaged rostral to the motor decussation. These images give the user the unique opportunity of seeing where corticospinal fibers are located at all levels of the human brainstem. Also, one is constantly reminded of: 1) the relationship of corticospinal fibers to other structures; 2) the deficits one can expect to see at representative levels due to this lesion; and 3) the general appearance of degenerated fibers in the human central nervous system. These images can be adapted to a wide range of instructional formats.

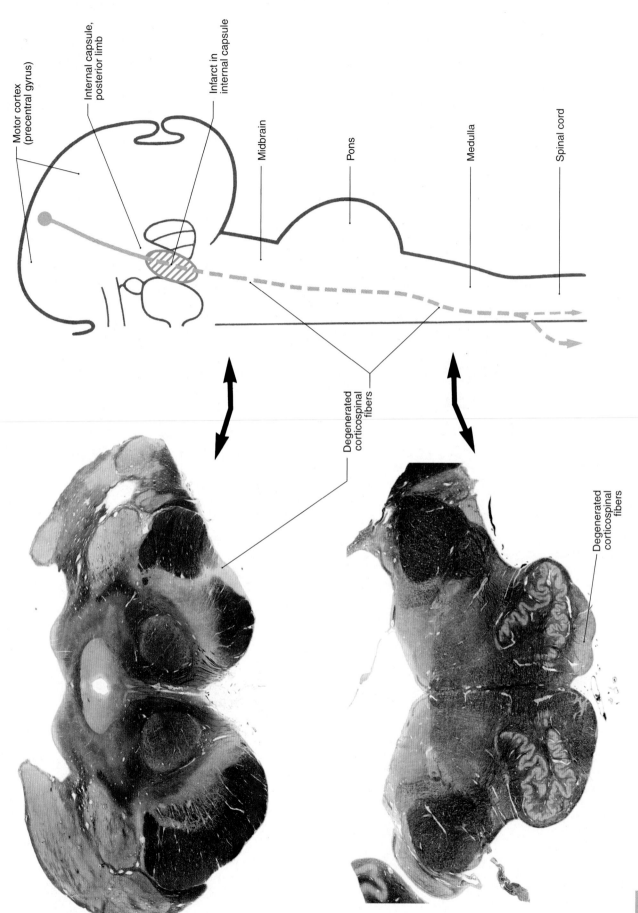

Motor cortex (precentral gyrus)

Internal capsule, posterior limb

Infarct in internal capsule

Midbrain

Pons

Medulla

Spinal cord

Degenerated corticospinal fibers

Degenerated corticospinal fibers

6-10A Transverse section of the medulla through the **motor decussation** (decussation of the pyramids [pyramidal decussation], crossing of corticospinal fibers). This is the level of the spinal cord–medulla transition. The corticospinal fibers have moved from their location in the lateral funiculus to the motor decussation (compare this image with Figure 6-7A, B) and will cross to form the pyramid on the opposite side.

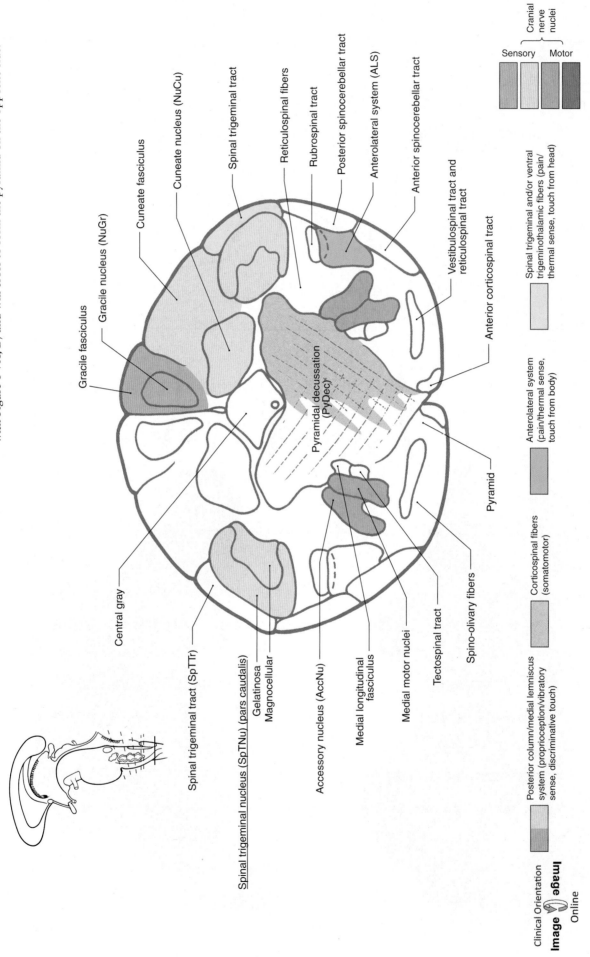

Gracile fasciculus

Gracile nucleus (NuGr)

Cuneate fasciculus

Cuneate nucleus (NuCu)

Spinal trigeminal tract

Reticulospinal fibers

Rubrospinal tract

Posterior spinocerebellar tract

Anterolateral system (ALS)

Anterior spinocerebellar tract

Vestibulospinal tract and reticulospinal tract

Anterior corticospinal tract

Pyramid

Spino-olivary fibers

Tectospinal tract

Medial motor nuclei

Medial longitudinal fasciculus

Accessory nucleus (AccNu)

Magnocellular

Gelatinosa

Spinal trigeminal nucleus (SpTNu) (pars caudalis)

Spinal trigeminal tract (SpTTr)

Central gray

Pyramidal decussation (PyDec)

Posterior column/medial lemniscus system (proprioception/vibratory sense, discriminative touch)

Anterolateral system (pain/thermal sense, touch from body)

Corticospinal fibers (somatomotor)

Spinal trigeminal and/or ventral trigeminothalamic fibers (pain/thermal sense, touch from head)

Sensory   Motor

Cranial nerve nuclei

Clinical Orientation

Image Online

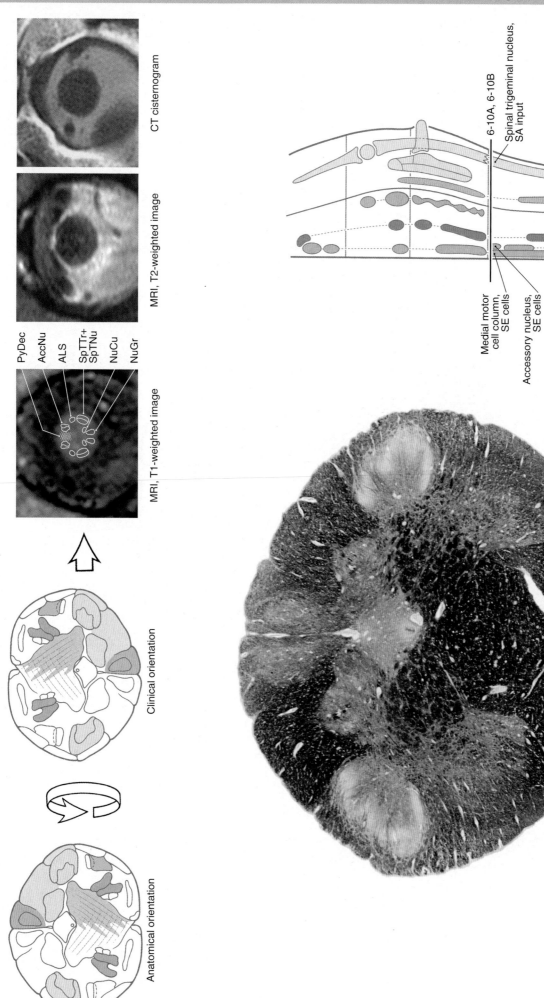

CT cisternogram

MRI, T2-weighted image

PyDec
AccNu
ALS
SpTTr+
SpTNu
NuCu
NuGr

MRI, T1-weighted image

Clinical orientation

Anatomical orientation

Spinal trigeminal nucleus,
SA input

6-10A, 6-10B

Medial motor
cell column,
SE cells

Accessory nucleus,
SE cells

Clinical Orientation
Image
Online

6-10B

6-11A Transverse section of the medulla through the **posterior column nuclei** (nucleus gracilis and nucleus cuneatus), caudal portions of the **hypoglossal nucleus,** caudal end of the **principal olivary nucleus,** and middle portions of the **sensory decussation** (crossing of internal arcuate fibers).

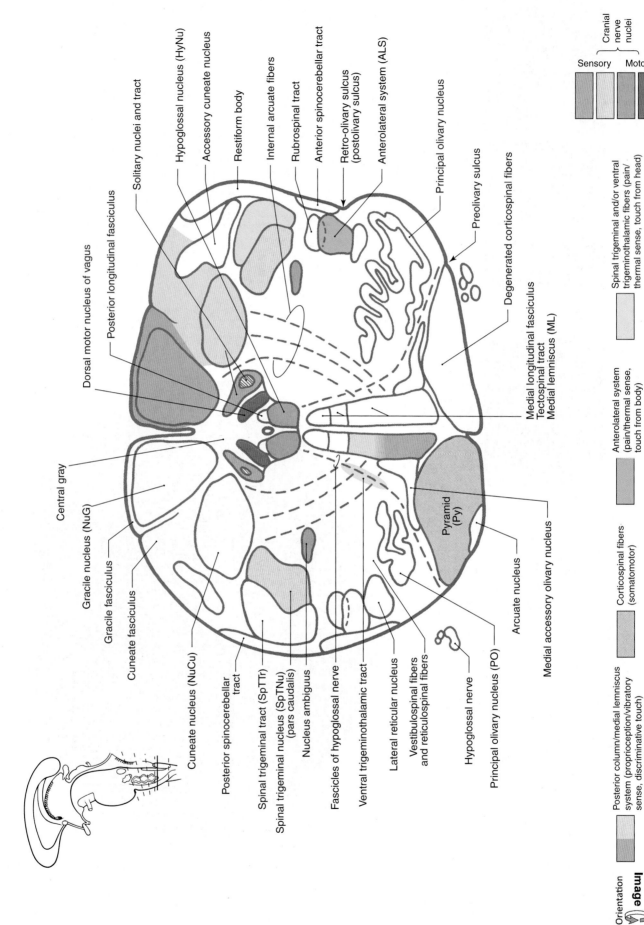

Solitary nuclei and tract
Hypoglossal nucleus (HyNu)
Accessory cuneate nucleus
Restiform body
Internal arcuate fibers
Rubrospinal tract
Anterior spinocerebellar tract
Retro-olivary sulcus (postolivary sulcus)
Anterolateral system (ALS)
Principal olivary nucleus
Preolivary sulcus
Degenerated corticospinal fibers

Posterior longitudinal fasciculus
Dorsal motor nucleus of vagus
Central gray
Gracile nucleus (NuG)
Gracile fasciculus
Cuneate fasciculus
Cuneate nucleus (NuCu)
Posterior spinocerebellar tract
Spinal trigeminal tract (SpTTr)
Spinal trigeminal nucleus (SpTNu) (pars caudalis)
Nucleus ambiguus
Fascicles of hypoglossal nerve
Ventral trigeminothalamic tract
Lateral reticular nucleus
Vestibulospinal fibers and reticulospinal fibers
Hypoglossal nerve
Principal olivary nucleus (PO)
Medial accessory olivary nucleus
Arcuate nucleus
Pyramid (Py)
Medial longitudinal fasciculus
Tectospinal tract
Medial lemniscus (ML)

Cranial nerve nuclei
Sensory   Motor

Spinal trigeminal and/or ventral trigeminothalamic fibers (pain/ thermal sense, touch from head)

Anterolateral system (pain/thermal sense, touch from body)

Corticospinal fibers (somatomotor)

Posterior column/medial lemniscus system (proprioception/vibratory sense, discriminative touch)

Clinical Orientation

Image Online

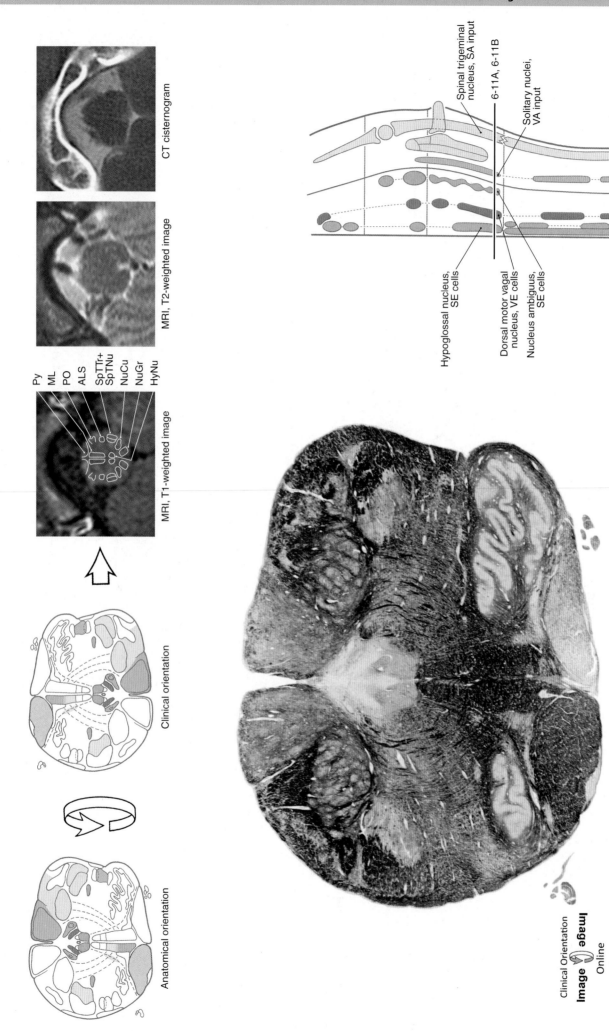

CT cisternogram

MRI, T2-weighted image

MRI, T1-weighted image

Py
ML
PO
ALS
SpTTr+
SpTNu
NuCu
NuGr
HyNu

Clinical orientation

Anatomical orientation

Spinal trigeminal
nucleus, SA input

6-11A, 6-11B

Solitary nuclei,
VA input

Hypoglossal nucleus,
SE cells

Dorsal motor vagal
nucleus, VE cells

Nucleus ambiguus,
SE cells

Clinical Orientation
Image
Image
Online

6-11B

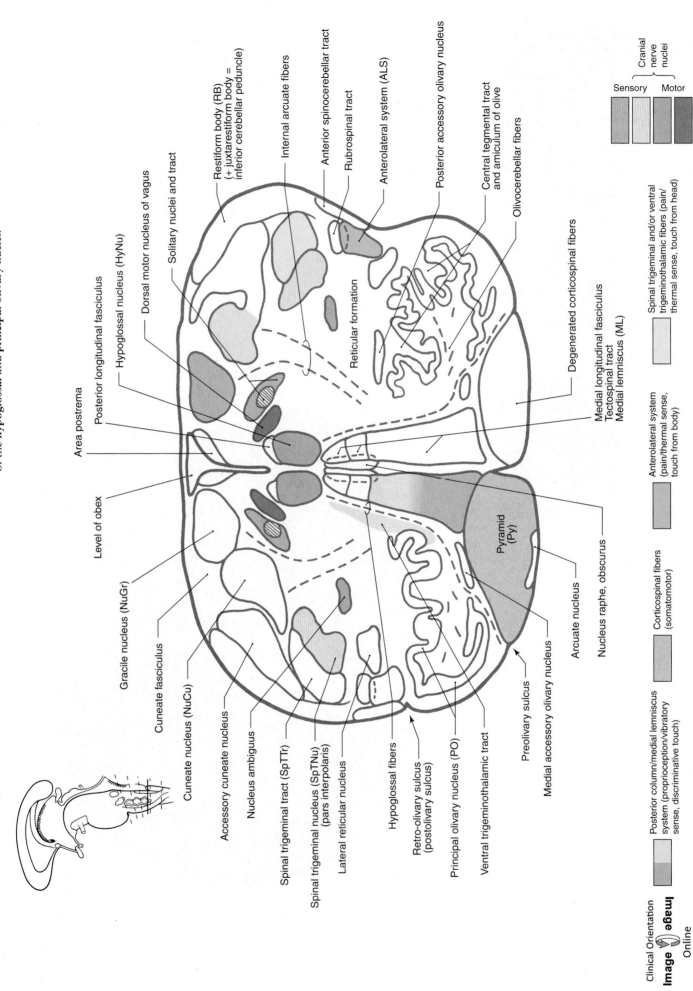

6-12A   Transverse section of the medulla through rostral portions of the **sensory decussation** (crossing of **internal arcuate fibers**), **obex**, and the caudal one-third of the **hypoglossal** and **principal olivary nuclei**.

Area postrema

Level of obex

Gracile nucleus (NuGr)

Cuneate fasciculus

Cuneate nucleus (NuCu)

Accessory cuneate nucleus

Nucleus ambiguus

Spinal trigeminal tract (SpTTr)

Spinal trigeminal nucleus (SpTNu)
(pars interpolaris)

Lateral reticular nucleus

Hypoglossal fibers

Retro-olivary sulcus
(postolivary sulcus)

Principal olivary nucleus (PO)

Ventral trigeminothalamic tract

Preolivary sulcus

Medial accessory olivary nucleus

Arcuate nucleus

Nucleus raphe, obscurus

Pyramid
(Py)

Posterior longitudinal fasciculus

Hypoglossal nucleus (HyNu)

Dorsal motor nucleus of vagus

Solitary nuclei and tract

Restiform body (RB)
(+ juxtarestiform body =
inferior cerebellar peduncle)

Internal arcuate fibers

Anterior spinocerebellar tract

Rubrospinal tract

Anterolateral system (ALS)

Posterior accessory olivary nucleus

Central tegmental tract
and amiculum of olive

Olivocerebellar fibers

Degenerated corticospinal fibers

Medial longitudinal fasciculus
Tectospinal tract
Medial lemniscus (ML)

Reticular formation

Clinical Orientation

Image
Online

Sensory   Motor

Cranial
nerve
nuclei

Spinal trigeminal and/or ventral
trigeminothalamic fibers (pain/
thermal sense, touch from head)

Anterolateral system
(pain/thermal sense,
touch from body)

Posterior column/medial lemniscus
system (proprioception/vibratory
sense, discriminative touch)

Corticospinal fibers
(somatomotor)

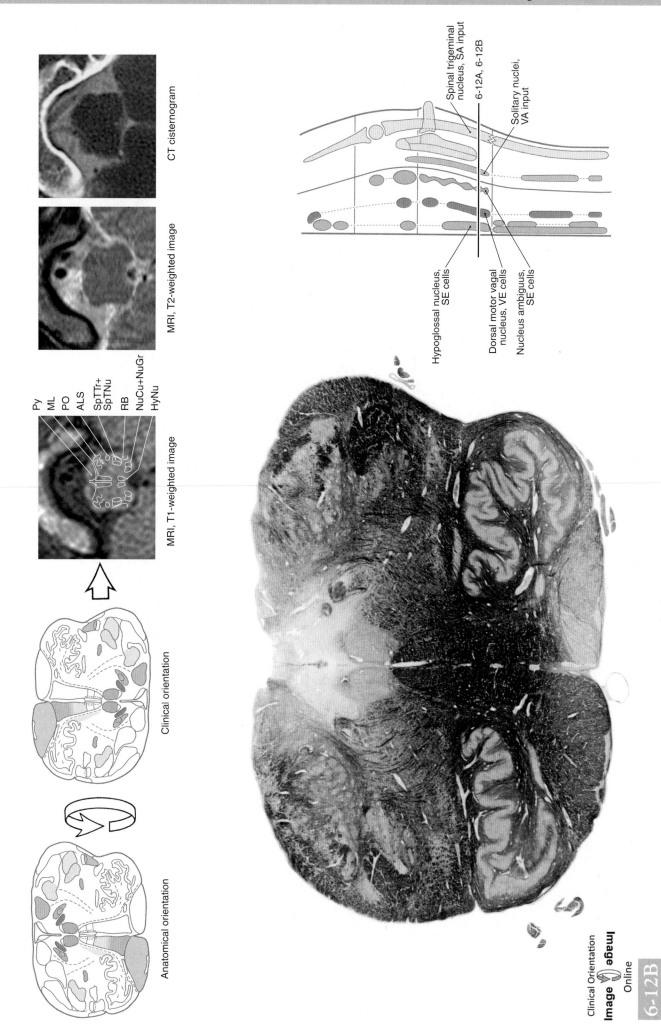

CT cisternogram

MRI, T2-weighted image

Py
ML
PO
ALS
SpTTr+
SpTNu
RB
NuCu+NuGr
HyNu

MRI, T1-weighted image

Clinical orientation

Anatomical orientation

Spinal trigeminal
nucleus, SA input

6-12A, 6-12B

Solitary nuclei,
VA input

Hypoglossal nucleus,
SE cells

Dorsal motor vagal
nucleus, VE cells

Nucleus ambiguus,
SE cells

Clinical Orientation
Image
Image
Online

6-12B

6-13A Transverse section of the medulla through rostral portions of the **hypoglossal nucleus** and the middle portions of the **principal olivary nucleus**. The fourth ventricle has flared open at this level, and the **restiform body** is enlarging to become a prominent structure on the dorsolateral aspect of the medulla.

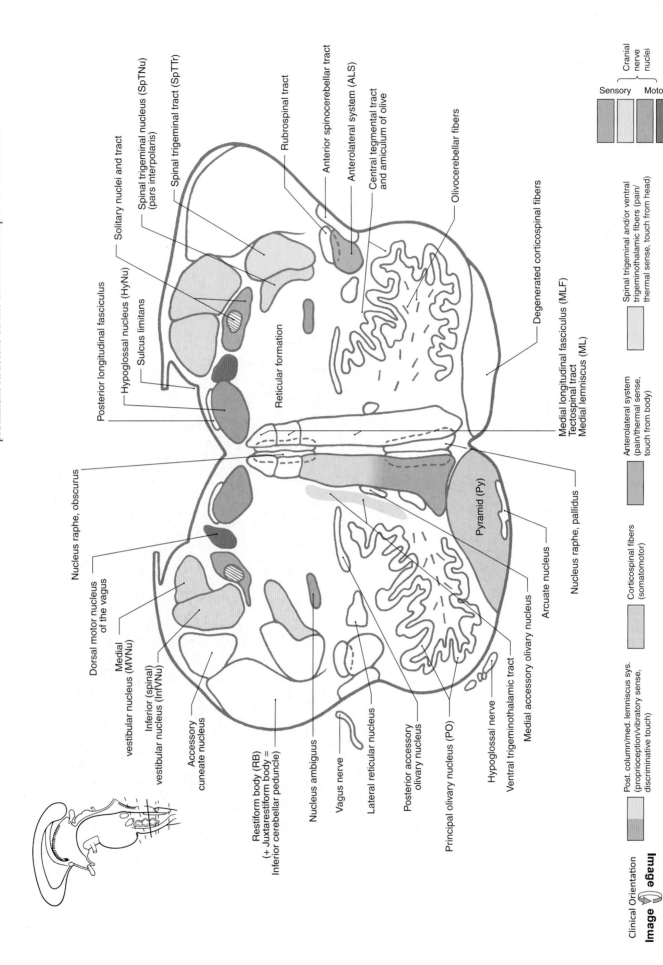

Solitary nuclei and tract

Spinal trigeminal nucleus (SpTNu) (pars interpolaris)

Spinal trigeminal tract (SpTr)

Rubrospinal tract

Anterior spinocerebellar tract

Anterolateral system (ALS)

Central tegmental tract and amiculum of olive

Olivocerebellar fibers

Posterior longitudinal fasciculus

Hypoglossal nucleus (HyNu)

Sulcus limitans

Reticular formation

Degenerated corticospinal fibers

Medial longitudinal fasciculus (MLF)
Tectospinal tract
Medial lemniscus (ML)

Nucleus raphe, obscurus

Pyramid (Py)

Nucleus raphe, pallidus

Arcuate nucleus

Dorsal motor nucleus of the vagus

Medial vestibular nucleus (MVNu)

Inferior (spinal) vestibular nucleus (InfVNu)

Accessory cuneate nucleus

Restiform body (RB) (+ Juxtarestiform body = Inferior cerebellar peduncle)

Nucleus ambiguus

Vagus nerve

Lateral reticular nucleus

Posterior accessory olivary nucleus

Principal olivary nucleus (PO)

Hypoglossal nerve

Ventral trigeminothalamic tract

Medial accessory olivary nucleus

Sensory

Cranial nerve nuclei

Motor

Spinal trigeminal and/or ventral trigeminothalamic fibers (pain/thermal sense, touch from head)

Anterolateral system (pain/thermal sense, touch from body)

Corticospinal fibers (somatomotor)

Post. column/med. lemniscus sys. (proprioception/vibratory sense, discriminative touch)

Clinical Orientation

Image Online

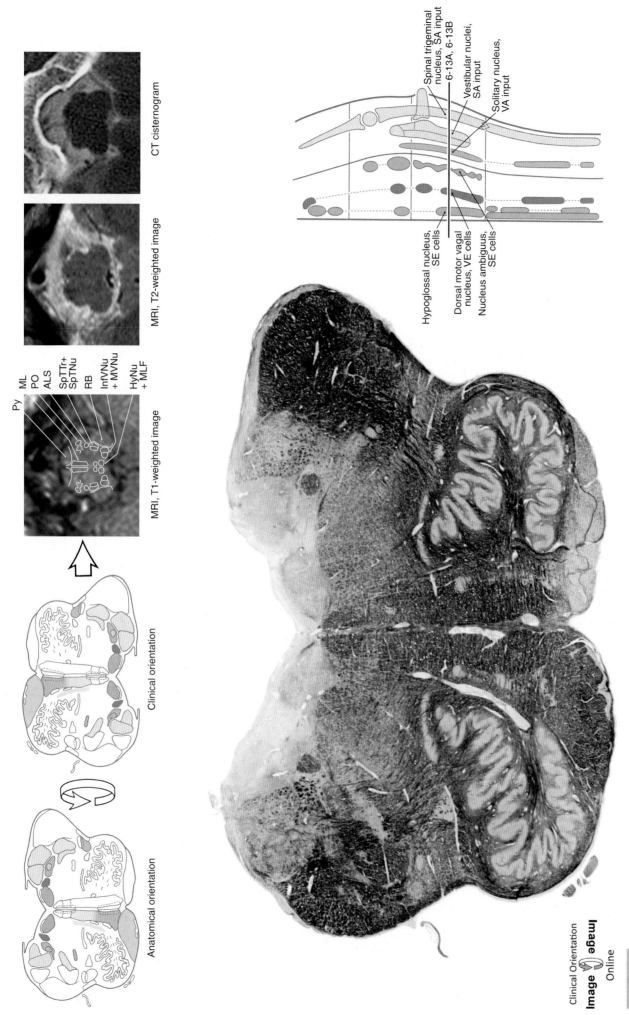

CT cisternogram

MRI, T2-weighted image

MRI, T1-weighted image

Py
ML
PO
ALS
SpTTr+
SpTNu
RB
InfVNu
+ MVNu
HyNu
+ MLF

Clinical orientation

Anatomical orientation

Spinal trigeminal nucleus, SA input
6-13A, 6-13B

Vestibular nuclei, SA input

Solitary nucleus, VA input

Hypoglossal nucleus, SE cells

Dorsal motor vagal nucleus, VE cells

Nucleus ambiguus, SE cells

Clinical Orientation
Image
Online

6-13B

6-14A Transverse section of the medulla through the posterior (dorsal) and anterior (ventral) cochlear nuclei and root of the glossopharyngeal nerve. This corresponds to approximately the rostral third to fourth of the principal olivary nucleus, to the location of the lateral recess of the fourth ventricle, and to the general area of the medulla–pons junction.

Anterior (ventral) cochlear nucleus

Posterior (dorsal) cochlear nucleus

Striae medullares of fourth ventricle

Inferior (or spinal) vestibular nucleus (InfVNu)

Medial vestibular nucleus (MVNu)

Nucleus prepositus (NuPre)

Posterior longitudinal fasciculus

Pontobulbar nucleus

Spinal trigeminal tract (SpTTr)

Spinal trigeminal nucleus (SpTNu) (pars oralis)

Rubrospinal tract

Nucleus ambiguus

Anterolateral system (ALS)

Central tegmental tract and amiculum of olive

Olivocerebellar fibers

Degenerated corticospinal fibers

Reticular formation

Nucleus raphe, pallidus

Medial longitudinal fasciculus (MLF)
Tectospinal tract
Medial lemniscus (ML)

Pyramid (Py)

Nucleus raphe, obscurus

Inferior salivatory nucleus

Solitary nuclei

Solitary tract

Restiform body (RB)

Cerebellum

Posterior (dorsal) cochlear nucleus

Anterior (ventral) cochlear nucleus

Cochlear nerve

Glossopharyngeal nerve

Anterior spinocerebellar tract

Reticulospinal fibers

Posterior accessory olivary nucleus

Principal olivary nucleus

Ventral trigeminothalamic tract

Medial accessory olivary nucleus

Arcuate nucleus

Sensory | Cranial nerve nuclei | **Motor**

Spinal trigeminal and/or ventral trigeminothalamic fibers (pain/thermal sense, touch from head)

Anterolateral system (pain/thermal sense, touch from body)

Corticospinal fibers (somatomotor)

Posterior column/medial lemniscus system (proprioception/vibratory sense, discriminative touch)

Clinical Orientation

Image Online

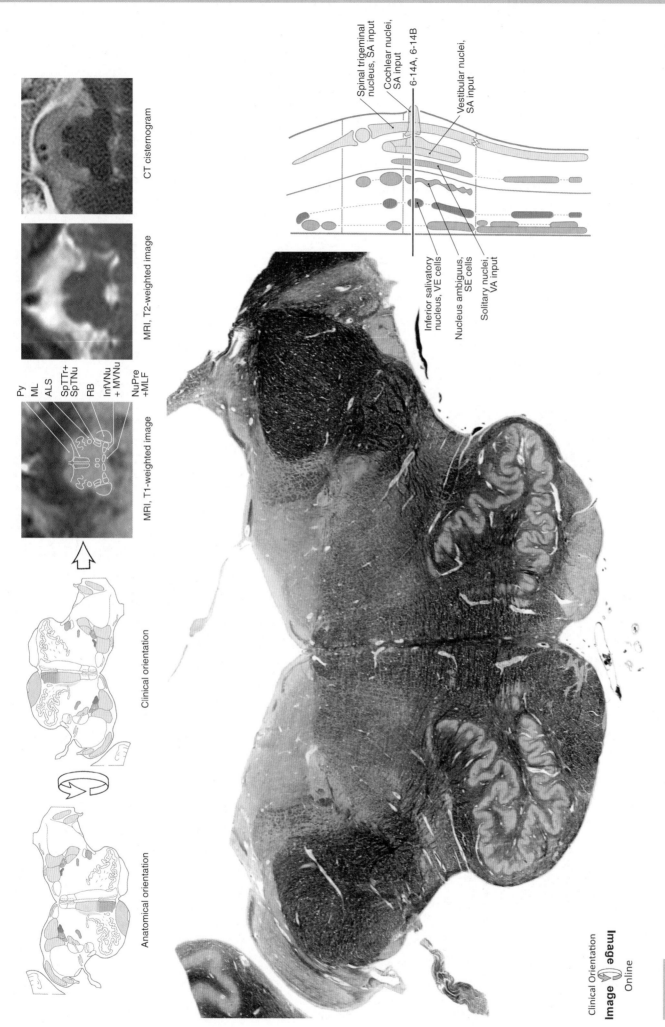

Spinal trigeminal nucleus, SA input

Cochlear nuclei, SA input

6-14A, 6-14B

Vestibular nuclei, SA input

Inferior salivatory nucleus, VE cells

Nucleus ambiguus, SE cells

Solitary nuclei, VA input

CT cisternogram

MRI, T2-weighted image

Py
ML
ALS
SpTTr+
SpTNu
RB
InfVNu
+ MVNu
NuPre
+MLF

MRI, T1-weighted image

Clinical orientation

Anatomical orientation

Clinical Orientation

Image

Online

6-14B

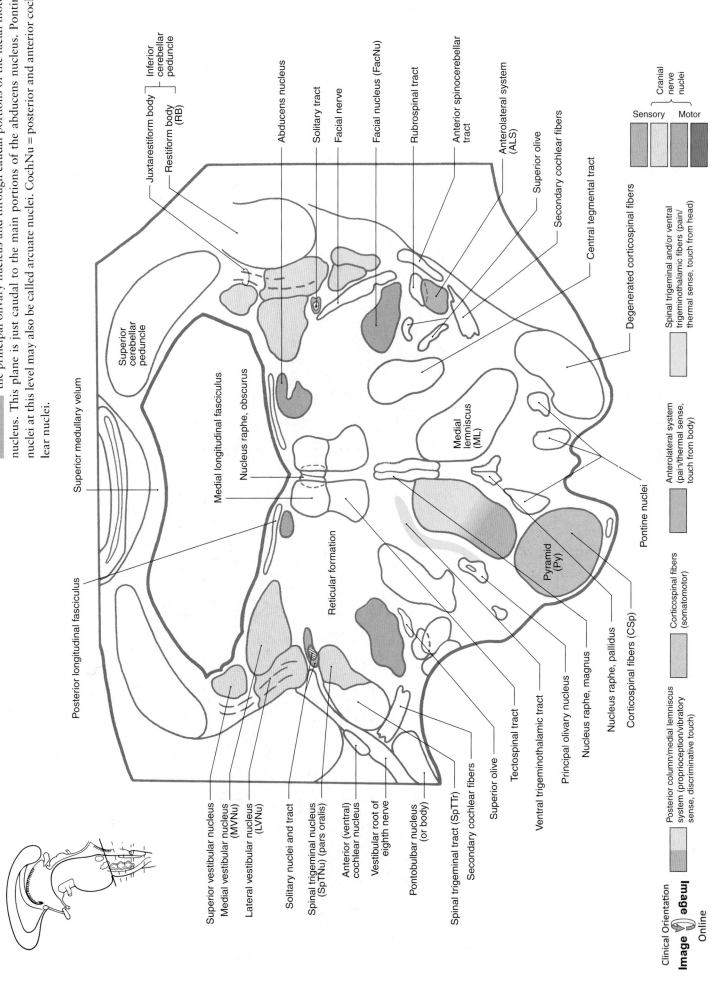

6-15A   Transverse section of the medulla–pons junction through the rostral pole of the principal olivary nucleus and through caudal portions of the facial motor nucleus. This plane is just caudal to the main portions of the abducens nucleus. Pontine nuclei at this level may also be called arcuate nuclei. CochNu = posterior and anterior cochlear nuclei.

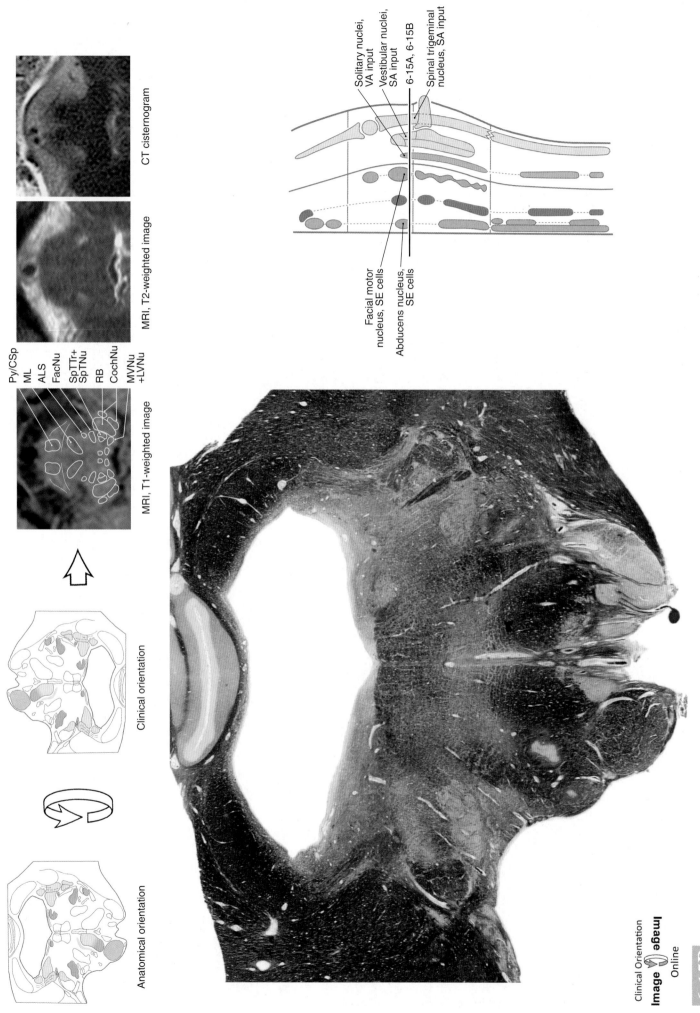

CT cisternogram

MRI, T2-weighted image

Py/CSp
ML
ALS
FacNu
SpTTr+
SpTNu
RB
CochNu
MVNu
+LVNu

MRI, T1-weighted image

Clinical orientation

Anatomical orientation

Solitary nuclei,
VA input

Vestibular nuclei,
SA input

6-15A, 6-15B

Spinal trigeminal
nucleus, SA input

Facial motor
nucleus, SE cells

Abducens nucleus,
SE cells

Clinical Orientation
Image Online

6-15B

6-16 Semi-diagrammatic representation of the internal distribution of arteries in the medulla oblongata. Selected main structures are labeled primarily on the left side of each section, and the general pattern of arterial distribution overlies these structures on the right side. The general distribution patterns of arteries in the medulla, as illustrated here, may vary from patient to patient. For example, the territories served by adjacent vessels may overlap to differing degrees at their margins, or the territory of a particular vessel may be smaller or larger than seen in the typical pattern.

ABBREVIATIONS

FCu	Cuneate fasciculus	Py	Pyramid
FGr	Gracile fasciculus	RB	Restiform body (+ juxtarestiform body = inferior cerebellar peduncle)
ML	Medial lemniscus		
NuCu	Cuneate nucleus	RetF	Reticular formation
NuGr	Gracile nucleus		

Vascular Syndromes or Lesions of the Medulla Oblongata

Medial Medullary Syndrome

This results from occlusion of branches of the anterior spinal artery.

Deficit	Structure Damage
• Contralateral hemiplegia of upper extremity (UE), trunk, and lower extremity (LE)	• Pyramid (corticospinal fibers)
• Contralateral loss of position sense, vibratory sense, and discriminative touch (UE, trunk, LE)	• Medial lemniscus
• Deviation of tongue to ipsilateral side when protruded; muscle atrophy and fasciculations	• Hypoglossal nerve in medulla or hypoglossal nucleus

The **medial medullary syndrome** (**Déjérine syndrome**) is rare compared to the more common occurrence of the lateral medullary syndrome. **Nystagmus** may result if the lesion involves the medial longitudinal fasciculus or the nucleus prepositus hypoglossi. The lesion may involve ventral trigeminothalamic fibers, but diminished pain and thermal sense from the contralateral side of the face is rarely seen. The combination of a **contralateral hemiplegia and ipsilateral deviation of the tongue** is called an inferior alternating hemiplegia when the lesion is at this level.

Lateral Medullary Syndrome

Results from occlusion of posterior inferior cerebellar artery (PICA), or branches of PICA, to the dorsolateral medulla (**PICA syndrome, Wallenberg syndrome**). In some cases, the lateral medullary syndrome may result from occlusion of the vertebral artery at the origin of the PICA with consequent loss of flow into PICA.

Deficit	Structure Damage
• Contralateral loss of pain and thermal sense on body	• Anterolateral system fibers
• Ipsilateral loss of pain and thermal sense on face	• Spinal trigeminal tract and nucleus
• Dysphagia, soft palate paralysis, hoarseness, diminished gag reflex	• Nucleus ambiguus, roots of 9th and 10th nerves
• Ipsilateral Horner syndrome (miosis, ptosis, anhidrosis, flushing of face)	• Descending hypothalamospinal fibers
• Nausea, diplopia, tendency to fall to ipsilateral side, nystagmus, vertigo	• Vestibular nuclei (mainly inferior and medial)
• Ataxia to the ipsilateral side	• Restiform body and spinocerebellar fibers

In addition to the preceding, involvement of the solitary tract and nucleus may (rarely) cause **dysgeusia. Dyspnea** and **tachycardia** may be seen in patients with damage to the dorsal motor nucleus of the vagus. It is also possible that damage to respiratory centers in the reticular formation or to the vagal motor nucleus may result in hiccup (**singultus**). Bilateral medullary damage may cause the syndrome of the "Ondine curse," an inability to breathe without willing it or "thinking about it"; the onset of this condition represents a medical emergency.

Tonsillar Herniation

Although the cerebellar tonsil is not part of the medulla, the herniation of this structure (**tonsillar herniation**) down through the **foramen magnum** has serious consequences for function of the medulla. Although the causes vary, such as a sudden increase in pressure in the posterior cranial fossa, or a shift in pressure in the cranial cavity (such as during a lumbar puncture in a patient with a mass lesion) in cases of **tonsillar herniation**, the cerebellar tonsils "cone" downward into and through the foramen magnum. The result is a compression of the medulla (mechanical damage to the medulla plus occlusion of vessels), damage to respiratory and cardiac centers, and **sudden respiratory and cardiac arrest**. This may constitute a medical emergency, especially if the onset is sudden, and must be addressed **immediately** or the patient may die. See Chapter 9 for further information on **tonsillar herniation**.

Syringobulbia

A cavitation within the brainstem (**syringobulbia**) may exist with **syringomyelia**, be independent of syringomyelia, or, in some cases, both may exist and communicate with each other. The cavity in syringobulbia is usually on one side of the midline of the medulla. Signs and symptoms of **syringobulbia** may include **weakness of tongue muscles** (hypoglossal nucleus or nerve), **weakness of pharyngeal, palatal, and vocal musculature** (ambiguus nuclei), **nystagmus** (vestibular nuclei), and **loss of pain and thermal sensation on the ipsilateral side of the face** (spinal trigeminal tract and nucleus, or crossing of trigeminothalamic fibers).

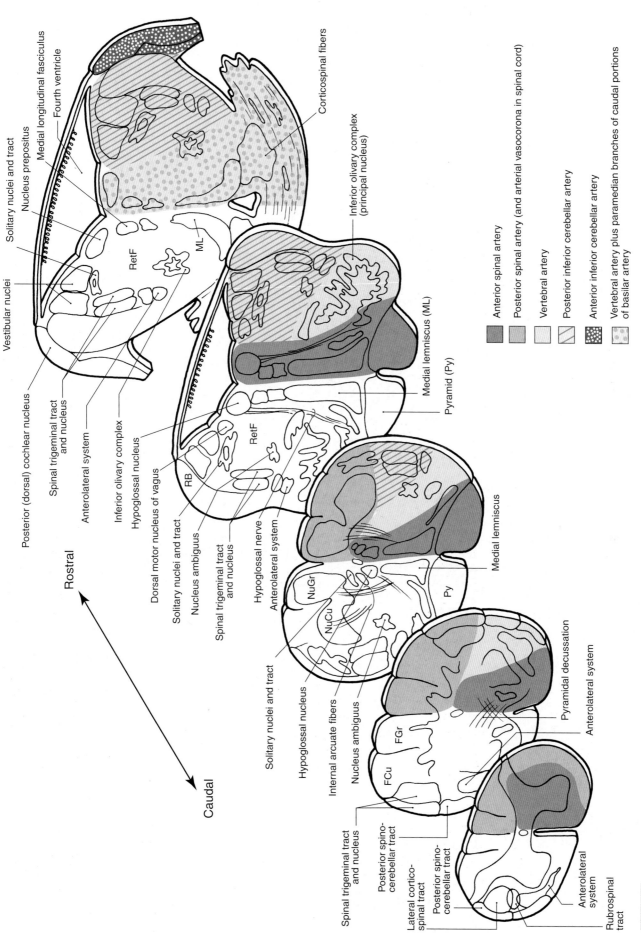

Rostral

Caudal

Fourth ventricle
Medial longitudinal fasciculus
Nucleus prepositus
Solitary nuclei and tract
Vestibular nuclei
Posterior (dorsal) cochlear nucleus
Spinal trigeminal tract and nucleus
Anterolateral system
Inferior olivary complex
Hypoglossal nucleus
Dorsal motor nucleus of vagus
Solitary nuclei and tract
Nucleus ambiguus
Spinal trigeminal tract and nucleus
Hypoglossal nerve
Anterolateral system
Solitary nuclei and tract
Hypoglossal nucleus
Internal arcuate fibers
Nucleus ambiguus
Spinal trigeminal tract and nucleus
Posterior spino-cerebellar tract
Lateral cortico-spinal tract
Posterior spino-cerebellar tract
Anterolateral system
Rubrospinal tract

Corticospinal fibers
Inferior olivary complex (principal nucleus)
Medial lemniscus (ML)
Pyramid (Py)
Medial lemniscus
Pyramidal decussation
Anterolateral system

RetF
ML
RetF
RB
NuGr
NuCu
Py
FGr
FCu

Anterior spinal artery
Posterior spinal artery (and arterial vasocorona in spinal cord)
Vertebral artery
Posterior inferior cerebellar artery
Anterior inferior cerebellar artery
Vertebral artery plus paramedian branches of caudal portions of basilar artery

6-16

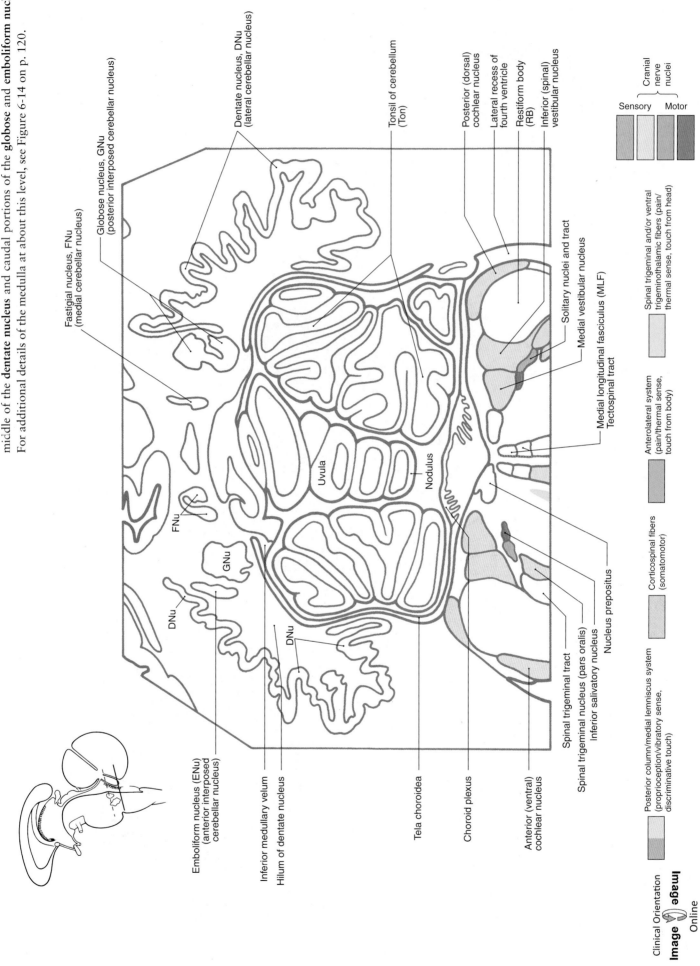

6-17A Transverse section through the dorsal aspects of the medulla at the level of the **cochlear nuclei** and the **cerebellar nuclei**. The plane corresponds to about the middle of the **dentate nucleus** and caudal portions of the **globose** and **emboliform nuclei**. For additional details of the medulla at about this level, see Figure 6-14 on p. 120.

Globose nucleus, GNu (posterior interposed cerebellar nucleus)

Dentate nucleus, DNu (lateral cerebellar nucleus)

Tonsil of cerebellum (Ton)

Posterior (dorsal) cochlear nucleus

Lateral recess of fourth ventricle

Restiform body (RB)

Inferior (spinal) vestibular nucleus

Fastigial nucleus, FNu (medial cerebellar nucleus)

Solitary nuclei and tract

Medial vestibular nucleus

Medial longitudinal fasciculus (MLF)
Tectospinal tract

Uvula

Nodulus

FNu

GNu

DNu

DNu

Spinal trigeminal tract

Spinal trigeminal nucleus (pars oralis)

Inferior salivatory nucleus

Nucleus prepositus

Emboliform nucleus (ENu) (anterior interposed cerebellar nucleus)

Inferior medullary velum

Hilum of dentate nucleus

Tela choroidea

Choroid plexus

Anterior (ventral) cochlear nucleus

Clinical Orientation

Sensory

Cranial nerve nuclei

Motor

Posterior column/medial lemniscus system (proprioception/vibratory sense, discriminative touch)

Corticospinal fibers (somatomotor)

Anterolateral system (pain/thermal sense, touch from body)

Spinal trigeminal and/or ventral trigeminothalamic fibers (pain/thermal sense, touch from head)

Image Online

MRI, T2-weighted image

MRI, T1-weighted image

MLF
RB
Ton
DNu
ENu
GNu

Clinical orientation

Anatomical orientation

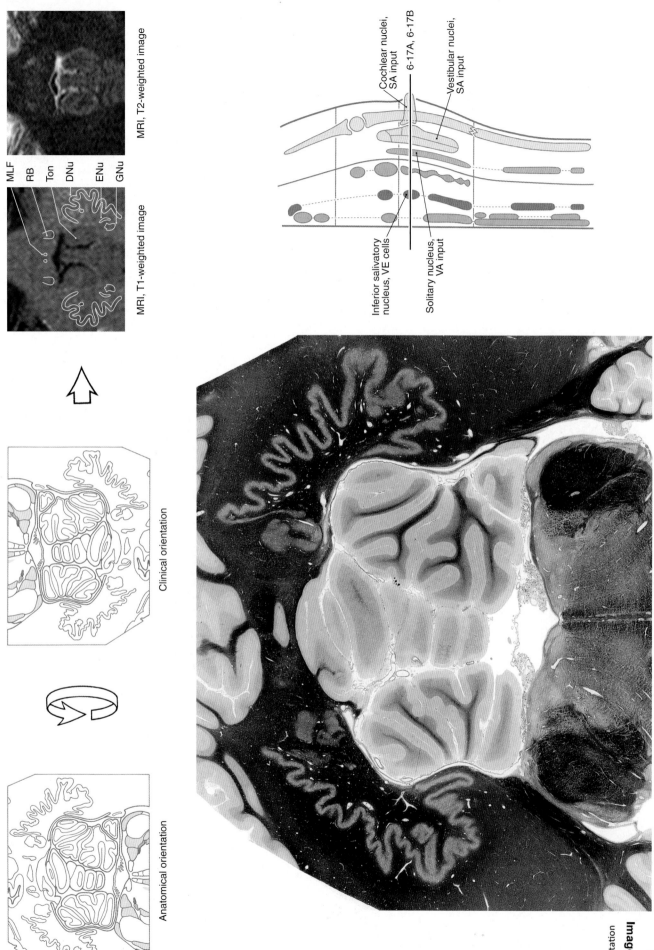

Cochlear nuclei,
SA input

6-17A, 6-17B

Vestibular nuclei,
SA input

Inferior salivatory
nucleus, VE cells

Solitary nucleus,
VA input

Clinical Orientation
Image
Online

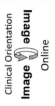

6-17B

6-18A Transverse section through dorsal portions of the pons at the level of the **abducens nucleus** (and **facial colliculus**) and through rostral portions of the **cerebellar nuclei**. For additional details of the pons at this level, see Figure 6-19 on p. 130.

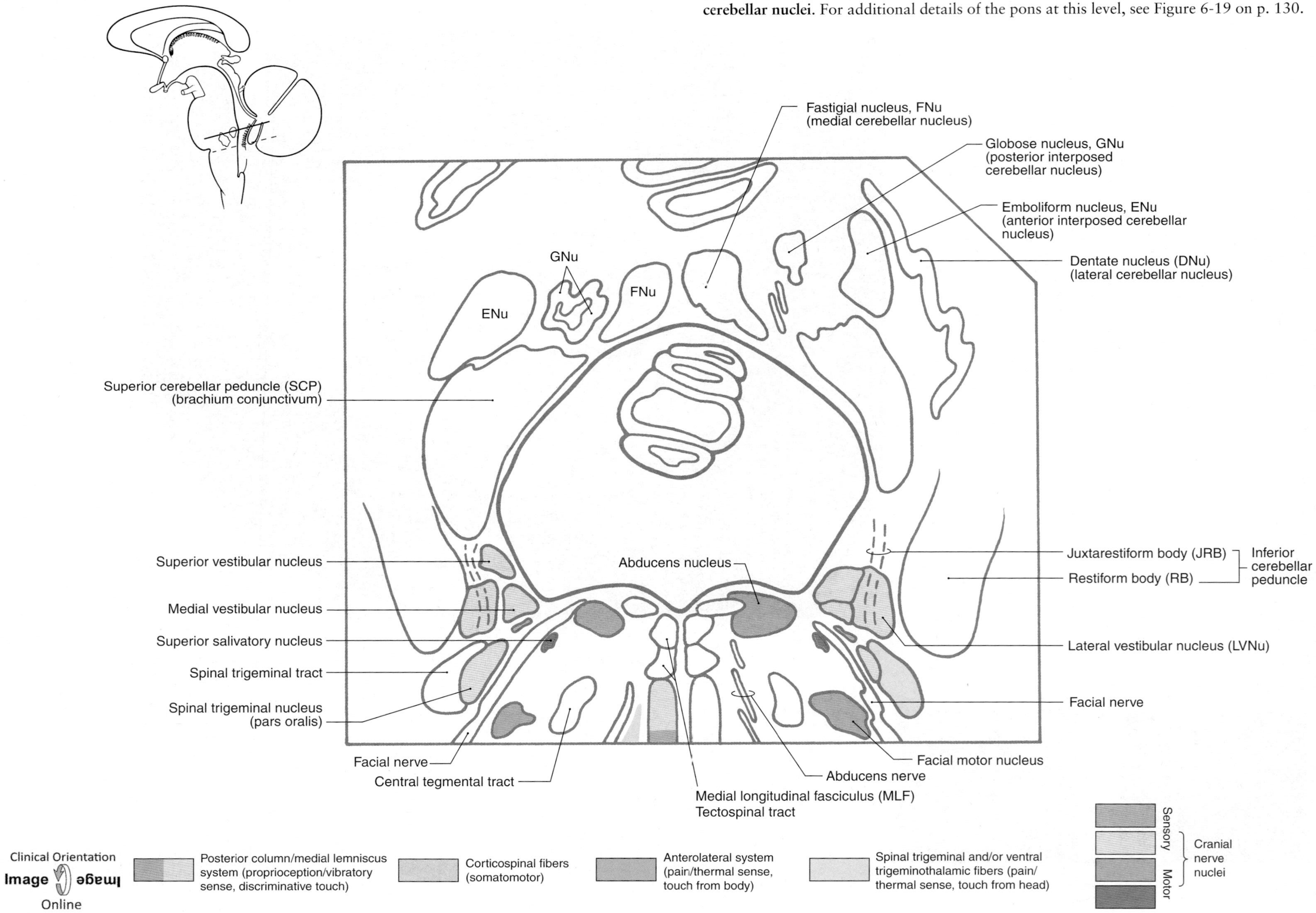

Fastigial nucleus, FNu (medial cerebellar nucleus)

Globose nucleus, GNu (posterior interposed cerebellar nucleus)

Emboliform nucleus, ENu (anterior interposed cerebellar nucleus)

Dentate nucleus (DNu) (lateral cerebellar nucleus)

Juxtarestiform body (JRB)
Restiform body (RB)
Inferior cerebellar peduncle

Lateral vestibular nucleus (LVNu)

Facial nerve

Facial motor nucleus

Abducens nerve

Medial longitudinal fasciculus (MLF)
Tectospinal tract

Abducens nucleus

FNu

GNu

ENu

Superior cerebellar peduncle (SCP) (brachium conjunctivum)

Superior vestibular nucleus

Medial vestibular nucleus

Superior salivatory nucleus

Spinal trigeminal tract

Spinal trigeminal nucleus (pars oralis)

Facial nerve

Central tegmental tract

Cranial nerve nuclei
Sensory   Motor

Spinal trigeminal and/or ventral trigeminothalamic fibers (pain/thermal sense, touch from head)

Anterolateral system (pain/thermal sense, touch from body)

Corticospinal fibers (somatomotor)

Posterior column/medial lemniscus system (proprioception/vibratory sense, discriminative touch)

Clinical Orientation

Image

Image

Online

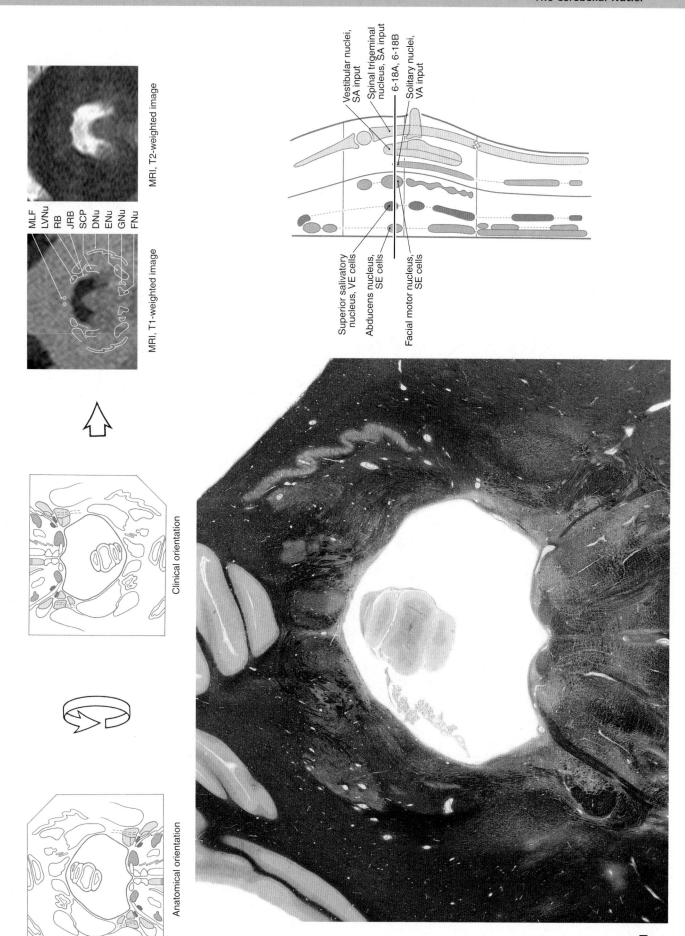

MRI, T2-weighted image

MRI, T1-weighted image

MLF
LVNu
RB
JRB
SCP
DNu
ENu
GNu
FNu

Clinical orientation

Anatomical orientation

Vestibular nuclei, SA input
Spinal trigeminal nucleus, SA input
6-18A, 6-18B
Solitary nuclei, VA input

Superior salivatory nucleus, VE cells
Abducens nucleus, SE cells
Facial motor nucleus, SE cells

Clinical Orientation
Image
Online

6-18B

6-19A   Transverse section of the caudal pons through the facial motor nucleus, abducens nucleus (and facial colliculus), and the intramedullary course of fibers of facial and abducens nerves.

Superior vestibular nucleus

Restiform body (RB)

Facial nerve, internal genu

Mesencephalic tract and nucleus

Superior salivatory nucleus, SSNu

Principal sensory nucleus

Trigeminal motor nucleus

Trigeminal nerve

Anterior spinocerebellar tract

Rubrospinal tract

Anterolateral system (ALS)

Central tegmental tract

Trapezoid body and nuclei

Pontocerebellar fibers

Pontine nuclei

Degenerated corticospinal fibers

Superior medullary velum

Medial longitudinal fasciculus (MLF)
Tectospinal tract

Superior cerebellar peduncle (SCP)

Reticular formation

Medial lemniscus (ML)

Nucleus raphe, magnus

Posterior longitudinal fasciculus

Abducens nucleus (AbdNu)

SSNu

Superior vestibular nucleus

Medial vestibular nucleus (MVNu)

Juxtarestiform body

Lateral vestibular nucleus (LVNu)

Solitary nuclei and tract

Spinal trigeminal tract (SpTTr)

Spinal trigeminal nucleus (SpTNu)(pars oralis)

Facial nerve

Facial motor nucleus (FacNu)

Corticospinal fibers (CSp)

Abducens nerve

Pontine nuclei

Superior olive

Lateral lemniscus

Ventral trigeminothalamic tract

Anterolateral system (pain/thermal sense, touch from body)

Corticospinal fibers (somatomotor)

Post. column/med. lemniscus sys. (proprioception/vibratory sense, discriminative touch)

Spinal trigeminal and/or ventral trigeminothalamic fibers (pain/thermal sense, touch from head)

Sensory   Cranial nerve nuclei   Motor

Clinical Orientation
Image
Image
Online

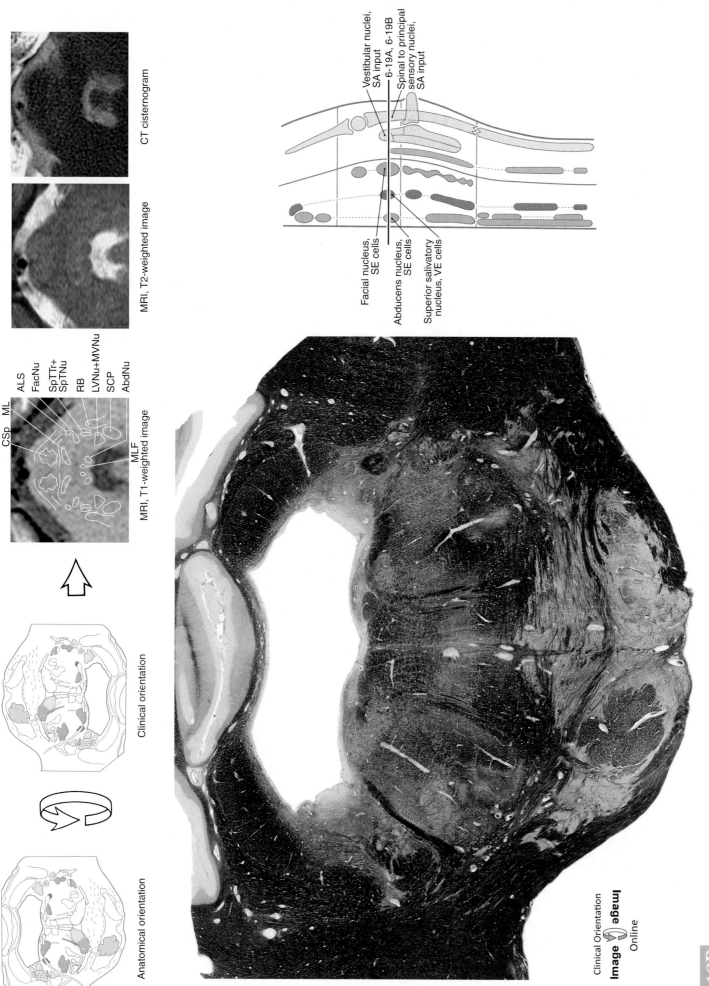

CT cisternogram

MRI, T2-weighted image

CSp ML

ALS
FacNu
SpTTr+
SpTNu
RB
LVNu+MVNu
SCP
AbdNu

MLF

MRI, T1-weighted image

Clinical orientation

Anatomical orientation

Vestibular nuclei,
SA input
6-19A, 6-19B
Spinal to principal
sensory nuclei,
SA input

Facial nucleus,
SE cells
Abducens nucleus,
SE cells
Superior salivatory
nucleus, VE cells

Clinical Orientation
Image Image
Online

6-19B

6-20A   Transverse section of the pons through the rostral pole of the **facial nucleus** and the internal **genu of the facial nerve** and rostral portions of the **abducens nucleus**.

Anterior spinocerebellar tract

Principal sensory nucleus (caudal part)

Trigeminal motor nucleus (caudal part)

Middle cerebellar peduncle

Trigeminal nerve

Anterolateral system (ALS)

Rubrospinal tract

Central tegmental tract

Mesencephalic nucleus and tract

Facial nerve, Internal genu (Fac,G)

Superior cerebellar peduncle (SCP)

Superior medullary velum

Reticular formation

Medial longitudinal fasciculus
Tectospinal tract

Posterior longitudinal fasciculus

Fac,G

Medial lemniscus (ML)

Pontine nuclei

Pontine nuclei

Pontocerebellar fibers

Degenerated corticospinal fibers

Trapezoid body

Nucleus raphe, magnus

Superior vestibular nucleus (SVNu)

Abducens nucleus (AbdNu)

Mesencephalic nucleus and tract

Superior salivatory nucleus

Spinal trigeminal nucleus and tract (SpTNu + Tr) (rostral end)

Facial nerve

Facial motor nucleus

Anterolateral system

Lateral lemniscus

Superior olive

Abducens nerve

Ventral trigeminothalamic tract

Corticospinal fibers (CSP)

Clinical Orientation

Sensory   Motor   Cranial nerve nuclei

Posterior column/medial lemniscus system (proprioception/vibratory sense, discriminative touch)

Anterolateral system (pain/thermal sense, touch from body)

Corticospinal fibers (somatomotor)

Spinal trigeminal and/or ventral trigeminothalamic fibers (pain/thermal sense, touch from head)

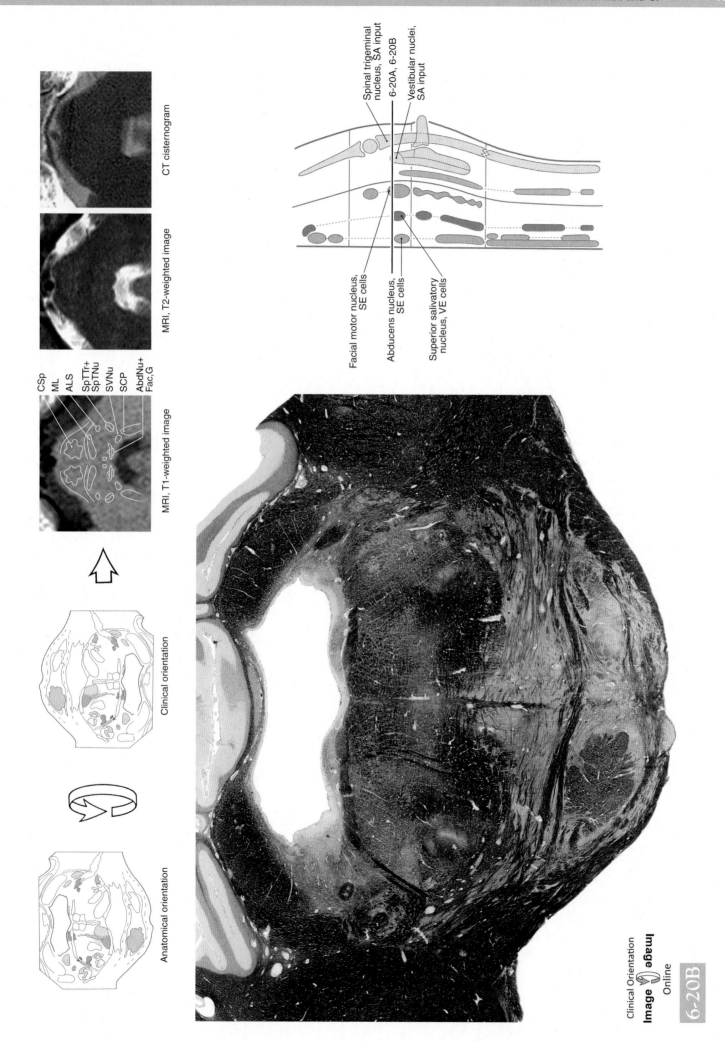

CT cisternogram

MRI, T2-weighted image

MRI, T1-weighted image

CSp
ML
ALS
SpTTr+
SpTNu
SVNu
SCP
AbdNu+
Fac,G

Clinical orientation

Anatomical orientation

Spinal trigeminal nucleus, SA input
6-20A, 6-20B
Vestibular nuclei, SA input

Facial motor nucleus, SE cells
Abducens nucleus, SE cells
Superior salivatory nucleus, VE cells

Clinical Orientation
Image
Online

6-20B

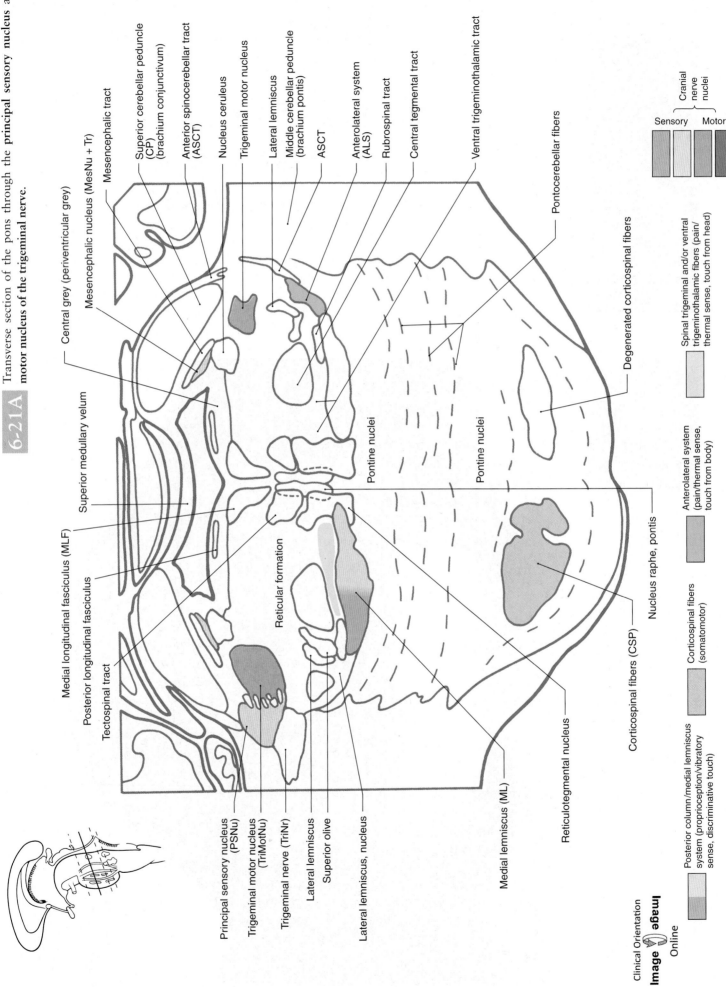

6-21A Transverse section of the pons through the **principal sensory nucleus and motor nucleus of the trigeminal nerve.**

Central grey (periventricular grey)

Mesencephalic nucleus (MesNu + Tr)

Mesencephalic tract

Superior cerebellar peduncle (CP) (brachium conjunctivum)

Anterior spinocerebellar tract (ASCT)

Nucleus ceruleus

Trigeminal motor nucleus

Lateral lemniscus

Middle cerebellar peduncle (brachium pontis)

ASCT

Anterolateral system (ALS)

Rubrospinal tract

Central tegmental tract

Ventral trigeminothalamic tract

Pontocerebellar fibers

Degenerated corticospinal fibers

Pontine nuclei

Pontine nuclei

Superior medullary velum

Medial longitudinal fasciculus (MLF)

Posterior longitudinal fasciculus

Tectospinal tract

Reticular formation

Nucleus raphe, pontis

Reticulotegmental nucleus

Corticospinal fibers (CSP)

Medial lemniscus (ML)

Lateral lemniscus, nucleus

Superior olive

Lateral lemniscus

Trigeminal nerve (TriNr)

Trigeminal motor nucleus (TriMotNu)

Principal sensory nucleus (PSNu)

Sensory

Cranial nerve nuclei

Motor

Posterior column/medial lemniscus system (proprioception/vibratory sense, discriminative touch)

Corticospinal fibers (somatomotor)

Anterolateral system (pain/thermal sense, touch from body)

Spinal trigeminal and/or ventral trigeminothalamic fibers (pain/thermal sense, touch from head)

Clinical Orientation

Image

Online

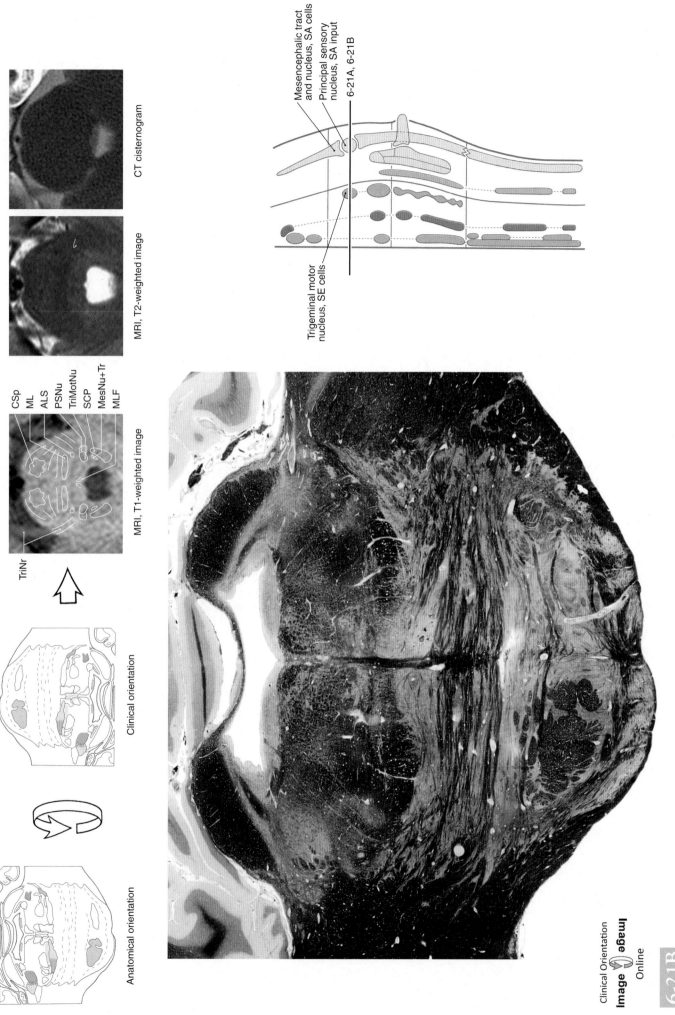

Mesencephalic tract and nucleus, SA cells

Principal sensory nucleus, SA input

6-21A, 6-21B

Trigeminal motor nucleus, SE cells

CT cisternogram

MRI, T2-weighted image

CSp
ML
ALS
PSNu
TriMotNu
SCP
MesNu+Tr
MLF

TriNr

MRI, T1-weighted image

Clinical orientation

Anatomical orientation

Clinical Orientation
Image
Online

6-21B

6-22A Transverse section of the rostral pons through the exit of the trochlear nerve and rostral portions of the exit of the trigeminal nerve. See also Figure 6-21 on p. 134.

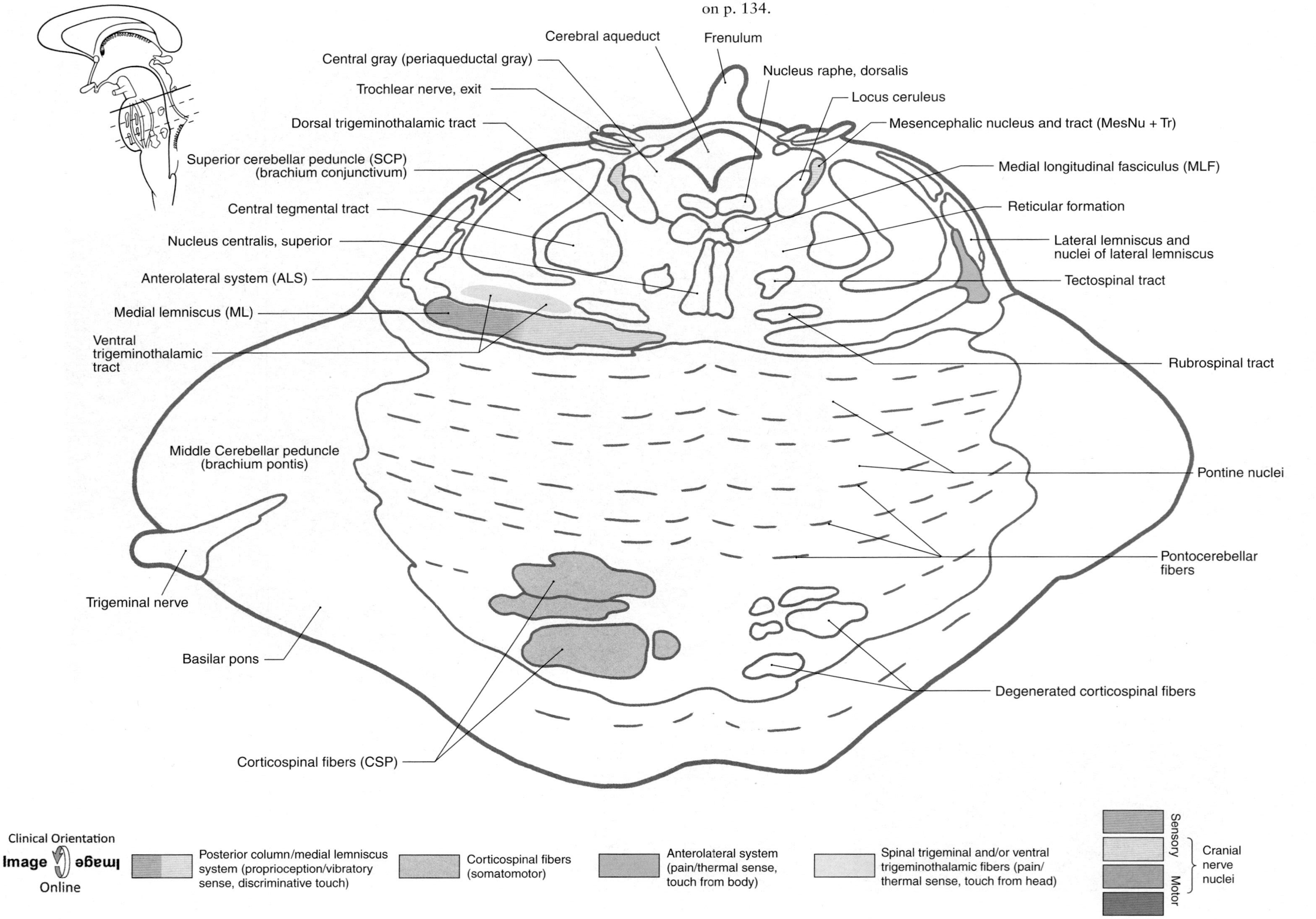

Frenulum

Nucleus raphe, dorsalis

Locus ceruleus

Mesencephalic nucleus and tract (MesNu + Tr)

Medial longitudinal fasciculus (MLF)

Reticular formation

Lateral lemniscus and nuclei of lateral lemniscus

Tectospinal tract

Rubrospinal tract

Pontine nuclei

Pontocerebellar fibers

Degenerated corticospinal fibers

Cerebral aqueduct

Central gray (periaqueductal gray)

Trochlear nerve, exit

Dorsal trigeminothalamic tract

Superior cerebellar peduncle (SCP) (brachium conjunctivum)

Central tegmental tract

Nucleus centralis, superior

Anterolateral system (ALS)

Medial lemniscus (ML)

Ventral trigeminothalamic tract

Middle Cerebellar peduncle (brachium pontis)

Basilar pons

Trigeminal nerve

Corticospinal fibers (CSP)

Clinical Orientation

Image Online

Sensory   Cranial nerve nuclei   Motor

Posterior column/medial lemniscus system (proprioception/vibratory sense, discriminative touch)

Corticospinal fibers (somatomotor)

Anterolateral system (pain/thermal sense, touch from body)

Spinal trigeminal and/or ventral trigeminothalamic fibers (pain/ thermal sense, touch from head)

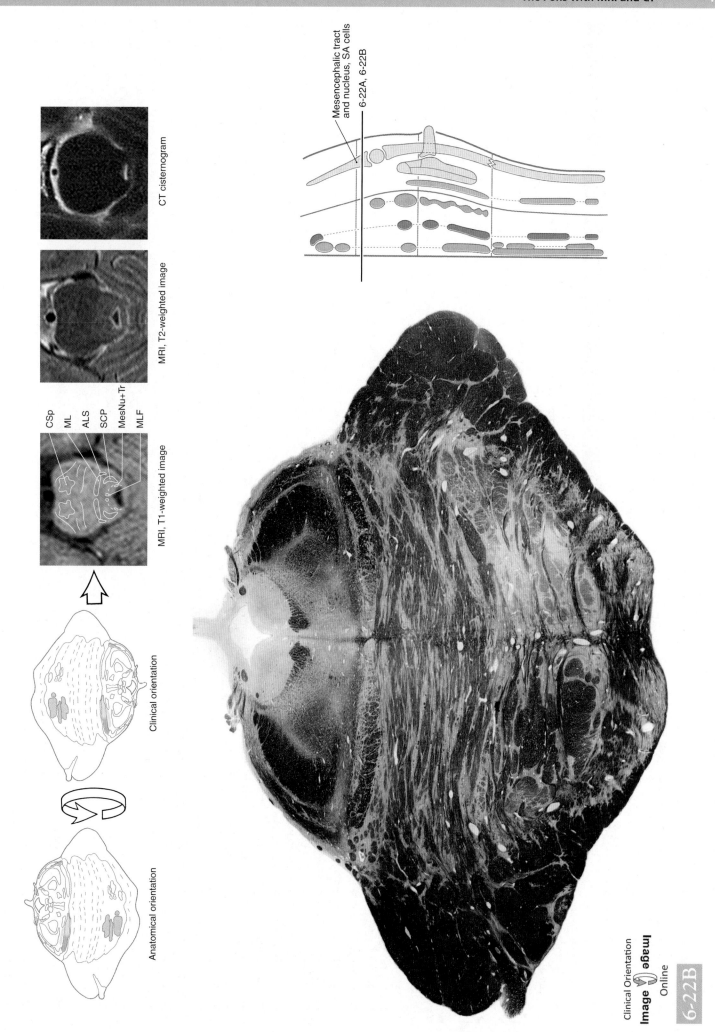

CT cisternogram

MRI, T2-weighted image

CSp
ML
ALS
SCP
MesNu+Tr
MLF

MRI, T1-weighted image

Clinical orientation

Anatomical orientation

Mesencephalic tract
and nucleus, SA cells

6-22A, 6-22B

Clinical Orientation

Image Online

6-22B

Vascular Syndromes or Lesions of the Pons

Medial Pontine Syndrome

This results from occlusion of paramedian branches of basilar artery.

Deficit	Structure Damage
• Contralateral hemiplegia of UE, trunk, and LE	• Corticospinal fibers in basilar pons
• Contralateral loss or decrease of position and vibratory sense and discriminative touch of UE, trunk, and LE	• Medial lemniscus
• Ipsilateral lateral rectus muscle paralysis	• Abducens nerve fibers or nucleus
• Paralysis of conjugate gaze toward side of lesion	• Paramedian pontine reticular formation (pontine gaze center)

The combination of **corticospinal deficits** on one side of the body coupled with a **cranial nerve motor deficit** on the opposite is called a **middle alternating hemiplegia** when the lesion is at this level. **Diplopia** will result (abducens nerve lesion) on gaze toward the side of the lesion. Involvement of the abducens nucleus may also result in an inability to adduct the contralateral medial rectus muscle (damage to abducens internuclear neurons).

At caudal levels, the lesion may extend lateral to involve the lateral lemniscus (**hypacusis**), parts of the middle cerebellar peduncle (some **ataxia**), the spinal trigeminal tract and nucleus (**ipsilateral facial paralysis**), the facial motor nucleus (**ipsilateral loss of pain and thermal sensation from the face**), and the anterolateral system (**contralateral loss of pain and thermal sensation from the body**).

At rostral pontine levels, the lesion may extend into the medial lemniscus or may involve only the arm fibers within this structure (**contralateral loss of vibratory sense, proprioception, and discriminative touch**), the motor nucleus of the trigeminal nerve (**ipsilateral paralysis of masticatory muscles**), or may damage the anterolateral system and rostral portions of the spinal trigeminal tract and nucleus (**loss of pain and thermal sensation from the body [contralateral] and from the face [ipsilateral]**).

Lesions in the medial pontine areas, especially at more caudal levels, may be known as the **Foville syndrome** or **Raymond syndrome**. The specifics of these syndromes are somewhat different but they may be used interchangeably. See Table 3-2 on p. 54 for more information on this point.

Lateral Pontine Syndrome

This results from occlusion of the long circumferential branches of the basilar artery.

Deficit	Structure Damage
• Ataxia, unsteady gait, fall toward side of lesion	• Middle and superior cerebellar peduncles (caudal and rostral levels)
• Vertigo, nausea, nystagmus, deafness, tinnitus, vomiting (at caudal levels)	• Vestibular and cochlear nerves and nuclei
• Ipsilateral paralysis of facial muscles	• Facial motor nucleus (caudal levels)
• Ipsilateral paralysis of masticatory muscles	• Trigeminal motor nucleus (midpontine levels)
• Ipsilateral Horner syndrome	• Descending hypothalamospinal fibers
• Ipsilateral loss of pain and thermal sense from face	• Spinal trigeminal tract and nucleus
• Contralateral loss of pain and thermal sense from UE, trunk, and LE	• Anterolateral system
• Paralysis of conjugate horizontal gaze	• Paramedian pontine reticular formation (at mid- to caudal levels)

The various combinations of these deficits may vary depending on whether the lesion is located in lateral pontine areas at caudal levels versus lateral pontine areas at rostral levels. As noted above, lesions located in lateral portions of the pontine tegmentum may also extend medial at either caudal or rostral levels and give rise to some of the deficits discussed above in the section on medial pontine syndrome.

Lesions that damage more lateral pontine areas generally are referred to as the **Gubler syndrome** (or the **Millard-Gubler syndrome**, although **Gubler** is preferred). In some instances, the term **midpontine base syndrome** is used to describe a basilar pontine lesion that involves the trigeminal root as well. Occlusion of the basilar artery may result in a **locked-in-syndrome**. This lesion is largely restricted to the basilar pons (damage to corticospinal and corticonuclear fibers) while sparing most of the major ascending sensory pathways in the brainstem. While the patient may perceive sensory stimuli, he/she is unable to respond with the exception of limited movements of the eyelids and/or eyes.

6-23 Semi-diagrammatic representation of the internal distribution of arteries in the pons. Selected main structures are labeled on the left side of each section; the general pattern of arterial distribution overlies these structures on the right side. Some patients may have variations of the general distribution patterns of arteries to the pons as shown here. For example, the adjacent territories served by vessels may overlap to differing degrees at their margins, or the territory of a particular vessel may be smaller or larger than seen in the general pattern.

ABBREVIATIONS

BP	Basilar pons	**MLF**	Medial longitudinal fasciculus
CSp	Corticospinal fibers	**RB**	Restiform body (+ juxtarestiform body = inferior cerebellar peduncle)
CTT	Central tegmental tract		
MCP	Middle cerebellar peduncle (brachium pontis)	**RetF**	Reticular formation
		SCP	Superior cerebellar peduncle (brachium conjunctivum)
ML	Medial lemniscus		

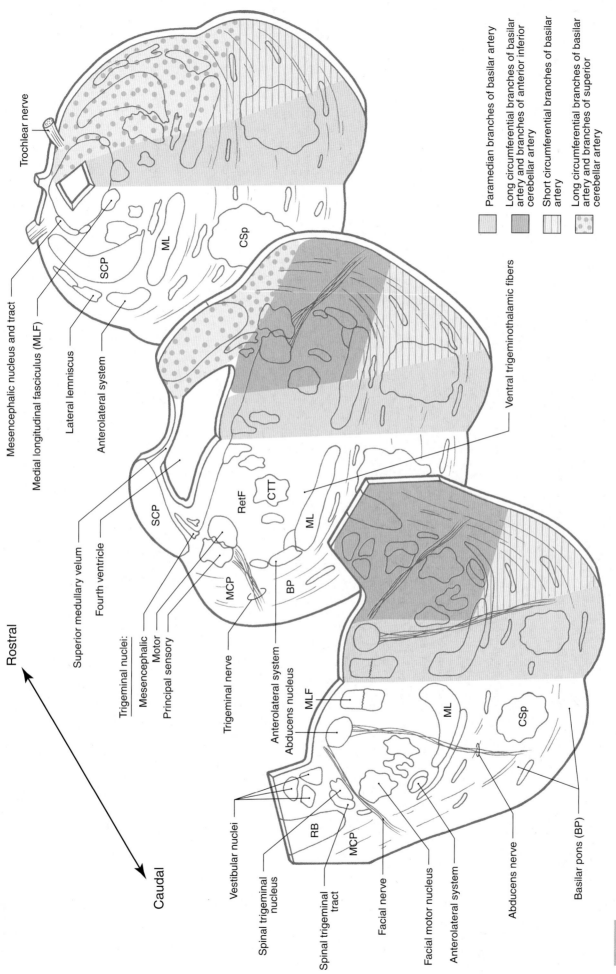

Rostral

Caudal

Trochlear nerve

Mesencephalic nucleus and tract

Medial longitudinal fasciculus (MLF)

Lateral lemniscus

Anterolateral system

SCP

ML

CSp

Ventral trigeminothalamic fibers

Superior medullary velum

Fourth ventricle

SCP

RetF

CTT

ML

Trigeminal nuclei:
  Mesencephalic
  Motor
  Principal sensory

Trigeminal nerve

MCP

BP

Anterolateral system

Abducens nucleus

MLF

ML

CSp

Vestibular nuclei

Spinal trigeminal nucleus

Spinal trigeminal tract

RB

MCP

Facial nerve

Facial motor nucleus

Anterolateral system

Abducens nerve

Basilar pons (BP)

Paramedian branches of basilar artery

Long circumferential branches of basilar artery and branches of anterior inferior cerebellar artery

Short circumferential branches of basilar artery

Long circumferential branches of basilar artery and branches of superior cerebellar artery

6-23

6-24A Transverse section of the brainstem at the pons–midbrain junction through the **inferior colliculus**, caudal portions of the decussation of the **superior cerebellar peduncle**, and rostral parts of the **basilar pons**. The plane of section is just caudal to the **trochlear nucleus**. IC = inferior colliculus on the cisternogram; the T1 and T2 are at a slightly different plane of section.

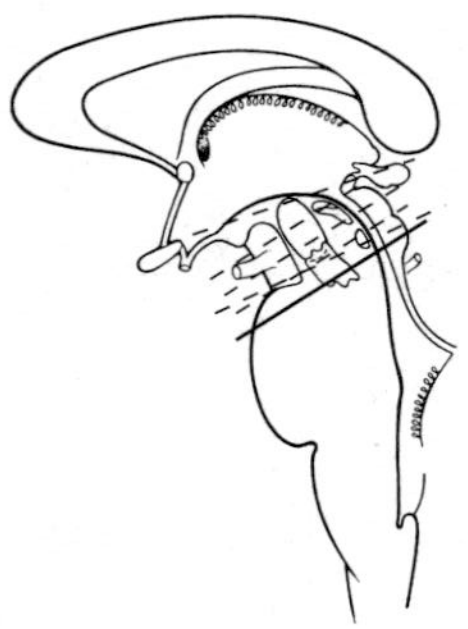

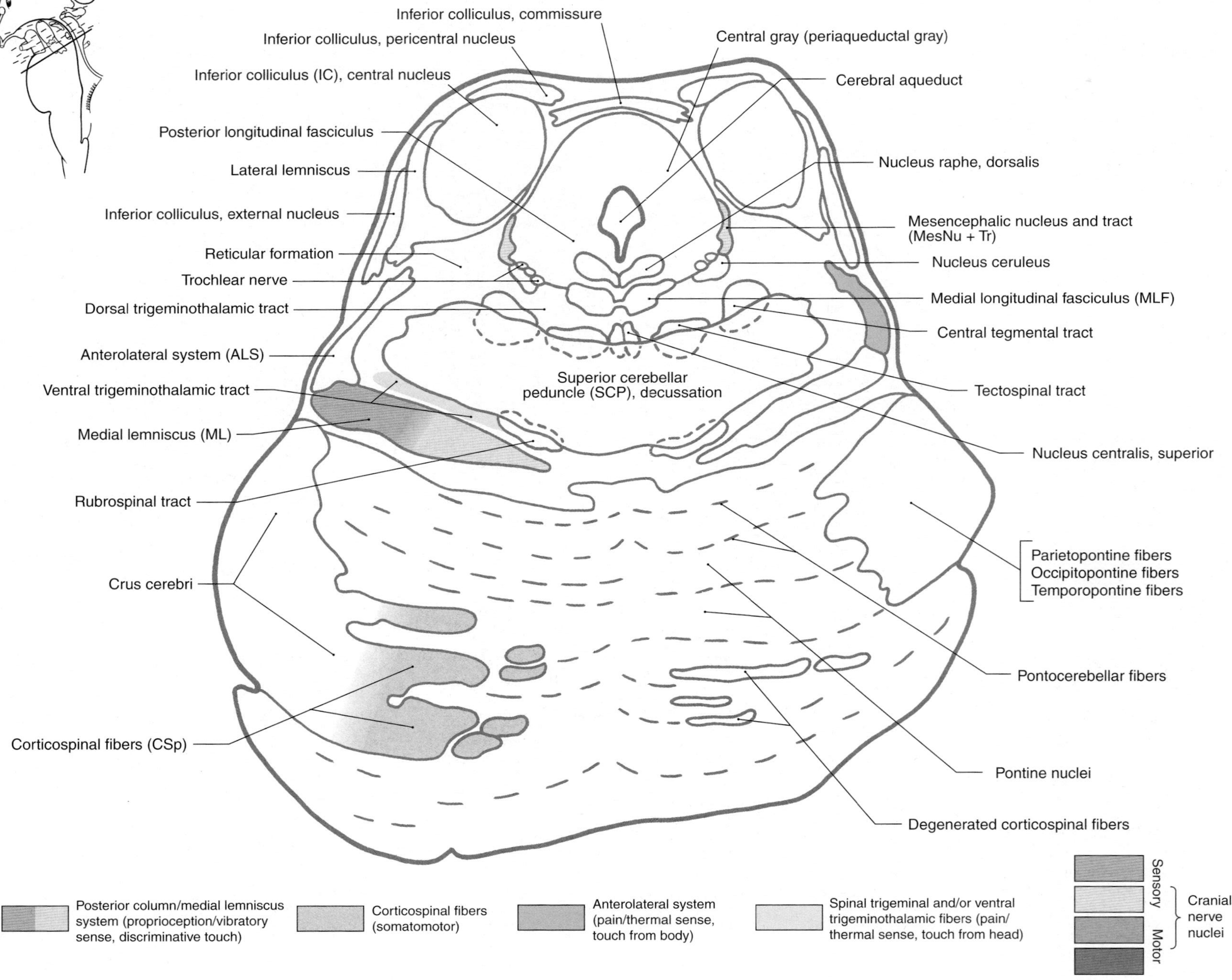

Mesencephalic nucleus and tract (MesNu + Tr)
Nucleus ceruleus
Medial longitudinal fasciculus (MLF)
Central tegmental tract
Tectospinal tract
Nucleus centralis, superior
Parietopontine fibers
Occipitopontine fibers
Temporopontine fibers
Pontocerebellar fibers
Pontine nuclei
Degenerated corticospinal fibers

Nucleus raphe, dorsalis
Cerebral aqueduct
Central gray (periaqueductal gray)

Inferior colliculus, commissure
Inferior colliculus, pericentral nucleus
Inferior colliculus (IC), central nucleus
Posterior longitudinal fasciculus
Lateral lemniscus
Inferior colliculus, external nucleus
Reticular formation
Trochlear nerve
Dorsal trigeminothalamic tract
Anterolateral system (ALS)
Ventral trigeminothalamic tract
Medial lemniscus (ML)
Rubrospinal tract
Crus cerebri
Corticospinal fibers (CSp)

Superior cerebellar peduncle (SCP), decussation

Sensory
Cranial nerve nuclei
Motor

Spinal trigeminal and/or ventral trigeminothalamic fibers (pain/thermal sense, touch from head)
Anterolateral system (pain/thermal sense, touch from body)
Corticospinal fibers (somatomotor)
Posterior column/medial lemniscus system (proprioception/vibratory sense, discriminative touch)

Clinical Orientation
Image Online

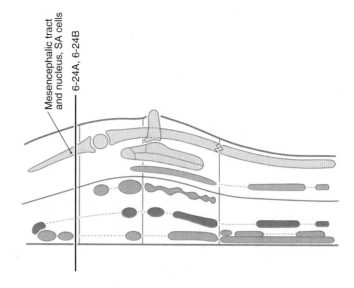

Mesencephalic tract and nucleus, SA cells

6-24A, 6-24B

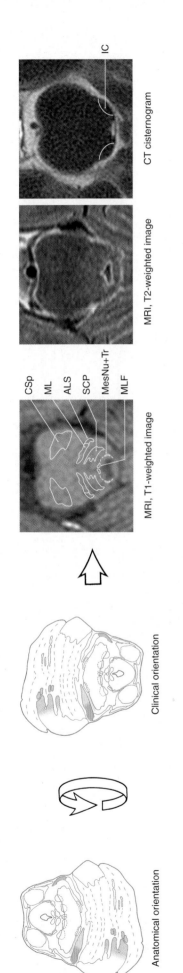

IC

CT cisternogram

MRI, T2-weighted image

CSp
ML
ALS
SCP
MesNu+Tr
MLF

MRI, T1-weighted image

Clinical orientation

Anatomical orientation

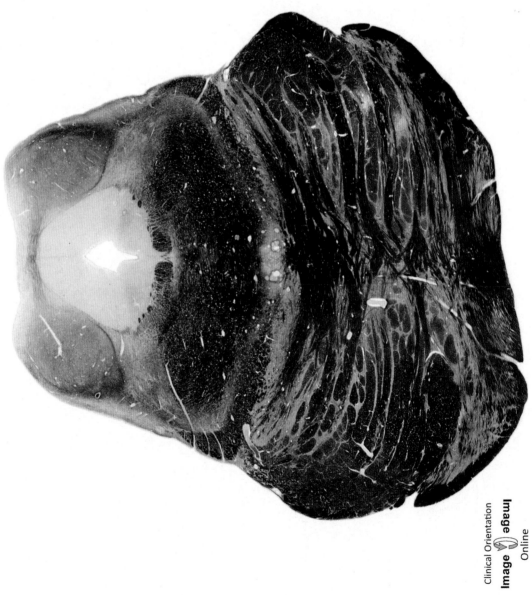

Clinical Orientation

Image Online

6-24B

6-25A   Transverse section of the brainstem showing structures specifically characteristic of the level of the inferior colliculus. These include the **nuclei of the inferior colliculus, trochlear nucleus, decussation of the superior cerebellar peduncle,** caudal aspects of the **substantia nigra,** and the **crus cerebri.** The plane of section also includes the most rostral tip of the basilar pons.

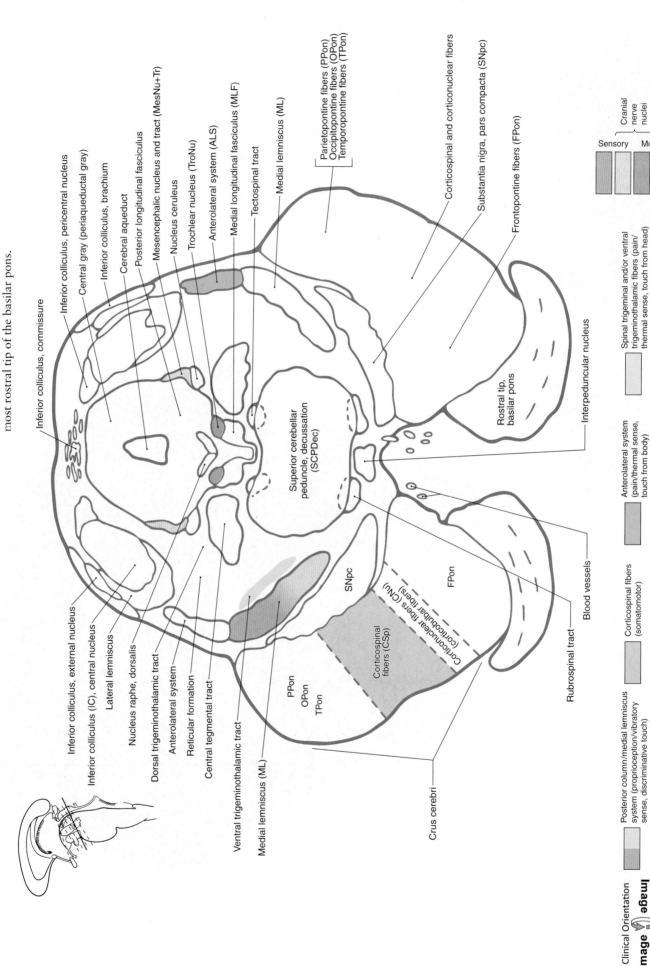

Inferior colliculus, commissure

Inferior colliculus, pericentral nucleus

Central gray (periaqueductal gray)

Inferior colliculus, brachium

Cerebral aqueduct

Posterior longitudinal fasciculus

Mesencephalic nucleus and tract (MesNu+Tr)

Nucleus ceruleus

Trochlear nucleus (TroNu)

Anterolateral system (ALS)

Medial longitudinal fasciculus (MLF)

Tectospinal tract

Medial lemniscus (ML)

Parietopontine fibers (PPon)
Occipitopontine fibers (OPon)
Temporopontine fibers (TPon)

Corticospinal and corticonuclear fibers

Substantia nigra, pars compacta (SNpc)

Frontopontine fibers (FPon)

Rostral tip,
basilar pons

Interpeduncular nucleus

Inferior colliculus, external nucleus

Inferior colliculus (IC), central nucleus

Lateral lemniscus

Nucleus raphe, dorsalis

Dorsal trigeminothalamic tract

Anterolateral system

Reticular formation

Central tegmental tract

Ventral trigeminothalamic tract

Medial lemniscus (ML)

Superior cerebellar
peduncle, decussation
(SCPDec)

SNpc

PPon
OPon
TPon

Corticonuclear fibers (CNu)
(corticobulbar fibers)

FPon

Corticospinal
fibers (CSp)

Blood vessels

Rubrospinal tract

Crus cerebri

Clinical Orientation

Image
Online

| Posterior column/medial lemniscus system (proprioception/vibratory sense, discriminative touch) | Corticospinal fibers (somatomotor) | Anterolateral system (pain/thermal sense, touch from body) | Spinal trigeminal and/or ventral trigeminothalamic fibers (pain/ thermal sense, touch from head) |

Sensory   Motor   Cranial nerve nuclei

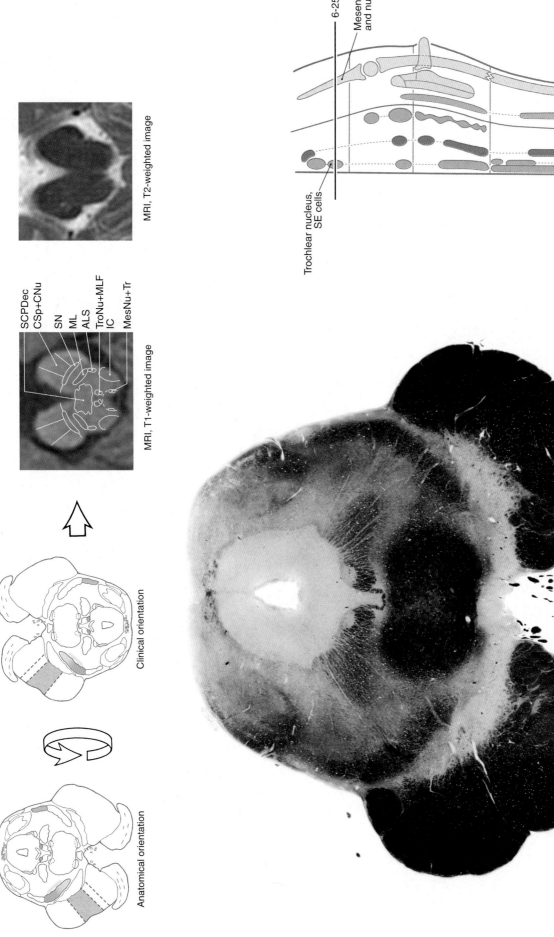

MRI, T2-weighted image

MRI, T1-weighted image

SCPDec
CSp+CNu
SN
ML
ALS
TroNu+MLF
IC
MesNu+Tr

Clinical orientation

Anatomical orientation

6-25A, 6-25B

Mesencephalic tract
and nucleus, SA cells

Trochlear nucleus,
SE cells

Clinical Orientation
Image
Online

6-25B

6-26A Transverse section of the midbrain through the **trochlear nucleus** and **decussation of the superior cerebellar peduncle**. The section also includes caudal parts of the **superior colliculus** and the rostral tip of the **basilar pons**. IC = inferior colliculus on the T1-weighted MRI; at the plane of this section, the T2-weighted MRI and cisternogram are at a slightly more caudal plane compared to the line drawing.

Posterior longitudinal fasciculus

Nucleus raphe, dorsalis

Trochlear nucleus (TroNu)

Spinotectal fibers

Spinothalamic fibers

Anterolateral system (ALS)

Tectospinal tract

Medial lemniscus (ML)

Substantia nigra (SN), pars compacta

Parietopontine fibers (PPon)
Occipitopontine fibers (OPon)
Temporopontine fibers (TPon)

Degenerated corticospinal fibers

Frontopontine fibers (FPon)

Interpeduncular nucleus

Interpeduncular fossa

Cerebral aqueduct

Central gray (periaqueductal gray)

Superior colliculus

Inferior colliculus, brachium

Mesencephalic nucleus and tract (MesNu + Tr)

Reticular formation

Dorsal trigeminothalamic tract

Medial longitudinal fasciculus (MLF)

Central tegmental tract

Ventral trigeminothalamic tract

Superior cerebellar peduncle, decussation (SCPDec)

Corticonuclear fibers (CNu) (corticobulbar fibers)

Corticospinal fibers (CSp)

PPon
OPon
TPon

FPon

Pontine nuclei

Rubrospinal tract

Crus cerebri

Clinical Orientation

Online

Sensory

Cranial nerve nuclei

Motor

Posterior column/medial lemniscus system (proprioception/vibratory sense, discriminative touch)

Corticospinal fibers (somatomotor)

Anterolateral system (pain/thermal sense, touch from body)

Spinal trigeminal and/or ventral trigeminothalamic fibers (pain/thermal sense, touch from head)

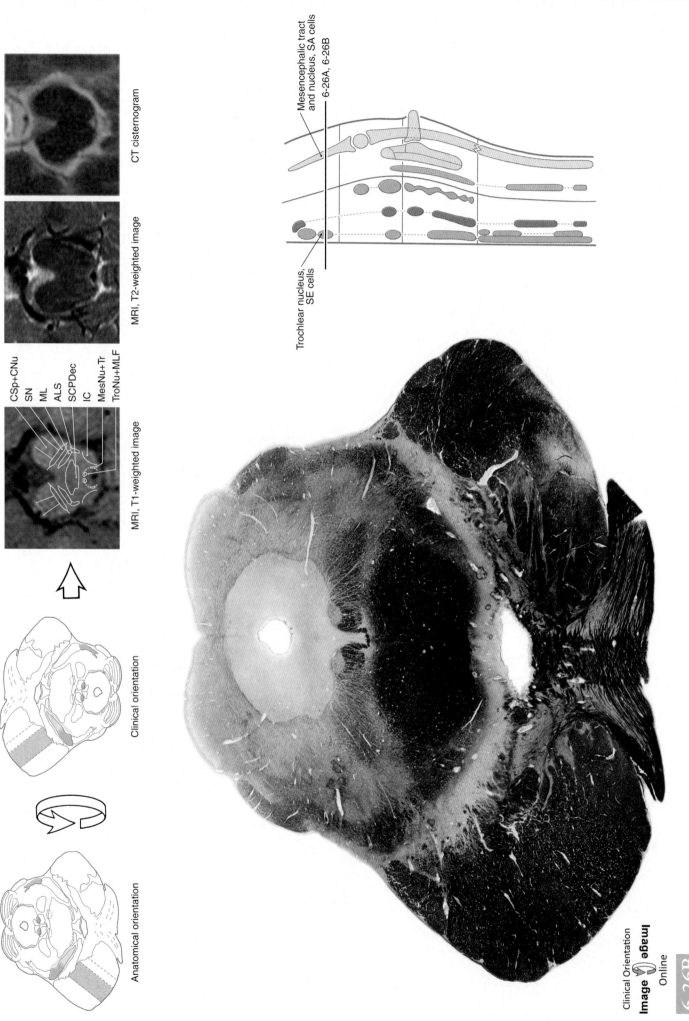

CT cisternogram

MRI, T2-weighted image

MRI, T1-weighted image

CSp+CNu
SN
ML
ALS
SCPDec
IC
MesNu+Tr
TroNu+MLF

Clinical orientation

Anatomical orientation

Mesencephalic tract
and nucleus, SA cells
6-26A, 6-26B

Trochlear nucleus,
SE cells

Clinical Orientation
Image Online

6-26B

6-27A Transverse section of the midbrain through the **superior colliculus**, caudal parts of the **oculomotor nucleus**, and caudal parts of the **red nucleus**. The plane of section is caudal to the **Edinger-Westphal complex** but includes rostral portions of the **decussation of the superior cerebellar peduncle**, which, at this level, are intermingled with the caudal part of the red nucleus. (LE = lower extremity; UE = upper extremity.) At this level, spinothalamic fibers are the main constituents of the bundle indicated as the anterolateral system at lower levels.

Posterior longitudinal fasciculus

Oculomotor nucleus (OcNu)

Mesencephalic nucleus and tract (MesNu + Tr)

Spinotectal tract

Medial longitudinal fasciculus (MLF)

Spinothalamic fibers (SpThF)

Central tegmental tract

Posterior (dorsal) tegmental decussation

Red nucleus

Substantia nigra pars compacta (SNpc)

Substantia nigra pars reticulata (SNpr)

Parietopontine fibers (PPon)
Occipitopontine fibers (OPon)
Temporopontine fibers (TPon)

Degenerated corticospinal fibers

Superior cerebellar peduncle, decussation (SCPDec)

Frontopontine fibers (FPon)

Rubrospinal tract

Anterior (ventral) tegmental decussation

Interpeduncular nucleus

Oculomotor nerve

Cerebral aqueduct

Central gray (periaqueductal gray)

Superior colliculus

Dorsal trigeminothalamic tract

Reticular formation

Inferior colliculus, brachium

Ventral trigeminothalamic tract

Medial geniculate nucleus

Pallidonigral fibers
Nigrostriatal fibers
Corticonigral fibers

Crus cerebri

Red nucleus (RNu), caudal aspect

Corticospinal fibers (CSp)

Corticonuclear fibers (CNu) (corticobulbar fibers)

LE
Trunk
UE

PPon
OPon
TPon

SNpc

SNpr

FPon

Medial lemniscus (ML)

Clinical Orientation

Image Online

Post. column/med. lemniscus sys. (proprioception/vibratory sense, discriminative touch)

Corticospinal fibers (somatomotor)

Anterolateral system (pain/thermal sense, touch from body)

Spinal trigeminal and/or ventral trigeminothalamic fibers (pain/thermal sense, touch from head)

Cranial nerve nuclei

Sensory   Motor

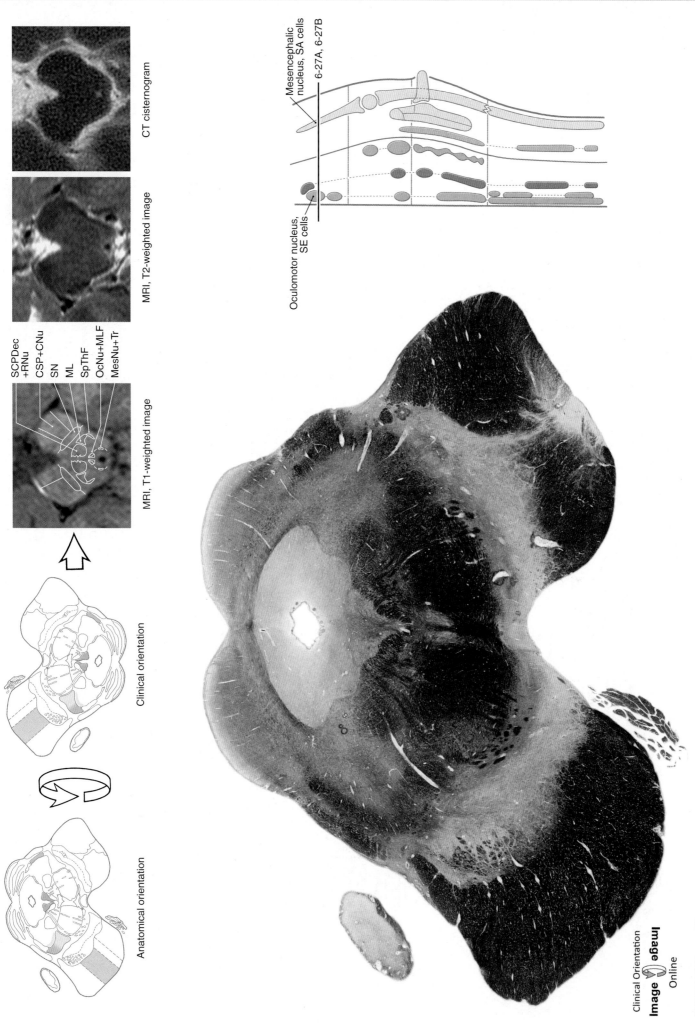

CT cisternogram

MRI, T2-weighted image

SCPDec
+RNu
CSP+CNu
SN
ML
SpThF
OcNu+MLF
MesNu+Tr

MRI, T1-weighted image

Clinical orientation

Anatomical orientation

Mesencephalic
nucleus, SA cells

6-27A, 6-27B

Oculomotor nucleus,
SE cells

Clinical Orientation
Image
Online

6-27B

6-28A   Transverse section of the midbrain through the **superior colliculus**, rostral portions of the **oculomotor nucleus**, including the **Edinger-Westphal complex**, and the exiting fibers of the **oculomotor nerve**. The plane of this section is also through caudal portions of the diencephalon including the **pulvinar nuclear complex** and the **medial and lateral geniculate nuclei.** LE = lower extremity; UE = upper extremity; CC = crus cerebri; OpTr = optic tract.

Parietopontine fibers (PPon)
Occipitopontine fibers (OPon)
Temporopontine fibers (TPon)

Inferior colliculus, brachium

Peripeduncular nucleus

Ventral trigeminothalamic tract

Dorsal trigeminothalamic tract

Spinotectal tract

Superior colliculus (SC)

Posterior longitudinal fasciculus

Degenerated corticospinal fibers

Cerebellorubral fibers and
cerebellothalamic fibers

Central tegmental tract

Medial longitudinal fasciculus (MLF)

Frontopontine fibers (FPon)

Habenulopeduncular tract

Oculomotor nuclei (OcNu)

Oculomotor nerve

SNpr

SNpc

Cerebral aqueduct

Superior colliculus, commissure

Central grey (periaqueductal grey)

Edinger-Westphal preganglionic nucleus (EWpgNu)

Edinger-Westphal centrally projecting nucleus

Mesencephalic tract and nucleus (MesNu + Tr)

Superior colliculus, brachium

Pulvinar nuclear complex

Medial geniculate nucleus (MGNu)

Spinothalamic fibers (SpThF)

Lateral geniculate nucleus (LGNu)

Medial lemniscus (ML)

Optic tract

Red nucleus (RNu)

Substantia nigra, pars compacta (SNpc)

Substantia nigra, pars reticulata (SNpr)

Corticonuclear fibers (CNu) (corticobulbar fibers)

Corticospinal fibers (CSp)

Corticonigral fibers
Pallidonigral fibers
Nigrostriatal fibers

FPon

LE
Trunk
UE

PPon

OPon

TPon

Cranial nerve nuclei
Sensory   Motor

Clinical Orientation

Image
Online

Posterior column/medial lemniscus system (proprioception/vibratory sense, discriminative touch)

Anterolateral system (pain/thermal sense, touch from body)

Corticospinal fibers (somatomotor)

Spinal trigeminal and/or ventral trigeminothalamic fibers (pain/thermal sense, touch from head)

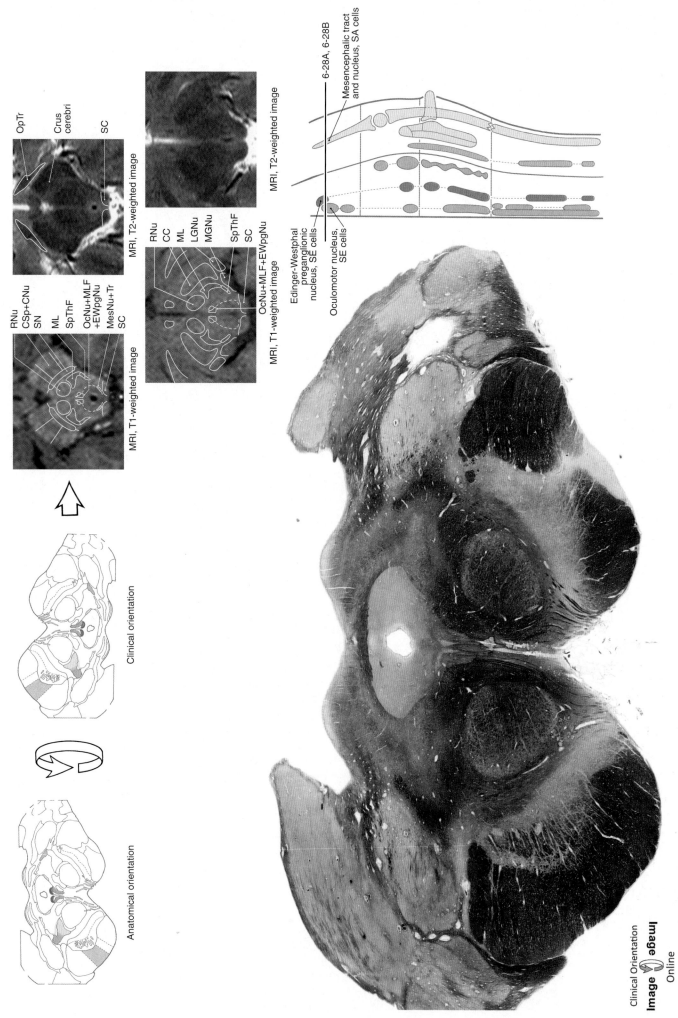

OpTr

Crus cerebri

SC

MRI, T2-weighted image

RNu
CSp+CNu
SN
ML
SpThF
OcNu+MLF
+EWpgNu
MesNu+Tr
SC

MRI, T1-weighted image

RNu
CC
ML
LGNu
MGNu
SpThF
SC
OcNu+MLF+EWpgNu

MRI, T1-weighted image

MRI, T2-weighted image

Clinical orientation

Anatomical orientation

6-28A, 6-28B

Mesencephalic tract and nucleus, SA cells

Edinger-Westphal preganglionic nucleus, SE cells

Oculomotor nucleus, SE cells

Clinical Orientation
Image
Online

6-28B

6-29A Slightly oblique section through the midbrain–diencephalon junction. The section passes through the **posterior commissure**, the rostral end of the **red nucleus**, and ends just dorsal to the **mammillary body**. At this level, the structure labeled **mammillothalamic tract** probably also contains some **mammillotegmental fibers**. Structures at the midbrain–thalamus junction are best seen in an MRI angled to accommodate that specific plane. To make the transition from drawing to stained section to MRI easy, selected structures in the MRI are labeled.

Brachium of superior colliculus

Spinothalamic fibers

Lateral geniculate nucleus (LGNu)

Medial lemniscus

Cerebellorubral fibers and Cerebellothalamic fibers

Transition from crus cerebri (CC) to internal capsule

Cerebral aqueduct

Central grey (periaqueductal grey)

Nucleus of Darkschewitsch

Nucleus of Cajal

Medial longitudinal fasciculus

Medial geniculate nucleus (MGNu)

Optic tract (OpTr)

Subthalamic nucleus

Supraoptic nucleus

Fornix (F)

Mammillothalamic tract (MTTr)

Red nucleus (RNu)

Pineal

Posterior commissure

Superior colliculus

Pretectal nuclei

Hypothalamus

Third ventricle

Dorsal trigeminothalamic tract

Pulvinar nuclear complex (Pul)

Corticospinal fibers

Central tegmental tract

Ventral trigemino-thalamic tract

Peripeduncular nucleus

Parietopontine fibers
Occipitopontine fibers
Temporopontine fibers

Corticonuclear fibers (corticobulbar fibers)

Frontopontine fibers

Habenulopeduncular tract

Clinical Orientation

Image Online

Posterior column/medial lemniscus system (proprioception/vibratory sense, discriminative touch)

Corticospinal fibers (somatomotor)

Anterolateral system (pain/thermal sense, touch from body)

Spinal trigeminal and/or ventral trigeminothalamic fibers (pain/thermal sense, touch from head)

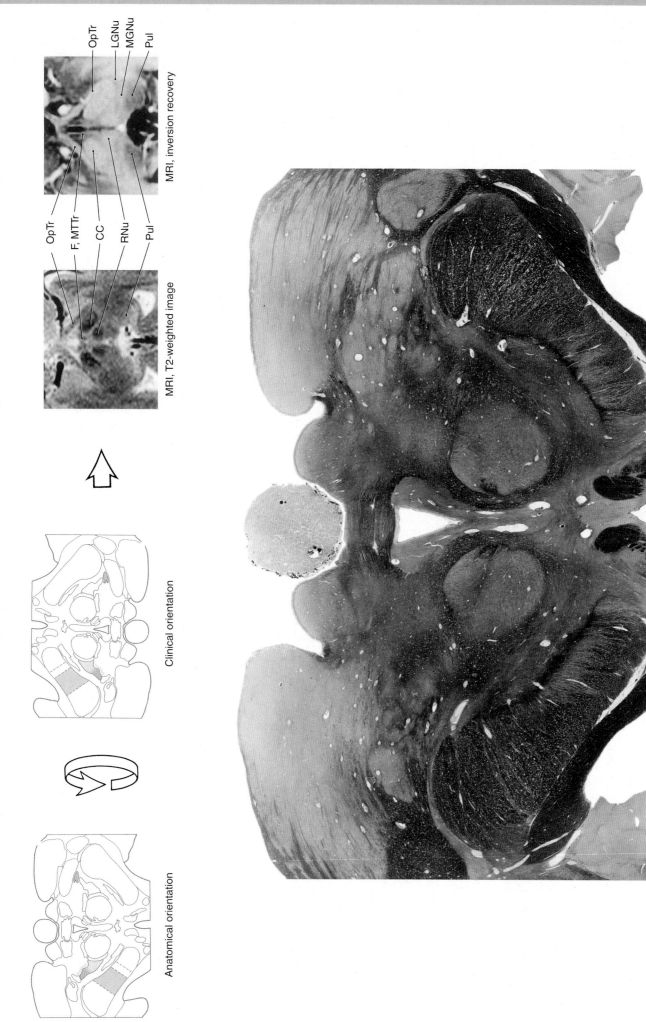

OpTr
LGNu
MGNu
Pul

MRI, inversion recovery

OpTr
F, MTTr
CC
RNu
Pul

MRI, T2-weighted image

Clinical orientation

Anatomical orientation

Clinical Orientation

Image Online

6-29B

6-30 Semi-diagrammatic representation of the internal distribution of arteries in the midbrain. Selected main structures are labeled on the left side of each section; the typical pattern of arterial distribution overlies these structures on the right side. The general distribution patterns of the vessels to the midbrain, as shown here, may vary somewhat from patient to patient. For example, the adjacent territories served by neighboring vessels may overlap to differing degrees at their margins, or the territory of a particular vessel may be larger or smaller than seen in the general pattern.

ABBREVIATIONS

BP	Basilar pons	MGNu	Medial geniculate nucleus
CC	Crus cerebri	ML	Medial lemniscus
DecSCP	Decussation of the superior cerebellar peduncle	RNu	Red nucleus
		SC	Superior colliculus
IC	Inferior colliculus	SCP	Superior cerebellar peduncle
LGNu	Lateral geniculate nucleus	SN	Substantia nigra

Vascular Syndromes or Lesions of the Midbrain

Medial Midbrain (Weber) Syndrome

This may result from occlusion of the paramedian branches of the P₁ segment of the posterior cerebral artery (PCA).

Deficit

- Contralateral hemiplegia of UE, trunk, and LE
- Ipsilateral paralysis of eye movement: eye oriented down and out and pupil dilated and fixed

Structure Damage

- Corticospinal fibers in crus cerebri
- Oculomotor nerve

This combination of motor deficits at this level of the brainstem is called a **superior alternating hemiplegia**. This pattern consists of **ipsilateral paralysis of eye movement (with pupil dilation)** and **contralateral hemiplegia** of the upper and lower extremities. Damage to the corticonuclear (corticobulbar) fibers in the crus cerebri may result in a partial deficit in tongue and facial movement on the contralateral side. These cranial nerve deficits are seen as a **deviation of the tongue to the side opposite the lesion on protrusion and a paralysis of the lower half of the facial muscles** on the contralateral side. Although parts of the substantia nigra are frequently involved, **akinesia and dyskinesia** are not frequently seen.

Central Midbrain Lesion (Claude Syndrome)

Deficit

- Ipsilateral paralysis of eye movement: eye oriented down and out and pupil dilated and fixed
- Contralateral ataxia and tremor of cerebellar origin

Structure Damage

- Oculomotor nerve
- Red nucleus and cerebellothalamic fibers

The lesion in this syndrome may extend laterally into the medial lemniscus and the dorsally adjacent ventral trigeminothalamic fibers. If this was the case, there could conceivably be a loss or diminution of position and vibratory sense and of discriminative touch from the contralateral arm and partial loss of pain and thermal sensation from the contralateral face.

Benedikt Syndrome

This results from a larger lesion of the midbrain that essentially involves both of the separate areas of Weber and Claude. The main deficits are **contralateral hemiplegia** of the extremities (corticospinal fibers), **ipsilateral paralysis of eye movement with dilated pupil** (oculomotor nerve), and **cerebellar** and rubral tremor and **ataxia** (red nucleus and cerebellothalamic fibers). Slight variations may be present based on the extent of the lesion.

Parinaud Syndrome

This syndrome is usually caused by a **tumor in the pineal region**, such as germinoma, astrocytoma, pineocytoma/pineoblastoma, or any of a variety of other tumors that impinge on the superior colliculi. The potential for occlusion at the cerebral aqueduct in these cases also indicates that hydrocephalus may be a component of this syndrome. The deficits in these patients consist of a **paralysis of upward gaze** (superior colliculi), **hydrocephalus** (occlusion of the cerebral aqueduct), and eventually a **failure of eye movement** due to pressure on the oculomotor and trochlear nuclei. These patients also may exhibit **nystagmus** due to involvement of the medial longitudinal fasciculus.

Uncal Herniation

Herniation of the uncus occurs in response to large and/or rapidly expanding lesions most frequently in the temporal lobe; this is a **supratentorial** location. **Uncal herniation** is an extrusion of the uncus through the **tentorial notch (tentorial incisura)** with resultant pressure on the **oculomotor nerve** and the **crus cerebri**. Initially, the pupils, unilaterally or bilaterally, may dilate or respond slowly to light, followed by weakness of oculomotor movement. As herniation progresses, the **pupils become fully dilated**, oculomotor movements may be slow or absent, and the eyes deviate slightly laterally because of the unopposed actions of the abducens nerves. There is usually weakness on the contralateral side of the body due to compression of corticospinal fibers in the crus cerebri. This combination of **ipsilateral oculomotor palsy and a contralateral hemiplegia** is also known as a **superior alternating hemiplegia.**

An alternative situation is when the pressure from the uncal herniation shifts the entire midbrain to the opposite side. In this case, the oculomotor root may be stretched or **avulsed** on the side of the herniation (the ipsilateral side), and the crus cerebri on the contralateral impaled against the edge of the tentorium cerebelli with consequent damage to corticospinal fibers within the crus. This patient presents with an **oculomotor palsy and a hemiplegia of the UE and LE both on the same side of the body.** This combination of deficits is called the **Kernohan syndrome** (or **Kernohan phenomenon).**

Especially large, or bilateral, **supratentorial** lesions may also result in **decorticate rigidity** (flexion of forearm, wrist, and fingers with adduction of UE; extension of LE with internal rotation and plantar flexion of foot). As the lesion descends through the tentorial notch into an **infratentorial** location, decorticate rigidity gives rise to **decerebrate rigidity** (UE and LE extended, toes pointed inward, forearm pronated, and head and neck extended—**opisthotonos**).

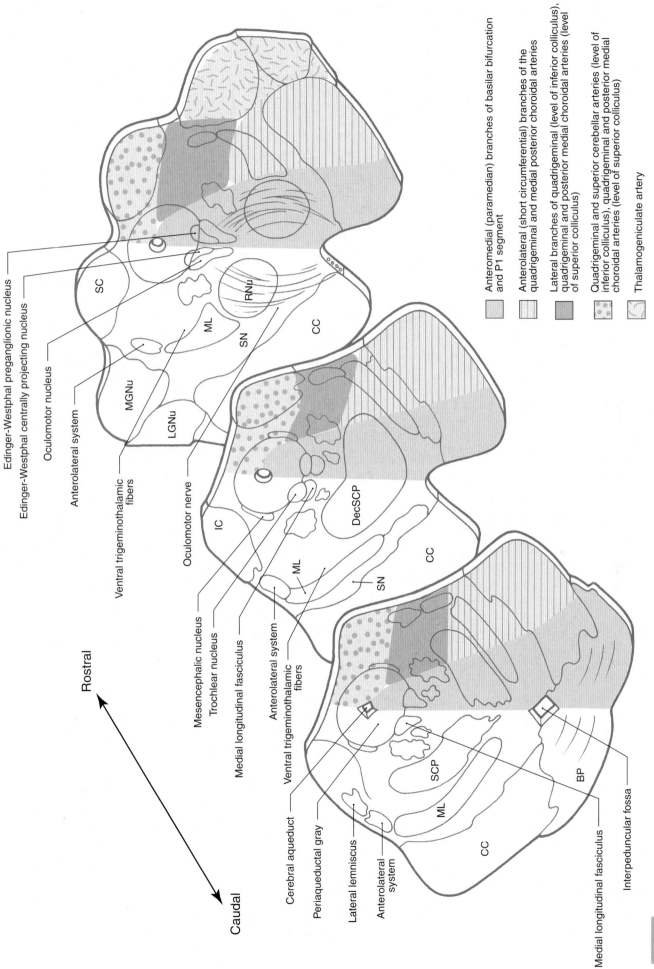

Rostral

Caudal

Edinger-Westphal preganglionic nucleus

Edinger-Westphal centrally projecting nucleus

Oculomotor nucleus

Anterolateral system

Ventral trigeminothalamic fibers

Oculomotor nerve

Mesencephalic nucleus

Trochlear nucleus

Medial longitudinal fasciculus

Anterolateral system

Ventral trigeminothalamic fibers

Cerebral aqueduct

Periaqueductal gray

Lateral lemniscus

Anterolateral system

Medial longitudinal fasciculus

Interpeduncular fossa

SC

RNu

ML

SN

CC

MGNu

LGNu

IC

ML

DecSCP

SN

CC

SCP

ML

BP

CC

Anteromedial (paramedian) branches of basilar bifurcation and P1 segment

Anterolateral (short circumferential) branches of the quadrigeminal and medial posterior choroidal arteries

Lateral branches of quadrigeminal (level of inferior colliculus), quadrigeminal and posterior medial choroidal arteries (level of superior colliculus)

Quadrigeminal and superior cerebellar arteries (level of inferior colliculus), quadrigeminal and posterior medial choroidal arteries (level of superior colliculus)

Thalamogeniculate artery

6-30

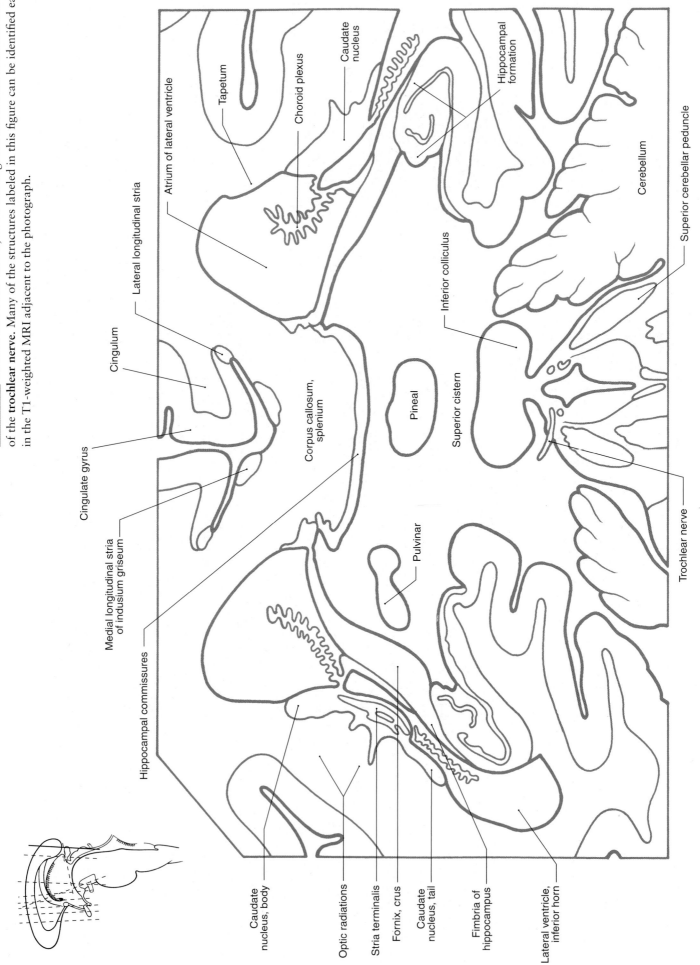

6-31A Coronal section of forebrain through the **splenium of the corpus callosum** and the **crus of the fornix**, and extending into the **inferior colliculus** and exit of the **trochlear nerve**. Many of the structures labeled in this figure can be identified easily in the T1-weighted MRI adjacent to the photograph.

Tapetum

Atrium of lateral ventricle

Choroid plexus

Caudate nucleus

Hippocampal formation

Cerebellum

Superior cerebellar peduncle

Lateral longitudinal stria

Cingulum

Inferior colliculus

Cingulate gyrus

Pineal

Superior cistern

Corpus callosum, splenium

Medial longitudinal stria of indusium griseum

Pulvinar

Trochlear nerve

Hippocampal commissures

Caudate nucleus, body

Optic radiations

Stria terminalis

Fornix, crus

Caudate nucleus, tail

Fimbria of hippocampus

Lateral ventricle, inferior horn

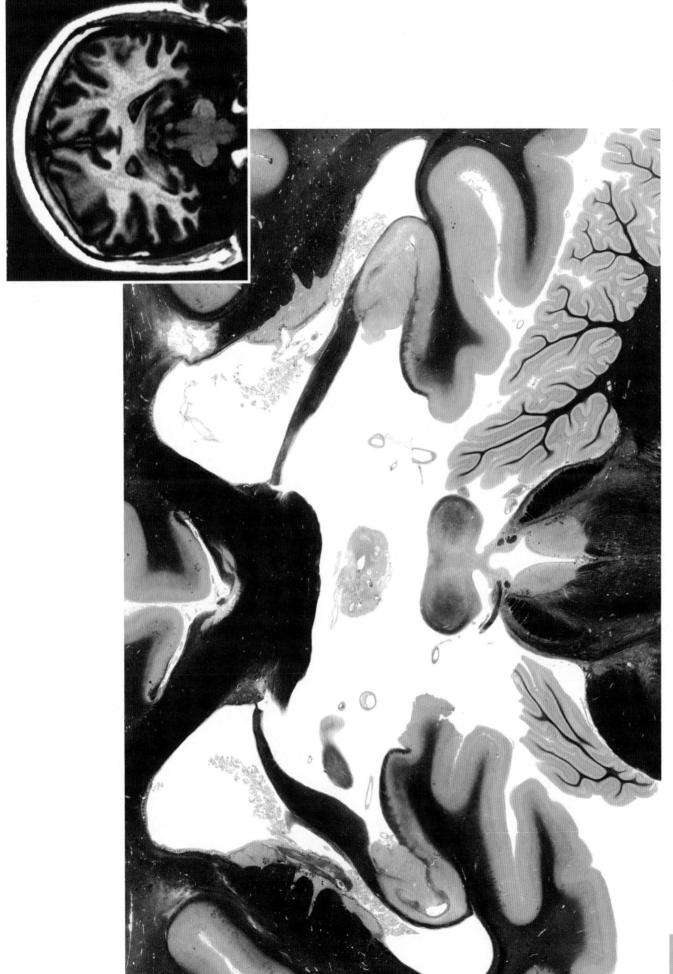

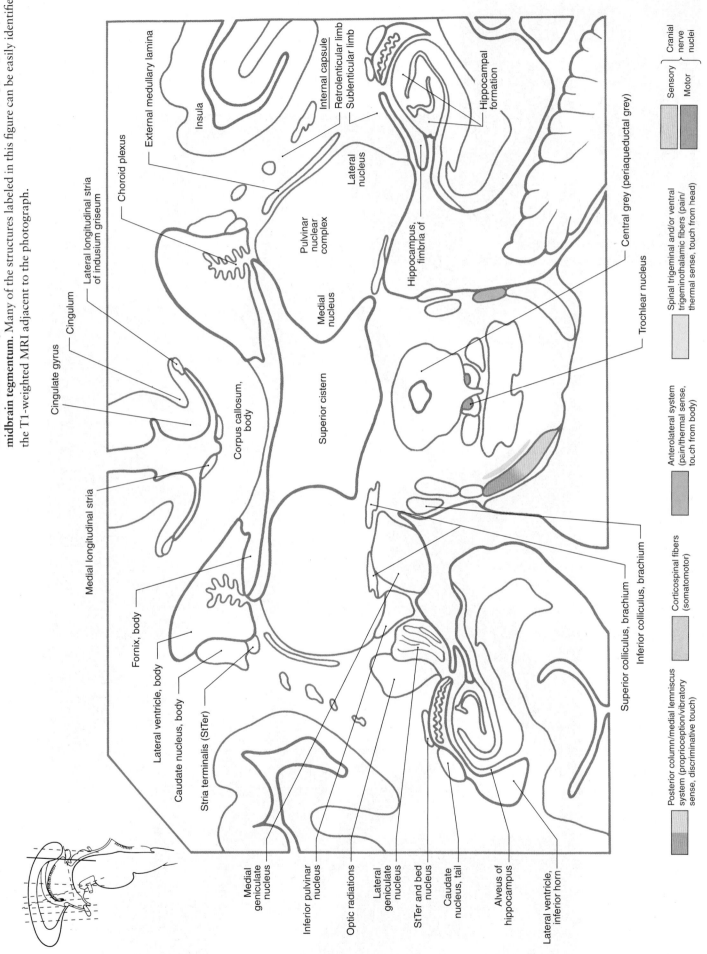

6-32A   Coronal section of the forebrain through the **pulvinar** and the **medial and lateral geniculate nuclei**. The section extends into upper portions of the **midbrain tegmentum**. Many of the structures labeled in this figure can be easily identified in the T1-weighted MRI adjacent to the photograph.

Cingulate gyrus

Cingulum

Lateral longitudinal stria
of indusium griseum

Choroid plexus

External medullary lamina

Insula

Internal capsule
Retrolenticular limb
Sublenticular limb

Hippocampal
formation

Lateral
nucleus

Pulvinar
nuclear
complex

Hippocampus,
fimbria of

Medial
nucleus

Superior cistern

Central grey (periaqueductal grey)

Trochlear nucleus

Superior colliculus, brachium

Inferior colliculus, brachium

Medial longitudinal stria

Corpus callosum,
body

Fornix, body

Lateral ventricle, body

Caudate nucleus, body

Stria terminalis (StTer)

Medial
geniculate
nucleus

Inferior pulvinar
nucleus

Optic radiations

Lateral
geniculate
nucleus

StTer and bed
nucleus

Caudate
nucleus, tail

Alveus of
hippocampus

Lateral ventricle,
inferior horn

Sensory ⎱ Cranial
Motor ⎰ nerve
nuclei

Spinal trigeminal and/or ventral
trigeminothalamic fibers (pain/
thermal sense, touch from head)

Anterolateral system
(pain/thermal sense,
touch from body)

Corticospinal fibers
(somatomotor)

Posterior column/medial lemniscus
system (proprioception/vibratory
sense, discriminative touch)

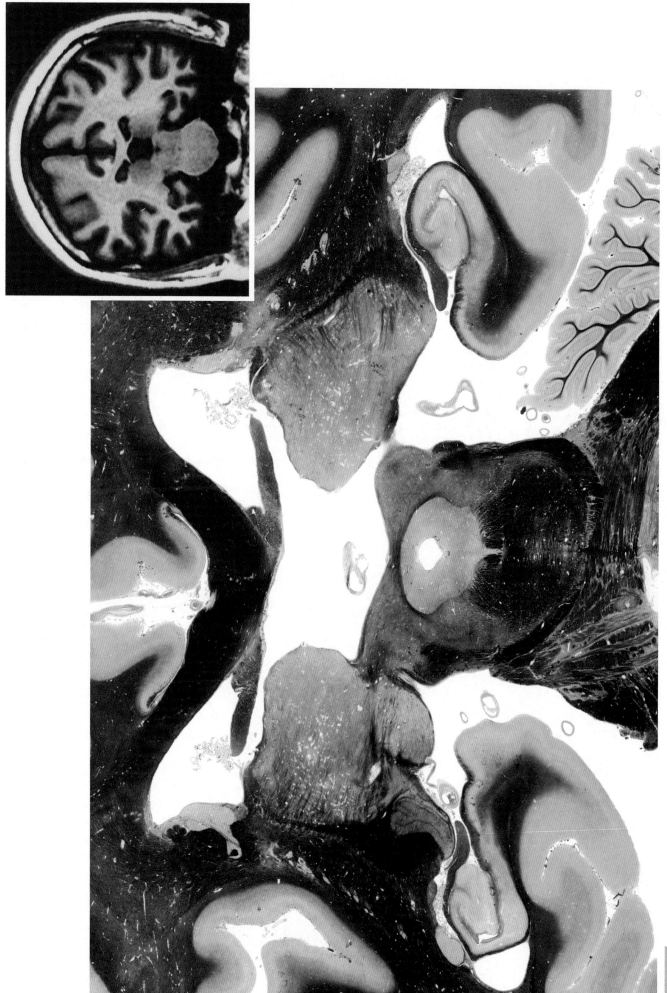

6-32B

6-33A   Slightly oblique section of the forebrain through the **pulvinar, ventral postero-medial,** and **ventral posterolateral nuclei** .The section extends rostrally through the **subthalamic nucleus** and ends in the **caudal hypothalamus**, just dorsal to the **mammillary bodies**, as seen by the position of the (postcommissural) fornix.

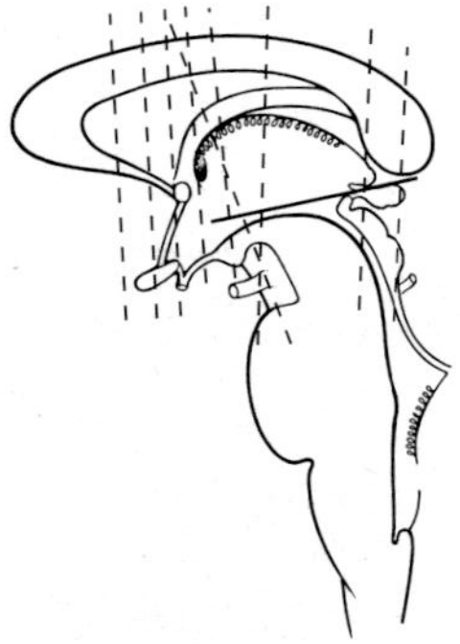

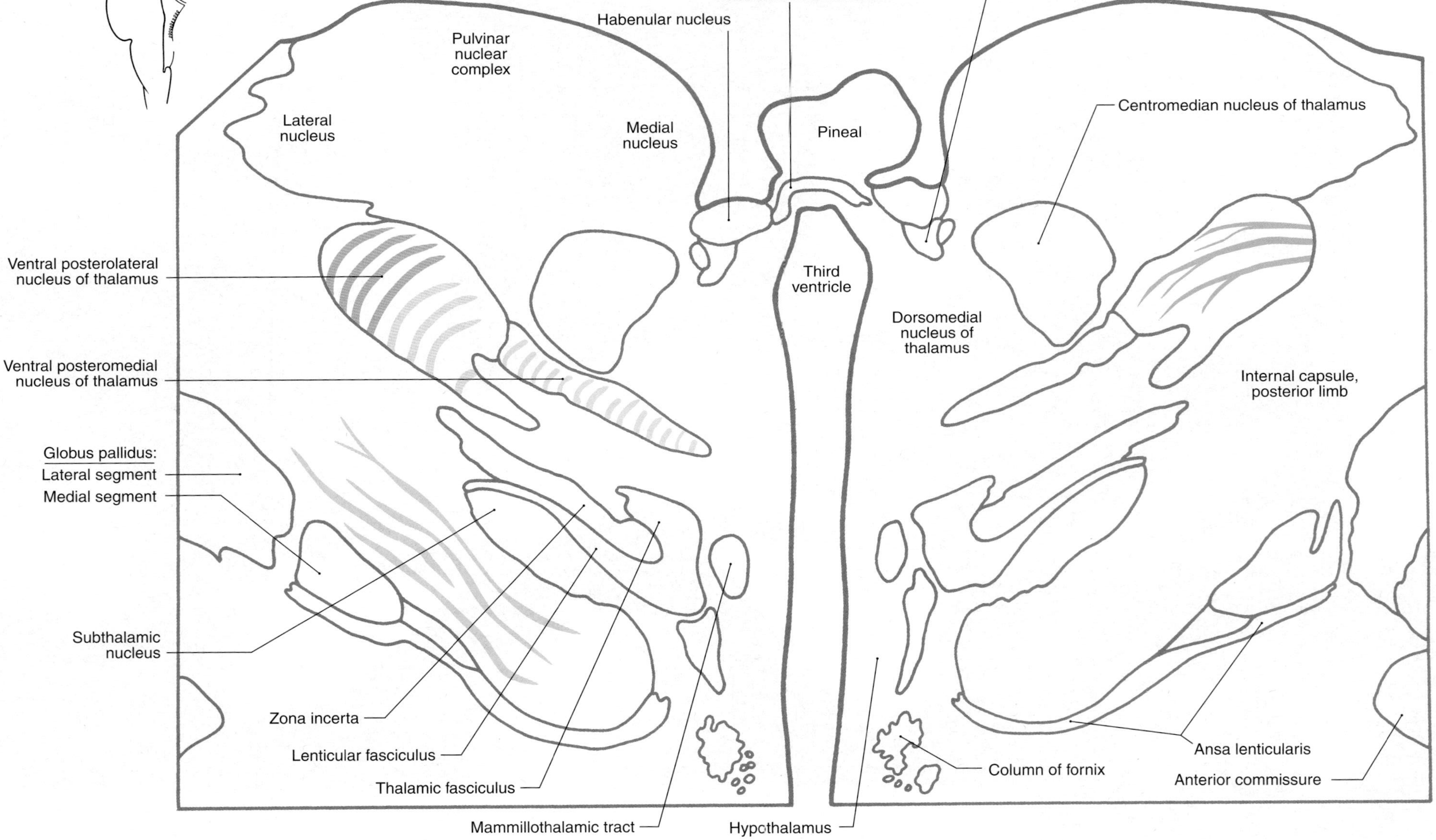

Habenulopeduncular tract

Centromedian nucleus of thalamus

Internal capsule, posterior limb

Ansa lenticularis

Anterior commissure

Habenular commissure

Pineal

Dorsomedial nucleus of thalamus

Column of fornix

Habenular nucleus

Third ventricle

Medial nucleus

Hypothalamus

Pulvinar nuclear complex

Mammillothalamic tract

Lateral nucleus

Zona incerta

Lenticular fasciculus

Thalamic fasciculus

Ventral posterolateral nucleus of thalamus

Ventral posteromedial nucleus of thalamus

Globus pallidus:
Lateral segment
Medial segment

Subthalamic nucleus

Clinical Orientation

Image Online

Posterior column/medial lemniscus system (proprioception/vibratory sense, discriminative touch)

Anterolateral system (pain/thermal sense, touch from body)

Corticospinal fibers (somatomotor)

Spinal trigeminal and/or ventral trigeminothalamic fibers (pain/thermal sense, touch from head)

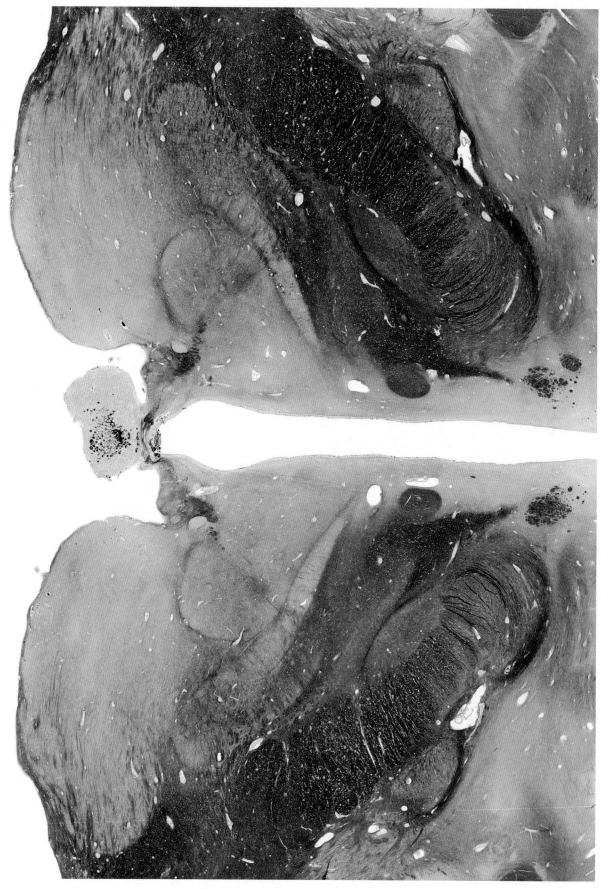

6-34A Coronal section of the forebrain through the **lateral dorsal nucleus, massa intermedia,** and **subthalamic nucleus.** Many of the structures labeled in this figure can be easily identified in the T1-weighted MRI adjacent to the photograph.

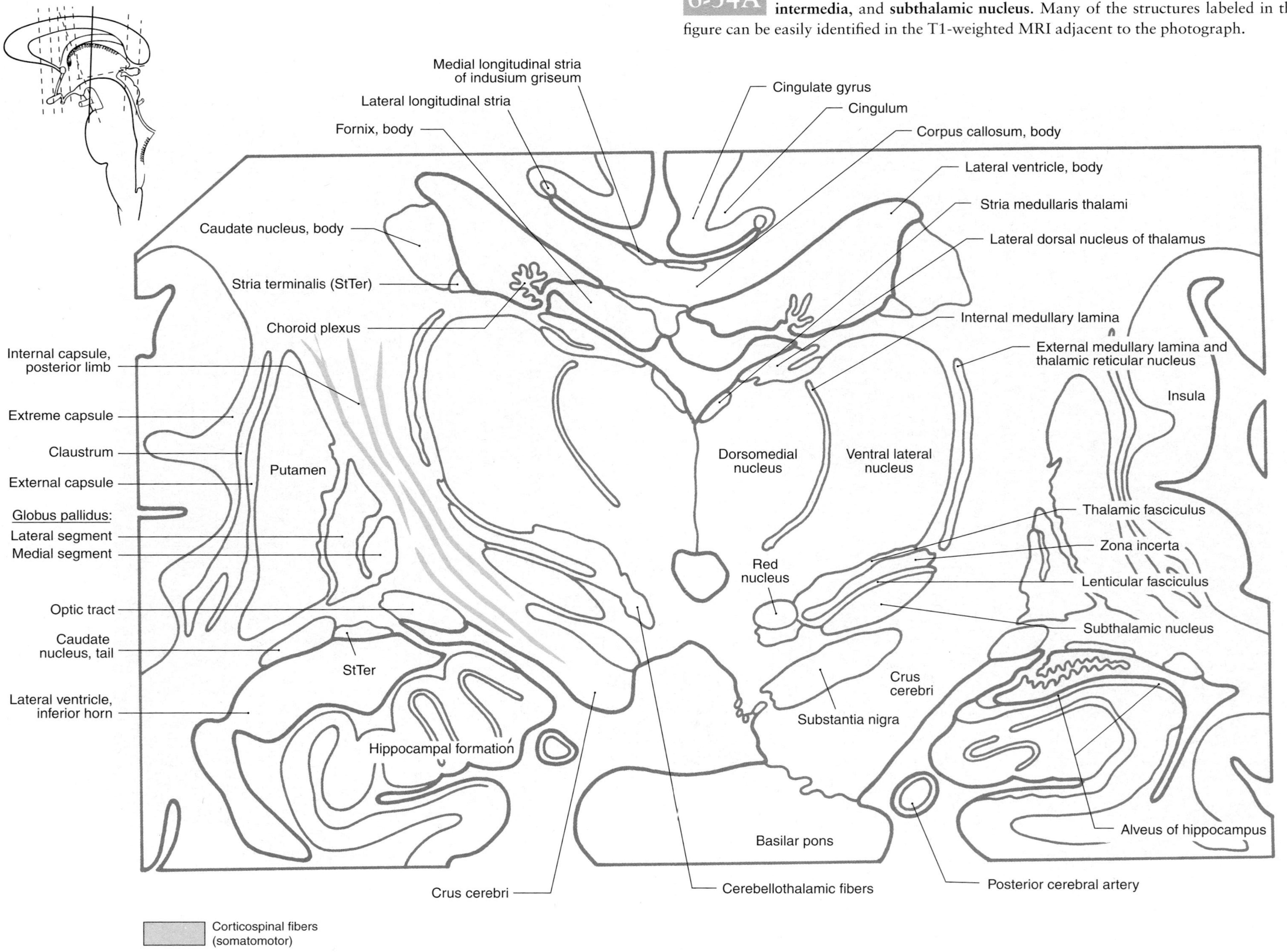

Cingulate gyrus

Cingulum

Corpus callosum, body

Lateral ventricle, body

Stria medullaris thalami

Lateral dorsal nucleus of thalamus

Internal medullary lamina

External medullary lamina and thalamic reticular nucleus

Insula

Thalamic fasciculus

Zona incerta

Lenticular fasciculus

Subthalamic nucleus

Alveus of hippocampus

Posterior cerebral artery

Ventral lateral nucleus

Crus cerebri

Dorsomedial nucleus

Red nucleus

Substantia nigra

Basilar pons

Cerebellothalamic fibers

Medial longitudinal stria of indusium griseum

Lateral longitudinal stria

Fornix, body

Caudate nucleus, body

Stria terminalis (StTer)

Choroid plexus

Internal capsule, posterior limb

Extreme capsule

Claustrum

External capsule

Globus pallidus:

Lateral segment

Medial segment

Optic tract

Caudate nucleus, tail

Lateral ventricle, inferior horn

Putamen

StTer

Hippocampal formation

Crus cerebri

Corticospinal fibers (somatomotor)

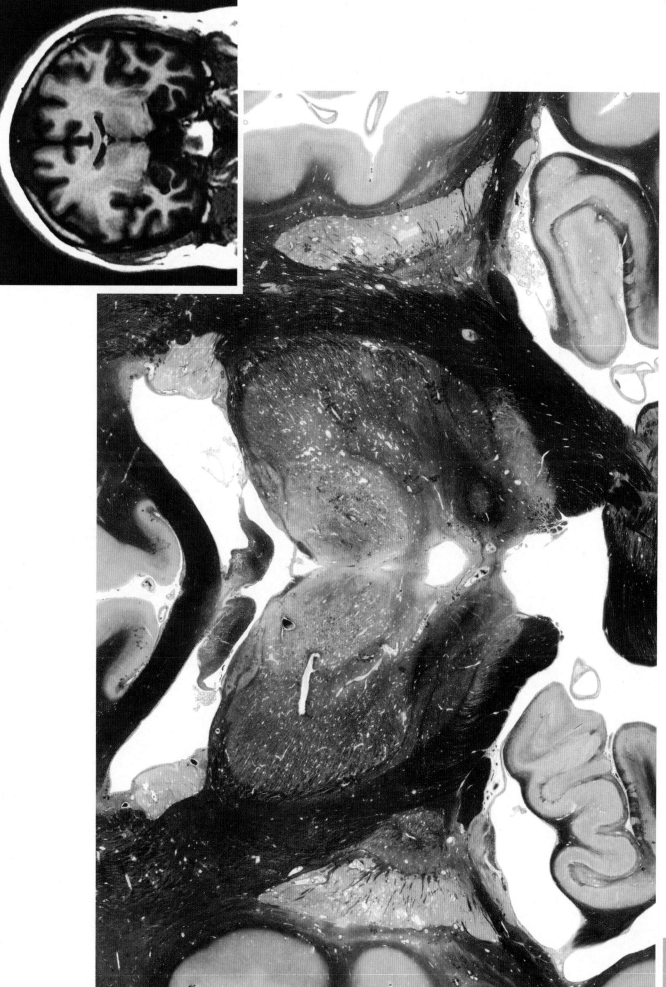

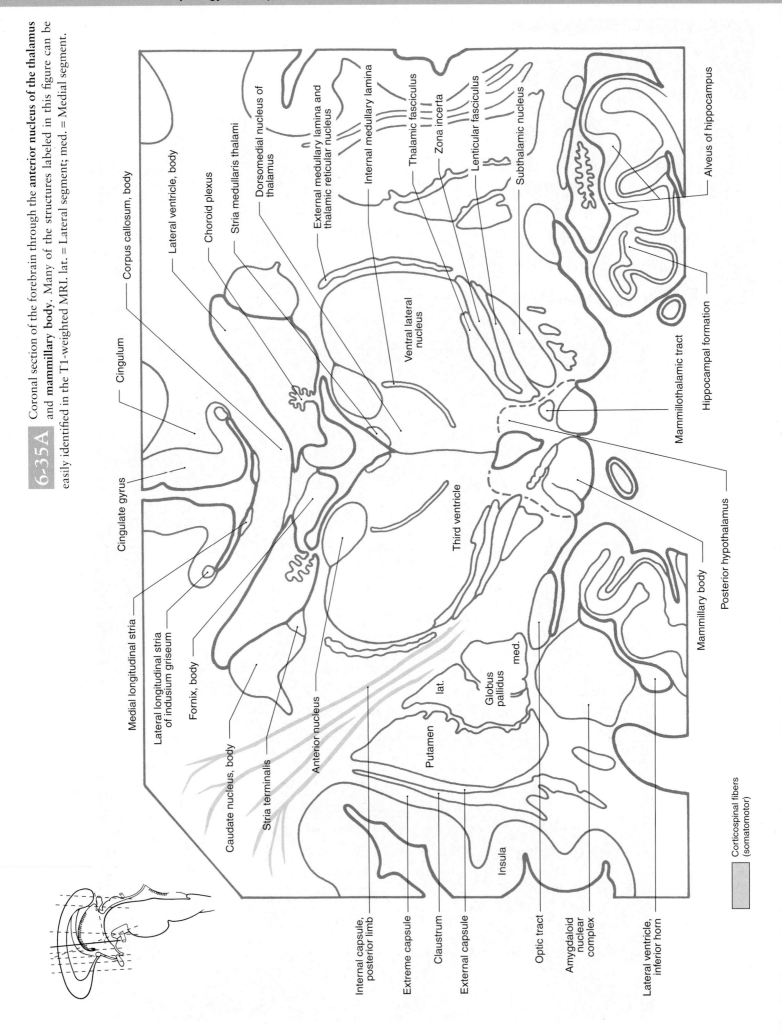

6-35A Coronal section of the forebrain through the **anterior nucleus of the thalamus** and **mammillary body**. Many of the structures labeled in this figure can be easily identified in the T1-weighted MRI. lat. = Lateral segment; med. = Medial segment.

Cingulate gyrus

Cingulum

Corpus callosum, body

Lateral ventricle, body

Choroid plexus

Stria medullaris thalami

Dorsomedial nucleus of thalamus

External medullary lamina and thalamic reticular nucleus

Internal medullary lamina

Thalamic fasciculus

Zona incerta

Lenticular fasciculus

Subthalamic nucleus

Alveus of hippocampus

Hippocampal formation

Mammillothalamic tract

Posterior hypothalamus

Mammillary body

Ventral lateral nucleus

Third ventricle

Medial longitudinal stria

Lateral longitudinal stria of indusium griseum

Fornix, body

Caudate nucleus, body

Stria terminalis

Anterior nucleus

Globus pallidus
lat.
med.

Putamen

Insula

Internal capsule, posterior limb

Extreme capsule

Claustrum

External capsule

Optic tract

Amygdaloid nuclear complex

Lateral ventricle, inferior horn

Corticospinal fibers (somatomotor)

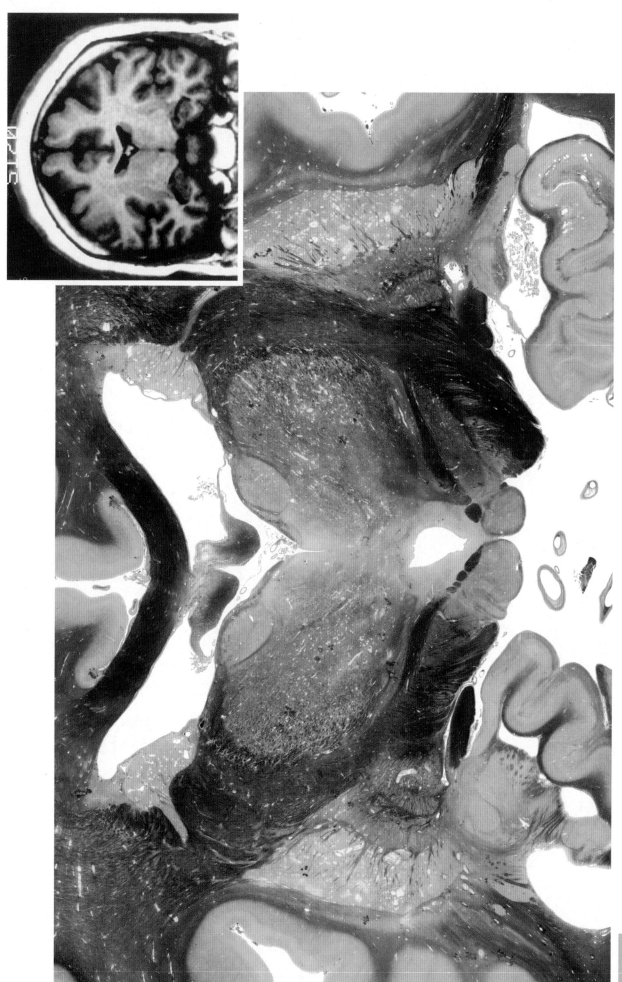

6-36A Slightly oblique section of the forebrain through the **anterior nucleus of the thalamus** and the **subthalamic nucleus.** The section also includes the rostral portion of the **midbrain tegmentum.** Many of the structures labeled in this figure can be easily identified in the T1-weighted MRI adjacent to the photograph. VL = ventral lateral nucleus of thalamus; VA = ventral anterior nucleus of thalamus.

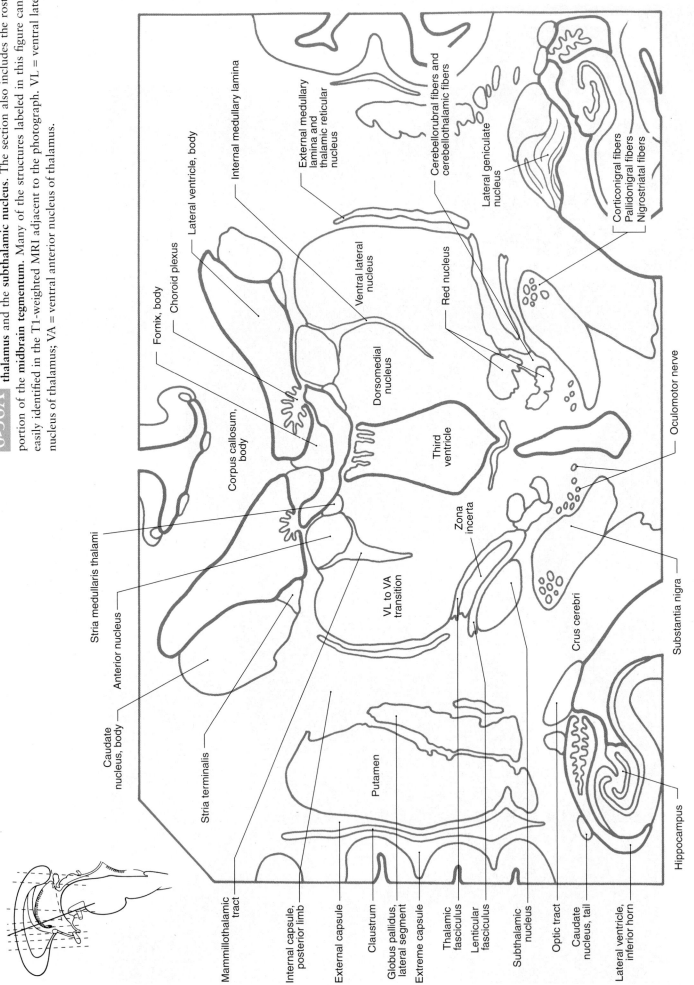

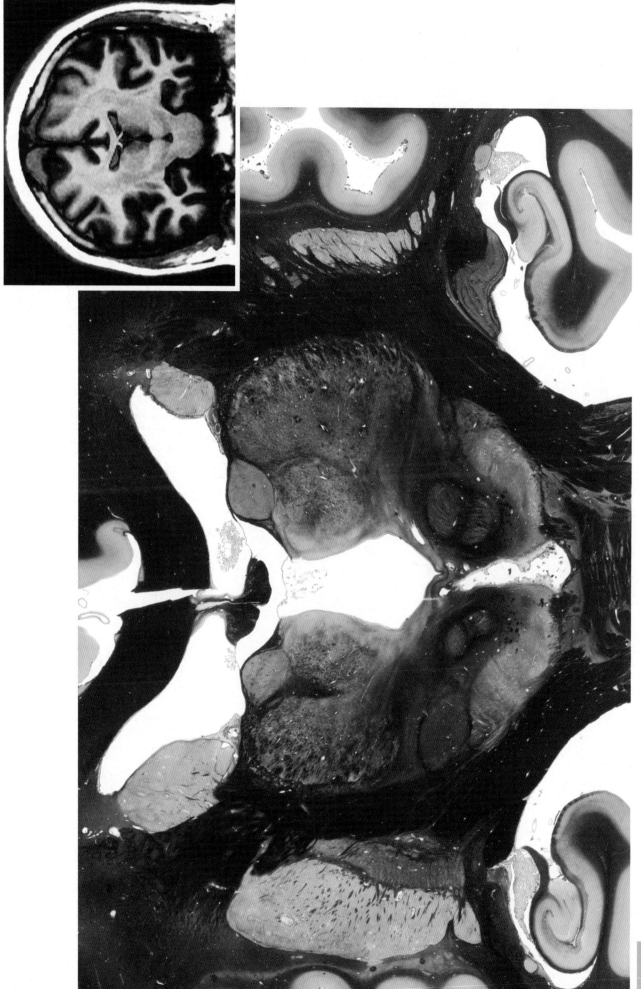

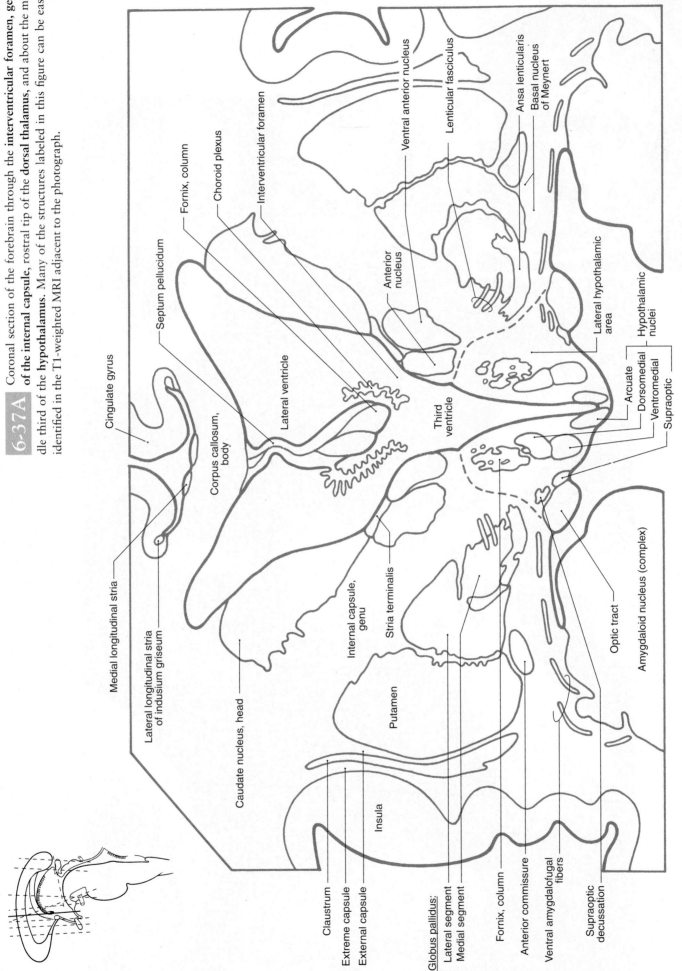

6-37A   Coronal section of the forebrain through the **interventricular foramen, genu of the internal capsule,** rostral tip of the **dorsal thalamus,** and about the middle third of the **hypothalamus.** Many of the structures labeled in this figure can be easily identified in the T1-weighted MRI adjacent to the photograph.

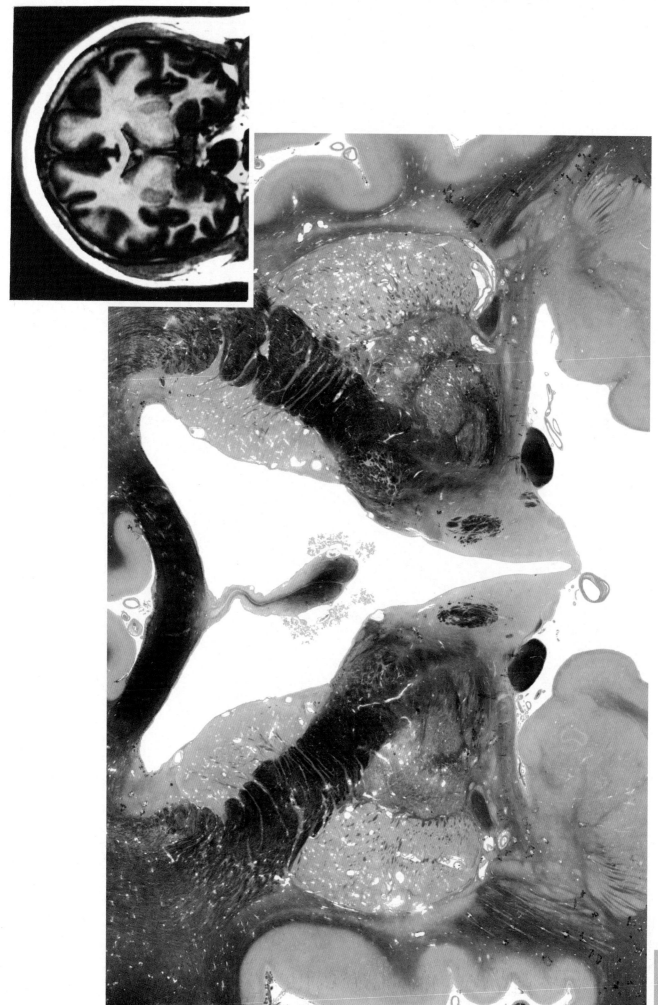

6-37B

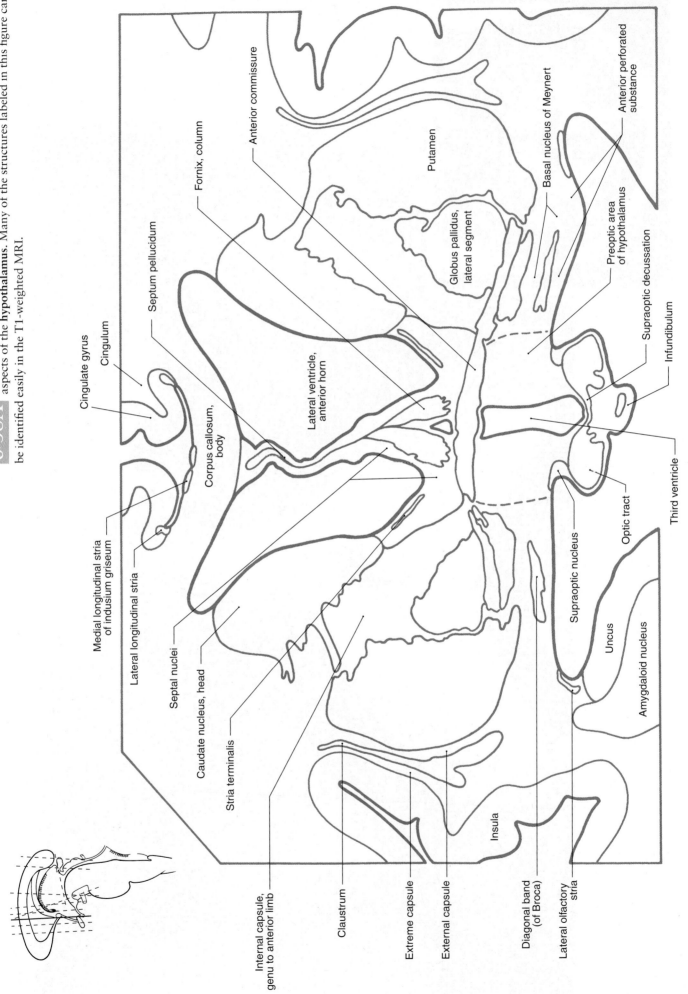

6-38A Coronal section of the forebrain through the **anterior commissure** and rostral aspects of the **hypothalamus.** Many of the structures labeled in this figure can be identified easily in the T1-weighted MRI.

Cingulate gyrus

Cingulum

Septum pellucidum

Fornix, column

Anterior commissure

Putamen

Globus pallidus, lateral segment

Basal nucleus of Meynert

Anterior perforated substance

Preoptic area of hypothalamus

Supraoptic decussation

Infundibulum

Lateral ventricle, anterior horn

Medial longitudinal stria of indusium griseum

Lateral longitudinal stria

Corpus callosum, body

Septal nuclei

Caudate nucleus, head

Stria terminalis

Supraoptic nucleus

Optic tract

Third ventricle

Uncus

Amygdaloid nucleus

Internal capsule, genu to anterior limb

Claustrum

Extreme capsule

External capsule

Insula

Diagonal band (of Broca)

Lateral olfactory stria

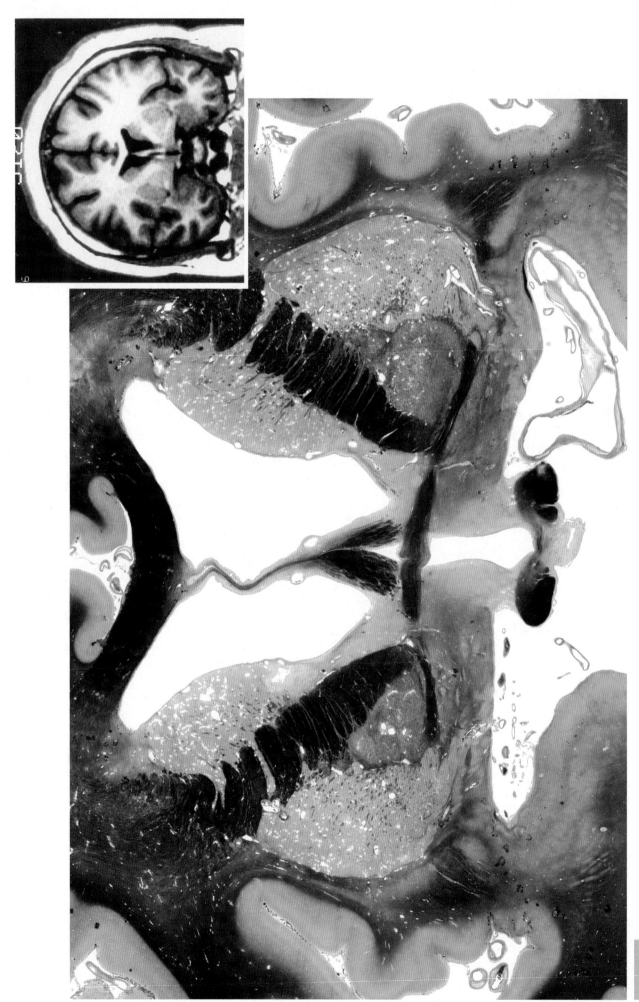

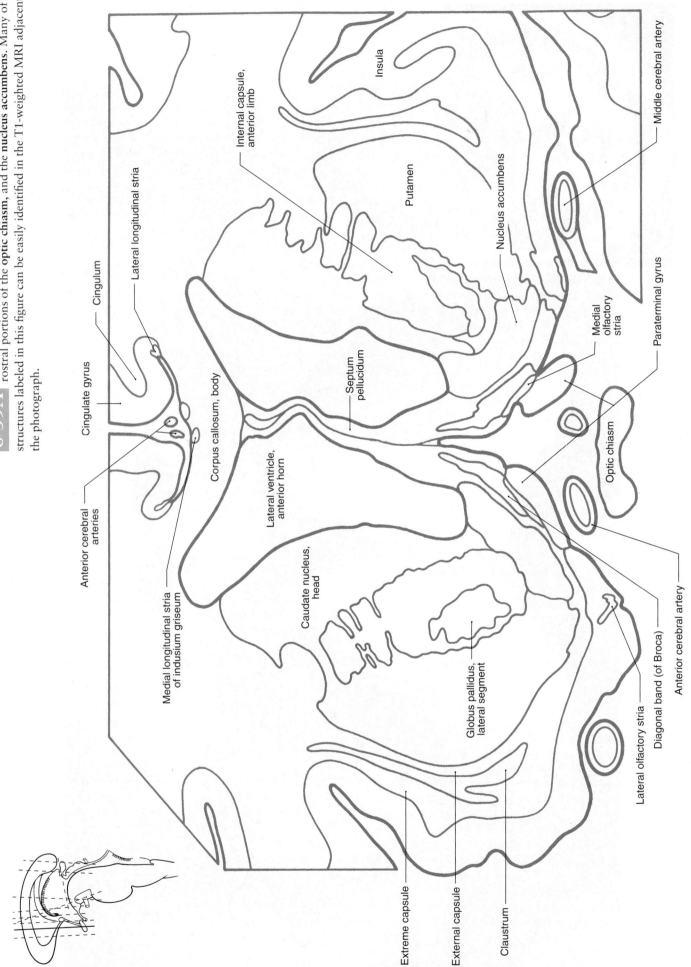

6-39A Coronal section of the forebrain through the **head of the caudate nucleus,** rostral portions of the **optic chiasm,** and the **nucleus accumbens.** Many of the structures labeled in this figure can be easily identified in the T1-weighted MRI adjacent to the photograph.

Cingulate gyrus

Cingulum

Lateral longitudinal stria

Insula

Internal capsule, anterior limb

Putamen

Nucleus accumbens

Medial olfactory stria

Paraterminal gyrus

Middle cerebral artery

Anterior cerebral arteries

Medial longitudinal stria of indusium griseum

Corpus callosum, body

Septum pellucidum

Lateral ventricle, anterior horn

Caudate nucleus, head

Globus pallidus, lateral segment

Extreme capsule

External capsule

Claustrum

Diagonal band (of Broca)

Lateral olfactory stria

Optic chiasm

Anterior cerebral artery

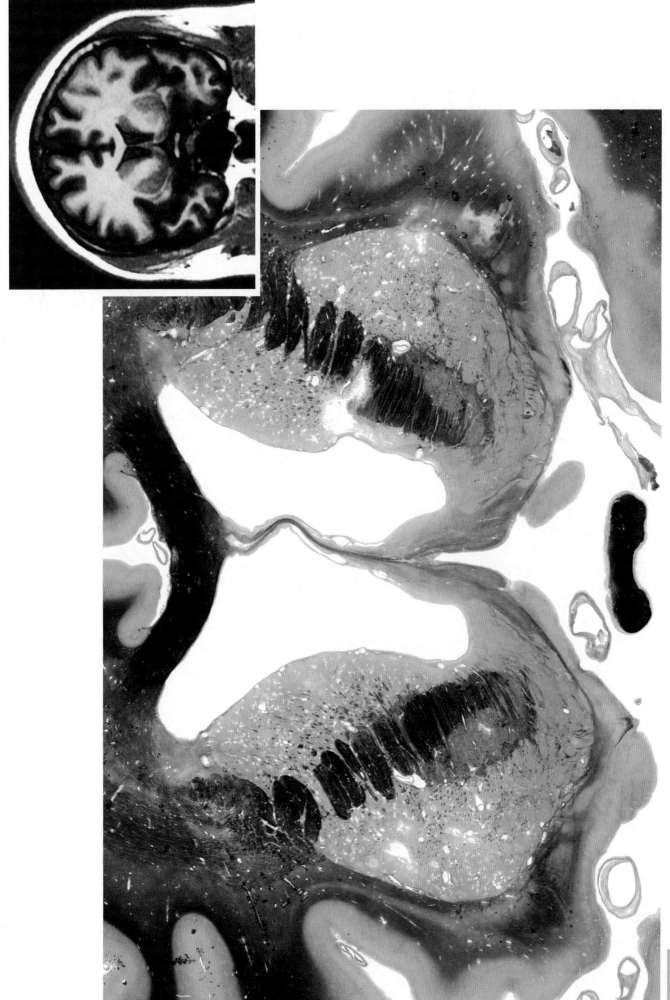

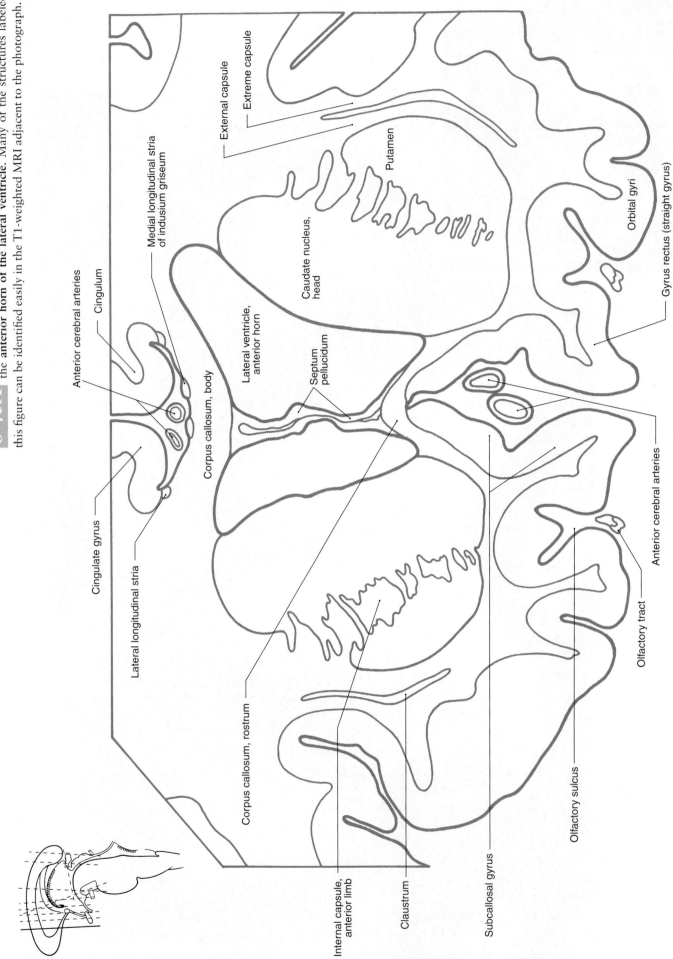

6-40A Coronal section of the forebrain through the **head of the caudate nucleus** and the **anterior horn of the lateral ventricle**. Many of the structures labeled in this figure can be identified easily in the T1-weighted MRI adjacent to the photograph.

External capsule

Extreme capsule

Putamen

Caudate nucleus, head

Medial longitudinal stria of indusium griseum

Cingulum

Anterior cerebral arteries

Orbital gyri

Gyrus rectus (straight gyrus)

Lateral ventricle, anterior horn

Corpus callosum, body

Septum pellucidum

Cingulate gyrus

Lateral longitudinal stria

Anterior cerebral arteries

Olfactory tract

Corpus callosum, rostrum

Internal capsule, anterior limb

Claustrum

Subcallosal gyrus

Olfactory sulcus

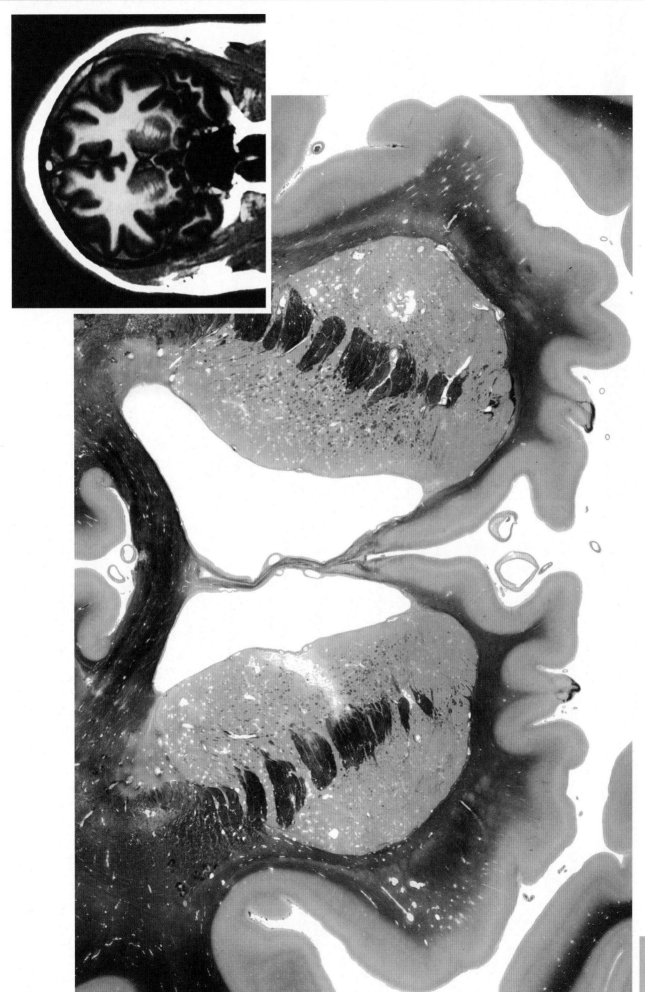

6-40B

6-41

Semi-diagrammatic representation of the internal distribution of arteries to the diencephalon, basal nuclei, and internal capsule. Selected structures are labeled on the left side of each section; the general pattern of arterial distribution overlies these structures on the right side. The general distribution patterns of arteries in the forebrain, as shown here, may vary from patient to patient. For example, the adjacent territories served by neighboring vessels may overlap to varying degrees at their margins or the territory of a particular vessel may be larger or smaller than seen in the general pattern.

ABBREVIATIONS

APS	Anterior perforated substance	HyTh	Hypothalamus
BCorCl	Body of corpus callosum	PulNu	Pulvinar nuclear complex
CC	Crus cerebri	Put	Putamen
CM	Centromedian nucleus of thalamus	SplCorCl	Splenium of the corpus callosum
		VA	Ventral anterior nucleus of thalamus
DMNu	Dorsomedial nucleus of thalamus	VL	Ventral lateral nucleus of thalamus
GP	Globus pallidus		

Vascular Syndromes or Lesions of the Forebrain

Forebrain vascular lesions result in a wide range of deficits that include motor and sensory losses and a variety of cognitive disorders. Forebrain vessels may be occluded by a **thrombus**. This is a structure (usually a clot) formed by blood products and frequently attached to the vessel wall. Deficits may appear slowly, or wax and wane, as the blood flow is progressively restricted.

Vessels may also be occluded by **embolization**. A foreign body, or **embolus** (fat, air, piece of thrombus, piece of sclerotic plaque, clump of bacteria, etc.), is delivered from some distant site into the cerebral circulation where it lodges in a vessel. Because this is a sudden event, deficits usually appear quickly and may progress rapidly. Interruption of blood supply to a part of the forebrain results in an **infarct** of the area served by the occluded vessel.

Lesion in the Subthalamic Nucleus

Small vascular lesions occur in the subthalamic nucleus, resulting in rapid and unpredictable flailing movements of the contralateral extremities (**hemiballismus**). Movements are more obvious in the upper extremity than in the lower extremity. The clinical expression of this lesion is through corticospinal fibers; therefore, these deficits are located on the side of the body contralateral to the lesion.

Occlusion of Lenticulostriate Branches to Internal Capsule

Damage to the internal capsule may result in **contralateral hemiplegia** (corticospinal fibers) and **a loss, or diminution, of sensory perception** (pain, thermal sense, proprioception) caused by damage to thalamocortical fibers traversing the posterior limb to the overlying sensory cortex. If the lesion extends into the genu of the capsule (damaging corticonuclear fibers), *a partial paralysis of facial muscles and tongue movement may also occur contralaterally.*

Infarction of Posterior Thalamic Nuclei

Occlusion of vessels to posterior thalamic regions results in either a **complete sensory loss** (pain/ thermal sense, touch, and vibratory and position sense) on the contralateral side of the body or **a dissociated sensory loss.** In the latter case, the patient may experience pain/thermal sensory losses but not position/vibratory losses, or vice versa. As the lesion resolves, the patient may experience intense persistent pain, **thalamic pain, or anesthesia dolorosa.**

Occlusion of Distal Branches of the Anterior or Middle Cerebral Arteries

Occlusion of distal branches of the anterior cerebral artery (ACA) results in **motor and sensory losses in the contralateral foot, leg, and thigh** owing to **damage to the anterior and posterior paracentral gyri (primary motor and sensory cortices for the lower extremity).** Occlusion of distal branches of the middle cerebral artery (MCA) results in **contralateral motor and sensory losses of the upper extremity, trunk, and face with sparing of the leg and foot,** and a consensual deviation of the eyes to the ipsilateral side. This represents damage to the precentral and postcentral gyri and the frontal eye fields.

Watershed Infarct

Sudden systemic hypotension, hypoperfusion, or embolic showers may result in infarcts at borders zones between the territories served by the ACA, MCA, and posterior cerebral artery (PCA). **Anterior watershed infarcts** (at the ACA–MCA junction) result in a contralateral hemiparesis (mainly the LE) and expressive language or behavioral changes. **Posterior watershed infarcts** (MCA–PCA interface) result in visual deficits and language problems.

Anterior Choroidal Artery Syndrome

Occlusion of the anterior choroidal artery may result from small emboli or small vessel disease. This syndrome may also occur as a complication of temporal lobectomy (removal of the temporal lobe to treat intractable epilepsy). The infarcted area usually includes the optic tract, lower portions of the basal nuclei, and lower aspects of the internal capsule.

The patient experiences a contralateral **homonymous hemianopia** (damage to the optic tract) and a contralateral **hemiplegia** (damage to corticospinal fibers at the transition of the internal capsule into the crus cerebri). If the infarct involves enough of the posterior limb to also damage thalamocortical fibers from the ventral posterolateral nucleus to the somatosensory cortex, the patient will also have a **hemianesthesia** (or possibly **hemihypesthesia**) on the same side of the body as the **hemiplegia.**

Parkinson Disease

Parkinson disease (paralysis agitans) results from a loss of the dopamine-containing cells in the substantia nigra. Although this part of the brain is located in the midbrain, the terminals of these nigrostriatal fibers are in the putamen and caudate nucleus. The classic signs and symptoms of this disease are a **stooped posture, resting tremor, rigidity, shuffling or festinating gait,** and difficulty initiating or maintaining movement (**akinesia, hypokinesia, or bradykinesia**). Initially, the tremor and walking difficulty may appear on one side of the body, but these signs usually spread to both sides with time. This is a neurodegenerative disease that has a **dementia** component in its later stages.

Transient Ischemic Attack

A **transient ischemic attack,** commonly called TIA, is a temporary (and frequently focal) neurological deficit that usually resolves within 10 to 40 minutes from the onset of symptoms. The cause is temporary occlusion of a vessel or inadequate perfusion of a restricted vascular territory. TIAs that last 60 minutes or more may result in some permanent deficits. This vascular event may take place anywhere in the central nervous system but is more common in the cerebral hemisphere.

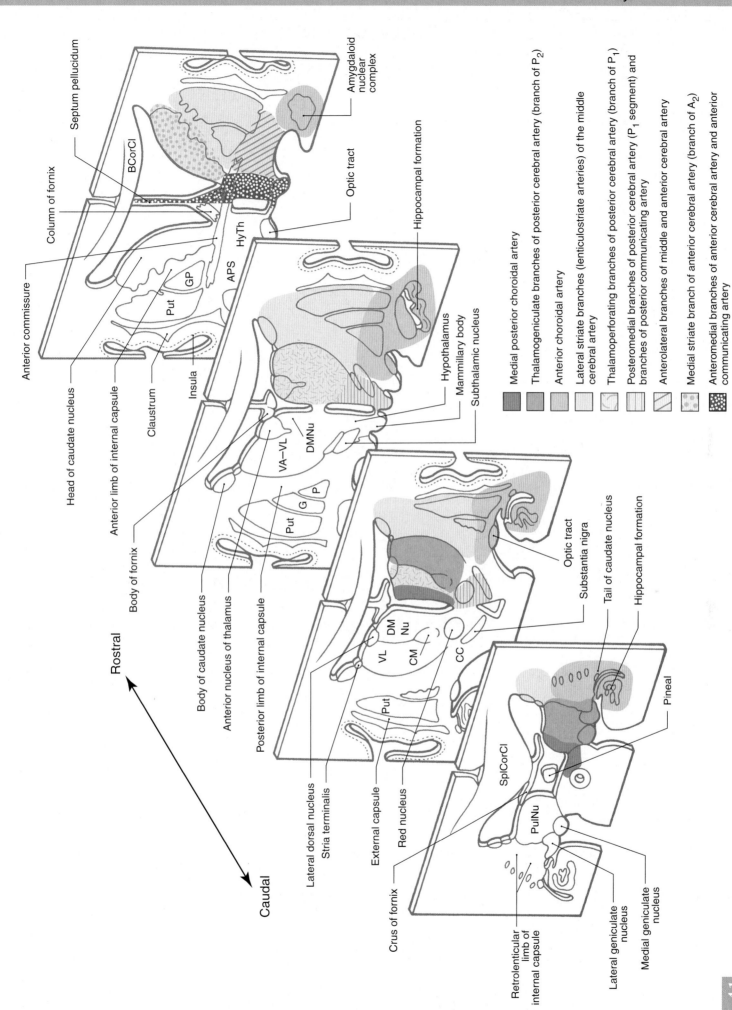

Rostral

Caudal

Septum pellucidum

Column of fornix

Anterior commissure

Head of caudate nucleus

Anterior limb of internal capsule

BCorCl

Claustrum

Insula

Put

GP

APS

HyTh

Optic tract

Amygdaloid nuclear complex

Hippocampal formation

Body of fornix

Body of caudate nucleus

Anterior nucleus of thalamus

Posterior limb of internal capsule

VA–VL

DMNu

Put

G

P

Hypothalamus

Mammillary body

Subthalamic nucleus

Lateral dorsal nucleus

Stria terminalis

External capsule

Red nucleus

Put

DM Nu

VL

CM

CC

Optic tract

Substantia nigra

Tail of caudate nucleus

Hippocampal formation

Crus of fornix

SplCorCl

PulNu

Pineal

Retrolenticular limb of internal capsule

Lateral geniculate nucleus

Medial geniculate nucleus

Medial posterior choroidal artery

Thalamogeniculate branches of posterior cerebral artery (branch of P$_2$)

Anterior choroidal artery

Lateral striate branches (lenticulostriate arteries) of the middle cerebral artery

Thalamoperforating branches of posterior cerebral artery (branch of P$_1$)

Posteromedial branches of posterior cerebral artery (P$_1$ segment) and branches of posterior communicating artery

Anterolateral branches of middle and anterior cerebral artery

Medial striate branch of anterior cerebral artery (branch of A$_2$)

Anteromedial branches of anterior cerebral artery and anterior communicating artery

6-41

NOTES

Internal Morphology of the Brain in Stained Sections: Axial–Sagittal Correlations with MRI

7

Although the general organization of Chapter 7 has been described in Chapter 1 (the reader may wish to refer back to this section), it is appropriate to reiterate its unique features at this point. Each set of facing pages has photographs of an axial stained section (left-hand page) and a sagittal stained section (right-hand page). In addition to individually labeled structures, a heavy red line appears on each photograph. This prominent line on the axial section represents the approximate plane of the sagittal section located on the facing page. On the sagittal section, this line signifies the approximate plane of the corresponding axial section. The reader can identify features in each photograph and then, using this line as a reference point, visualize structures that are located either above or below that plane (axial-to-sagittal comparison) or medial or lateral to that plane (sagittal-to-axial comparison). This method of presentation provides a useful format that will form the basis for a three-dimensional understanding of structures and relationships within the central nervous system.

The magnetic resonance image (MRI) placed on every page in this chapter gives the reader an opportunity to compare internal brain anatomy, as seen in stained sections, with those structures as visualized in clinical images generated in the same plane. Even a general comparison reveals that many features, as seen in the stained section, can be readily identified in the adjacent MRI.

This chapter is also organized so that one can view structures in either the axial or the sagittal plane only. Axial images appear on left-hand pages and are sequenced from dorsal to ventral (odd-numbered Figures 7-1 through 7-9), whereas sagittal images are on the right-hand pages and progress from medial to lateral (even-numbered Figures 7-2 through 7-10). Consequently, the user can identify and follow structures through an axial series by simply flipping through the left-hand pages or through a sagittal series by flipping through the right-hand pages. The inherent flexibility in this chapter should prove useful in a wide variety of instructional/learning situations. The drawings shown in the following illustrate the axial and sagittal planes of the photographs in this chapter.

Axial planes

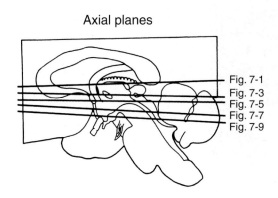

Fig. 7-1
Fig. 7-3
Fig. 7-5
Fig. 7-7
Fig. 7-9

Fig. 7-6
Fig. 7-4 Fig. 7-8
Fig. 7-2   Fig. 7-10

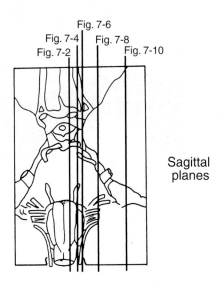

Sagittal planes

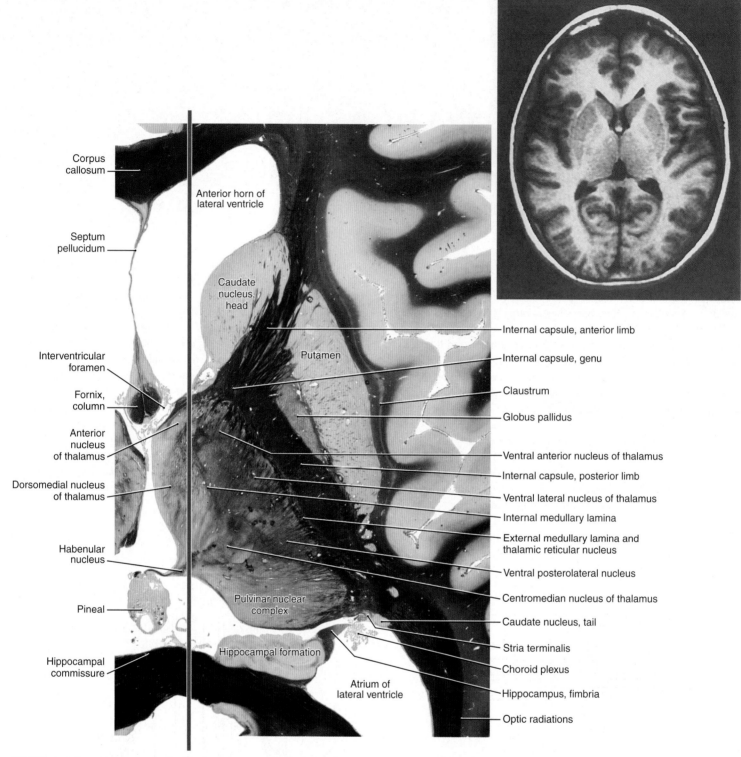

Corpus callosum

Anterior horn of lateral ventricle

Septum pellucidum

Caudate nucleus, head

Putamen

Interventricular foramen

Fornix, column

Anterior nucleus of thalamus

Dorsomedial nucleus of thalamus

Habenular nucleus

Pineal

Pulvinar nuclear complex

Hippocampal commissure

Hippocampal formation

Atrium of lateral ventricle

Internal capsule, anterior limb

Internal capsule, genu

Claustrum

Globus pallidus

Ventral anterior nucleus of thalamus

Internal capsule, posterior limb

Ventral lateral nucleus of thalamus

Internal medullary lamina

External medullary lamina and thalamic reticular nucleus

Ventral posterolateral nucleus

Centromedian nucleus of thalamus

Caudate nucleus, tail

Stria terminalis

Choroid plexus

Hippocampus, fimbria

Optic radiations

7-1 Axial section through the **head of the caudate nucleus** and several key **thalamic nuclei** (anterior, centromedian, pulvinar, and habenular). In this plane of section, the **internal medullary lamina**, separates the **dorsomedial nucleus** from a lateral row comprising the **ventral anterior, ventral lateral,** and **ventral posterolateral nuclei.** Rostrally, the internal medullary lamina encompasses the **anterior nucleus of the thalamus,** and the pulvinar is located caudal to the centromedian and ventral posterolateral nuclei. Collectively the anterior nucleus and the pulvinar form the rostral and caudal extents, respectively, of the dorsal thalamus in this axial section. The **centromedian nucleus** is located within the internal medullary lamina and is the largest of the intralaminar nuclei. The heavy red line represents the approximate plane of the sagittal section shown in Figure 7-2 (facing page). Many of the structures labeled in this photograph can be clearly identified in the adjacent T1-weighted MRI.

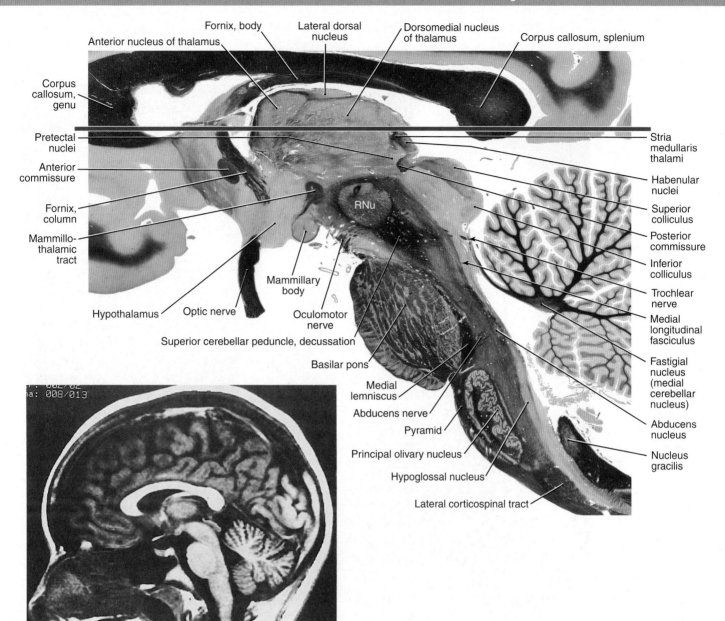

Fornix, body

Lateral dorsal nucleus

Dorsomedial nucleus of thalamus

Anterior nucleus of thalamus

Corpus callosum, splenium

Corpus callosum, genu

Pretectal nuclei

Stria medullaris thalami

Anterior commissure

Habenular nuclei

Fornix, column

Superior colliculus

Mammillo-thalamic tract

Posterior commissure

Inferior colliculus

Trochlear nerve

Medial longitudinal fasciculus

RNu

Hypothalamus

Optic nerve

Mammillary body

Oculomotor nerve

Fastigial nucleus (medial cerebellar nucleus)

Superior cerebellar peduncle, decussation

Basilar pons

Abducens nucleus

Medial lemniscus

Abducens nerve

Nucleus gracilis

Pyramid

Principal olivary nucleus

Hypoglossal nucleus

Lateral corticospinal tract

7-2 Sagittal section through the **column of the fornix, anterior thalamic nucleus, red nucleus**, and medial portions of the **pons (abducens nucleus), cerebellum (fastigial nucleus)**, and **medulla (nucleus gracilis)**. As the **fornix** (body to column) arches around the anterior thalamic nucleus, the space formed between the column of the fornix and the anterior thalamic nucleus is the **interventricular foramen** (see Figure 7-1 on the facing page). The column of the fornix continues immediately caudal to the anterior commissure, as the postcommissural fornix, to end in the **mammillary body**. Note the relative positions of the red nucleus and decussation of the superior cerebellar peduncle within the midbrain.

In this sagittal plane, the general structures seen at the level of the superior and inferior colliculi can be fully appreciated. A cross-section through the midbrain at the level of the superior colliculus contains the oculomotor nucleus and roots, red nucleus, substantia nigra, and crus cerebri. A cross-section of midbrain at the level of the inferior colliculus is characterized by the trochlear nucleus, decussation of the superior cerebellar peduncle, substantia nigra, and crus cerebri. The heavy red line represents the approximate plane of the axial section shown in Figure 7-1 (facing page). Many of the structures labeled in this photograph can be clearly identified in the adjacent T1-weighted MRI (RNu = red nucleus).

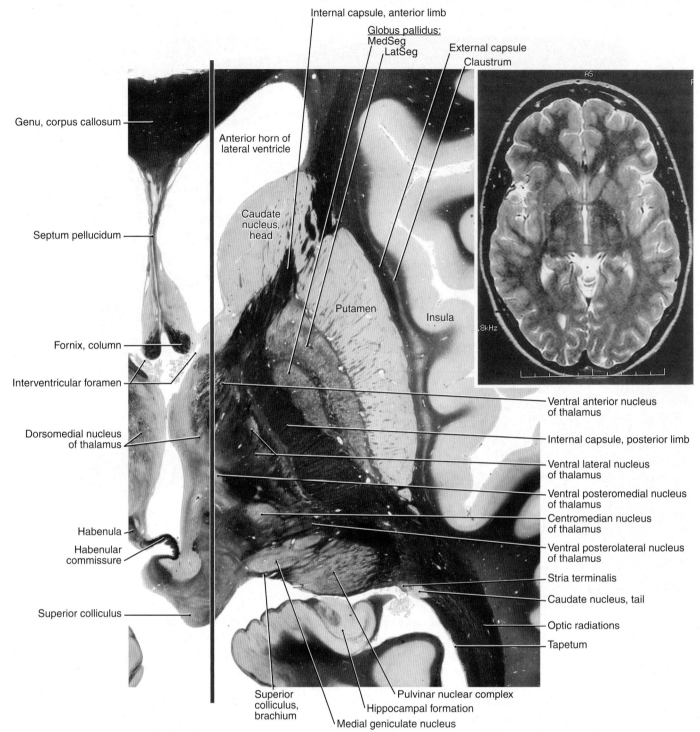

Genu, corpus callosum

Septum pellucidum

Fornix, column

Interventricular foramen

Dorsomedial nucleus
of thalamus

Habenula

Habenular
commissure

Superior colliculus

Internal capsule, anterior limb

Globus pallidus:
MedSeg
LatSeg

External capsule
Claustrum

Anterior horn of
lateral ventricle

Caudate
nucleus,
head

Putamen

Insula

.8kHz

Ventral anterior nucleus
of thalamus

Internal capsule, posterior limb

Ventral lateral nucleus
of thalamus

Ventral posteromedial nucleus
of thalamus

Centromedian nucleus
of thalamus

Ventral posterolateral nucleus
of thalamus

Stria terminalis

Caudate nucleus, tail

Optic radiations

Tapetum

Superior
colliculus,
brachium

Pulvinar nuclear complex

Hippocampal formation

Medial geniculate nucleus

7-3 Axial section through the **head of the caudate nucleus, centro-median nucleus, medial geniculate body,** and **superior colliculus.** In this more inferior plane of section, the anterior-to-posterior relationship of the **ventral anterior, ventral lateral,** and **ventral postero-lateral nuclei** are evident as is the relative position of the **centromedian nucleus** to the **ventral posterolateral, medial geniculate,** and the pulvinar nuclei. As seen here, and in Figures 7-1 and 7-5, the four major portions of the internal capsule are obvious in the axial plane, these being the **anterior limb, genu, posterior limb,** and the **retrolenticular limb.** The heavy red line represents the approximate plane of the sagittal section shown in Figure 7-4 (facing page). Many of the structures labeled in this photograph can be clearly identified in the adjacent T2-weighted MRI (MedSeg = Medial segment of globus pallidus; LatSeg = Lateral segment of globus pallidus).

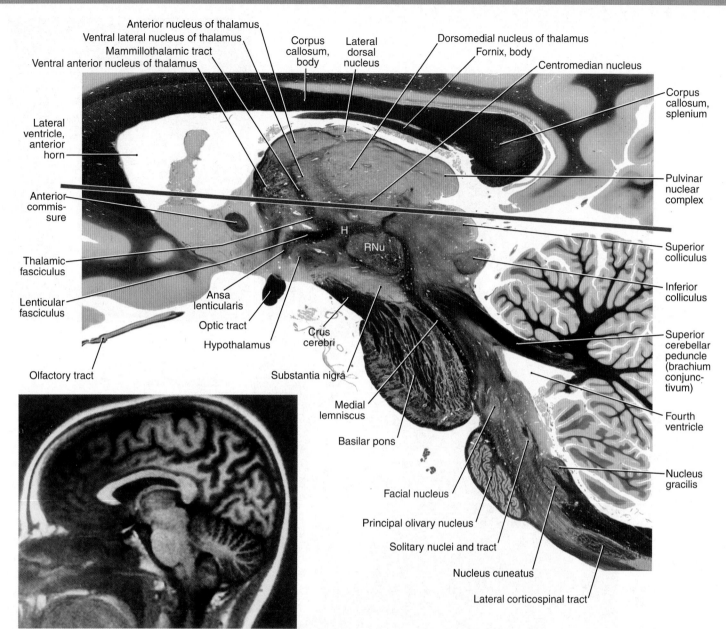

7-4 Sagittal section through **anterior** and **ventral anterior thalamic nuclei, red nucleus,** and central areas of the **pons, cerebellum** (and **superior peduncle**), and **medulla** (**solitary nuclei and tract**). Note the position of the **facial motor nucleus** at the pons–medulla junction. In this sagittal plane, several of the thalamic nuclei are clearly demarcated, and the important relationships between the **red nucleus, substantia nigra,** and **crus cerebri** are seen. Note that the fibers of the **crus cerebri** traverse the basilar pons and that the **medial lemniscus** is located at the interface of the basilar pons and the pontine tegmentum.

The teardrop shape of the anterior thalamic nucleus, which is clearly seen in this image, illustrates how the anterior nucleus may be seen in some coronal sections that also include the ventral lateral thalamic nucleus (see Figure 6-35A, B). Many clinically significant structures in the brainstem also stand out. The heavy red line represents the approximate plane of the axial section shown in Figure 7-3 (facing page). Many of the structures labeled in this photograph can be clearly identified in the adjacent T1-weighted MRI (H = Forel field H [prerubral area]; RNu = red nucleus).

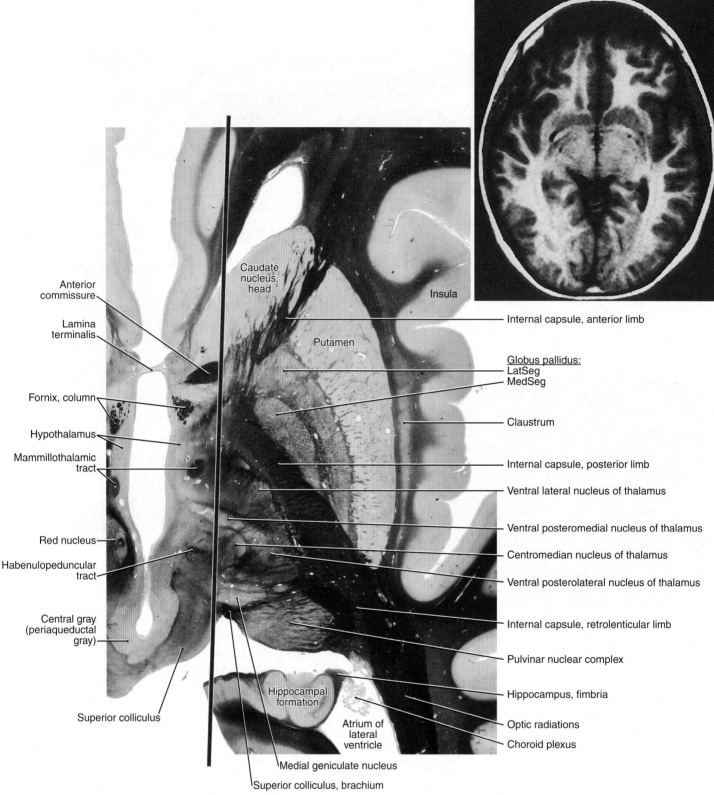

Anterior commissure

Lamina terminalis

Fornix, column

Hypothalamus

Mammillothalamic tract

Red nucleus

Habenulopeduncular tract

Central gray (periaqueductal gray)

Superior colliculus

Caudate nucleus, head

Putamen

Insula

Hippocampal formation

Atrium of lateral ventricle

Medial geniculate nucleus

Superior colliculus, brachium

Internal capsule, anterior limb

Globus pallidus:
LatSeg
MedSeg

Claustrum

Internal capsule, posterior limb

Ventral lateral nucleus of thalamus

Ventral posteromedial nucleus of thalamus

Centromedian nucleus of thalamus

Ventral posterolateral nucleus of thalamus

Internal capsule, retrolenticular limb

Pulvinar nuclear complex

Hippocampus, fimbria

Optic radiations

Choroid plexus

7-5   Axial section through the **head of the caudate nucleus, ventral posteromedial nucleus, medial geniculate body,** and ventral parts of the **pulvinar.** This axial section is through the upper portions of the **hypothalamus** and the lower, and widest, portions of the lenticular nucleus. The anterior limb of the internal capsule is beginning to disappear (the caudate head and putamen will join), and inferior portions of the **ventral lateral, ventral posterolateral,** and **pulvinar nuclei** are still present.

The **column of the fornix,** which lies immediately caudal to the **anterior commissure,** arches caudally to enter in the mammillary nuclei, and

the **mammillothalamic tract** arises from the mammillary nuclei and ascends to the anterior thalamic nucleus. Note the relative rostrocaudal position of these tracts within the stained section and within the MRI. The heavy red line represents the approximate plane of the sagittal section shown in Figure 7-6 (facing page). Many of the structures labeled in this photograph can be clearly identified in the adjacent T1-weighted MRI (MedSeg = Medial segment of globus pallidus; LatSeg = Lateral segment of globus pallidus).

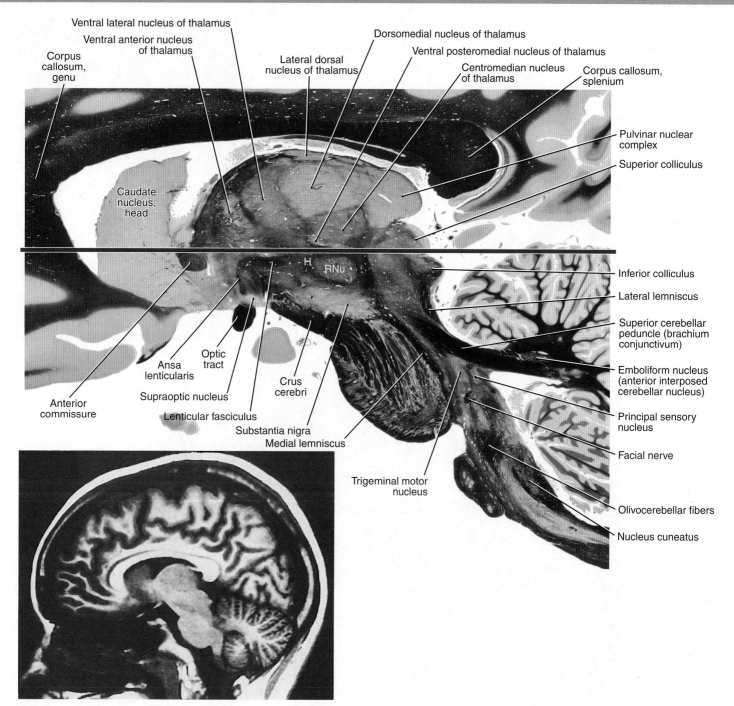

Ventral lateral nucleus of thalamus

Ventral anterior nucleus of thalamus

Corpus callosum, genu

Dorsomedial nucleus of thalamus

Ventral posteromedial nucleus of thalamus

Lateral dorsal nucleus of thalamus

Centromedian nucleus of thalamus

Corpus callosum, splenium

Pulvinar nuclear complex

Superior colliculus

Caudate nucleus, head

H

RNu

Inferior colliculus

Lateral lemniscus

Superior cerebellar peduncle (brachium conjunctivum)

Emboliform nucleus (anterior interposed cerebellar nucleus)

Principal sensory nucleus

Facial nerve

Olivocerebellar fibers

Nucleus cuneatus

Ansa lenticularis

Optic tract

Supraoptic nucleus

Crus cerebri

Anterior commissure

Lenticular fasciculus

Substantia nigra

Medial lemniscus

Trigeminal motor nucleus

7-6 Sagittal section through central regions of the **diencephalon** (**centromedian nucleus**) and **midbrain** (**red nucleus**), and through lateral areas of the **pons** (**trigeminal motor nucleus**) and **medulla** (**nucleus cuneatus**). A clear separation of the thalamic nuclei is seen in this sagittal plane along with the characteristics of the interface of midbrain structures with the diencephalon. Note how the fibers of the **crus cerebri** splay out into the basilar pons (see also Figure 7-4), the characteristic position of the medial lemniscus, and the clarity of the **crus cerebri** and **substantia nigra** in the MRI. The heavy red line represents the approximate plane of the axial section shown in Figure 7-5 (facing page). Many of the structures labeled in this photograph can be clearly identified in the adjacent T1-weighted MRI (H = Forel field H [prerubral area]; RNu = red nucleus).

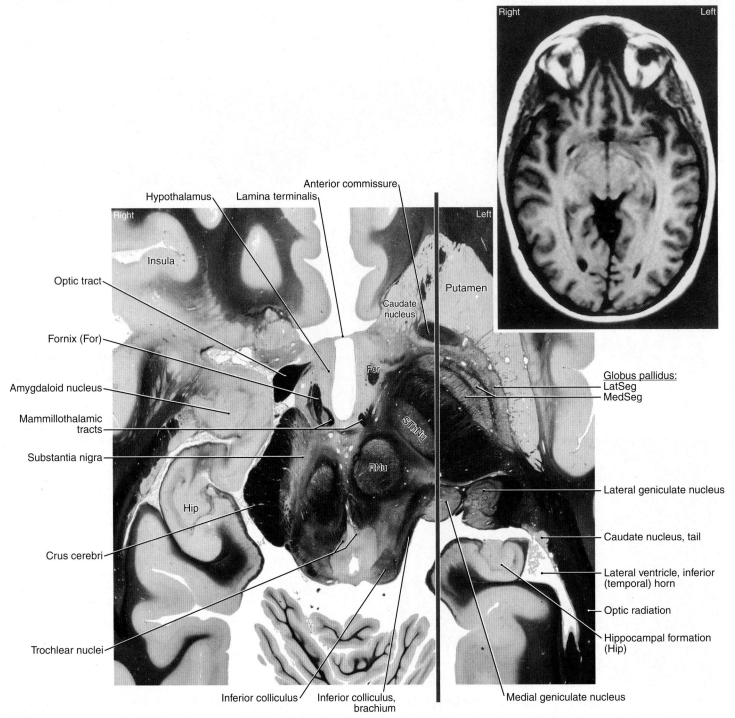

7-7 Axial section through the **hypothalamus, red nucleus, inferior colliculus,** and the **medial** and **lateral geniculate nuclei.** This axial section is slightly tilted; *the sides (right/left) of the stained section are considered the same as the sides (right/left) in the adjacent MRI.* The right side is more ventral and shows the **optic tract** in close proximity to the crus cerebri, the junction of the fornix and mammillothalamic tract at the mammillary body, and the amygdaloid nucleus and hippocampus in the medial temporal horn. The left side is more dorsal and contains the **fornix** and **mammillothalamic tract** separate within the hypothalamus (see also Figure 7-5), the **subthalamic nucleus** adjacent to the crus, the **red nucleus,** and junction of the caudate and putamen. The geniculate nuclei are also seen on the patient's left; the **trochlear nuclei** are present on both sides.

The **optic tract** is always located on the surface of the crus cerebri (see also Figure 7-8 on the facing page) no matter what the plane of

section. Also note the thin membranous nature of the lamina terminalis (see also Figures 7-5 and 7-9) separating the cistern of the lamina terminalis (rostral to it) from the space of the third ventricle (caudal to it). This structure frequently separates blood within the cistern from a lack of blood within the third ventricle (see Figure 4-7 on p. 65), or blood within the third ventricle from a lack of blood within the cistern (see Figure 4-13 on p. 71).

The heavy red line represents the approximate plane of the sagittal section shown in Figure 7-8 (facing page). The axial plane through the hemisphere, when continued into the midbrain, represents a slightly oblique section through the mesencephalon. Compare the appearance of the midbrain in this axial section with that in Figures 6-24 to 6-29 on pp. 140 to 151. Many of the structures labeled in this photograph can be clearly identified in the adjacent T1-weighted MRI (MedSeg = Medial segment of globus pallidus; LatSeg = Lateral segment of globus pallidus).

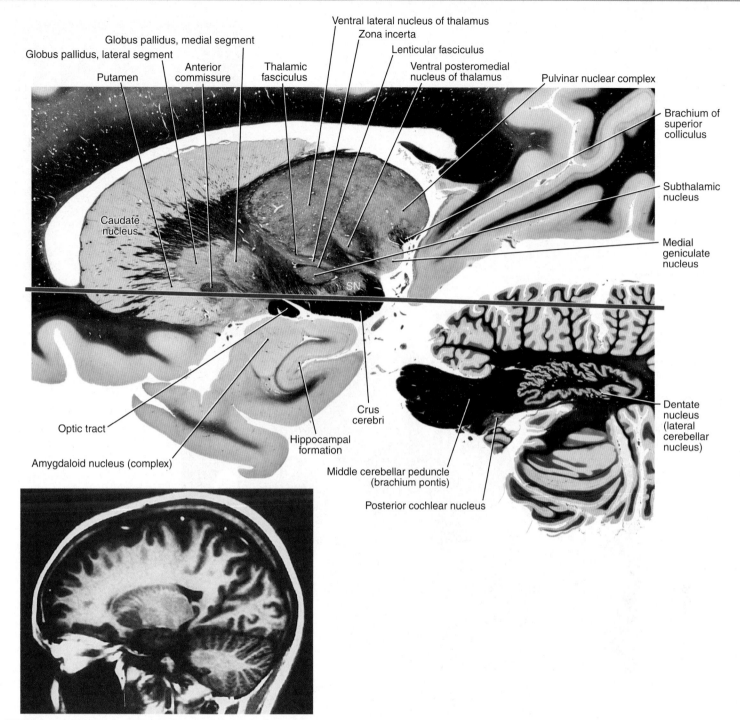

Globus pallidus, medial segment
Globus pallidus, lateral segment
Putamen
Anterior commissure
Thalamic fasciculus
Ventral lateral nucleus of thalamus
Zona incerta
Lenticular fasciculus
Ventral posteromedial nucleus of thalamus
Pulvinar nuclear complex
Brachium of superior colliculus
Subthalamic nucleus
Medial geniculate nucleus
Caudate nucleus
Optic tract
Amygdaloid nucleus (complex)
Hippocampal formation
Crus cerebri
Middle cerebellar peduncle (brachium pontis)
Posterior cochlear nucleus
Dentate nucleus (lateral cerebellar nucleus)

7-8 Sagittal section through the **caudate nucleus**, central parts of the **diencephalon** (**ventral posteromedial nucleus**), lateral portions of the **pons, middle cerebellar peduncle, cochlear nuclei,** and the **cerebellum** (**dentate nucleus**). In this sagittal plane, several important relationships are seen. First, the head of the caudate and putamen coalesce in the rostral and ventral area of the hemisphere. Second, the important structures in the immediate vicinity of the **zona incerta** and **subthalamic nucleus** are obvious. Third, the **medial** geniculate nucleus is characteristically located just inferior to the **pulvinar** and separated from it by the **brachium of the superior colliculus**. As noted in other figures in this chapter, the **optic tract** has an intimate apposition to the **crus cerebri** regardless of the plane of section. The heavy red line represents the approximate plane of the axial section shown in Figure 7-7 (facing page). Many of the structures labeled in this photograph can be clearly identified in the adjacent T1-weighted MRI.

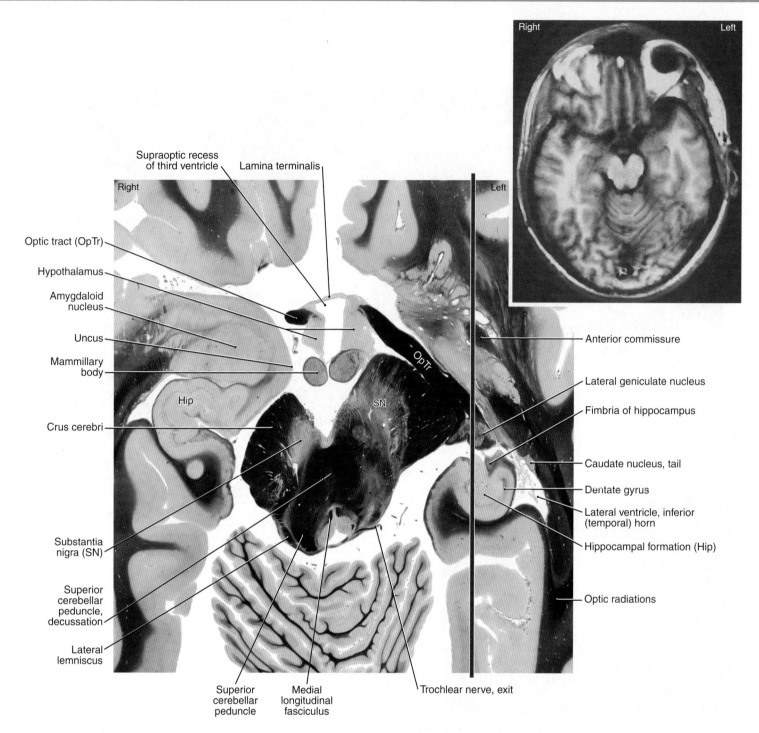

7-9 Axial section through ventral portions of the hypothalamus (**supraoptic recess** and **mammillary body**) and forebrain (**amygdaloid nucleus, hippocampal formation**), and through the **superior cerebellar peduncle decussation** in the midbrain. This axial section is slightly tilted through the lowest portions of the **hypothalamus** as evidenced by the presence of the **supraoptic recess**, a relatively small portion of the hypothalamus (especially on the right), lower parts of the mammillary bodies, and part of the supraoptic nucleus.

Note the close relationship of the **uncus** to the **crus cerebri** (also in the MRI), particularly on the right side, and the fact that the amygdaloid nucleus is internal to the uncus in the rostral wall of the temporal horn of the lateral ventricle (also on the right). This close apposition

of the uncus to the crus is the anatomical basis for damage to midbrain structures in cases of **uncal herniation** when there is impingement on, or shifting of, the midbrain structures resultant to enlarging temporal lobe lesions (see also Chapter 9). Also note, on the left, that the optic tract is located directly adjacent to the crus and ends in the lateral geniculate nucleus. The **tail of the caudate** is in the lateral wall of the ventricle, and the **hippocampus** is medially located.

The heavy red line represents the approximate plane of the sagittal section shown in Figure 7-10 (facing page). The axial plane through the hemisphere, when continued into the midbrain, represents a slightly oblique section through the mesencephalon. Many of the structures labeled in this photograph can be clearly identified in the adjacent T1-weighted MRI.

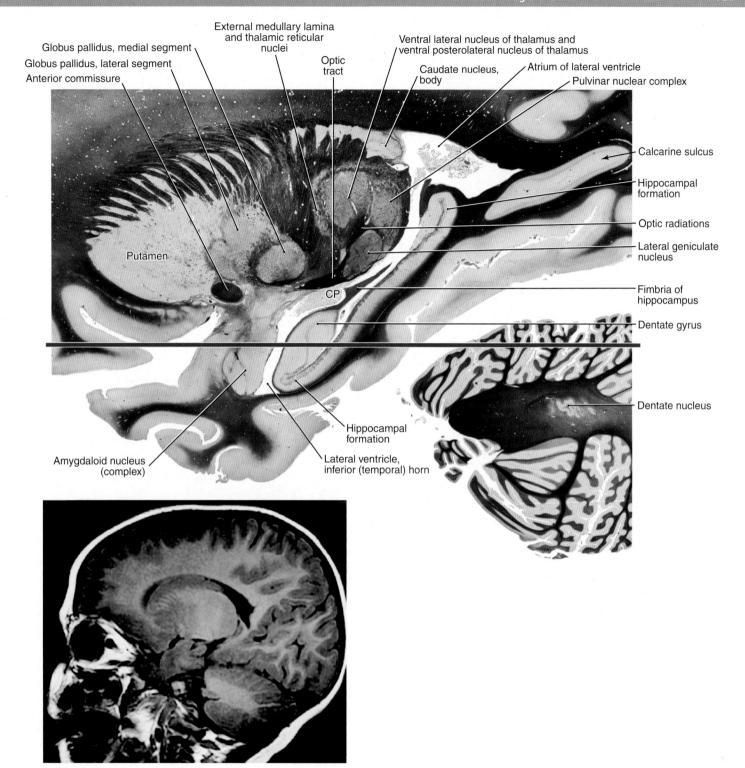

Globus pallidus, medial segment
Globus pallidus, lateral segment
Anterior commissure
External medullary lamina and thalamic reticular nuclei
Optic tract
Ventral lateral nucleus of thalamus and ventral posterolateral nucleus of thalamus
Caudate nucleus, body
Atrium of lateral ventricle
Pulvinar nuclear complex
Calcarine sulcus
Hippocampal formation
Optic radiations
Lateral geniculate nucleus
Fimbria of hippocampus
Dentate gyrus
Dentate nucleus
Putamen
CP
Hippocampal formation
Lateral ventricle, inferior (temporal) horn
Amygdaloid nucleus (complex)

7-10 Sagittal section through the **putamen, amygdaloid nucleus,** and **hippocampus** and through the most lateral portions of the **diencephalon** (**external medullary lamina** and **ventral posterolateral nucleus**). The relationship of the **amygdaloid nucleus**, anterior to the space of the temporal horn within the rostromedial portion of the temporal lobe, is clearly seen. In this sagittal section, the **optic tract** is seen entering the **lateral geniculate nucleus** which, as was the case for its medial counterpart (see Figure 7-8), is also located immediately inferior to the **pulvinar**. This plane also passes through the long axis of the **hippocampal formation**. The heavy red line represents the approximate plane of the axial section shown in Figure 7-9 (facing page). Many of the structures labeled in this photograph can be clearly identified in the adjacent T1-weighted MRI.

NOTES

Tracts, Pathways, and Systems in Anatomical and Clinical Orientation

8

The study of **regional neurobiology** (brain structures in gross specimens, brain slices, stained sections, and MRI and CT) is the basis for the study of **systems neurobiology** (tracts, pathways, and cranial nerves and their functions), which in turn is the basis for understanding and diagnosing the neurologically impaired patient. Building on the concepts learned in earlier chapters, this chapter explores **systems neurobiology,** with a particular emphasis on clinical relevance and correlations.

The modifications made in this chapter recognize an essential reality for users of this book who are preparing for a career in medicine, as broadly defined. Although it is common to teach the anatomy of the brain in an **Anatomical Orientation** (e.g., in the medulla, the pyramid is "down" in the image and the fourth ventricle is "up"), this information will be **viewed and used,** in the clinical years and beyond, in a **Clinical Orientation** (pyramid "up" in the image, fourth ventricle "down"). Therefore, it is essential to present systems information in a format that resembles, as closely as reasonably possible, how these systems (and dysfunctions thereof) are viewed in the clinical setting. To this end, selected systems are illustrated in the **Clinical Orientation.**

Anatomical Orientation

Major pathways, including those essential to diagnosis of the neurologically compromised patient, are illustrated in line drawings in an **Anatomical Orientation.** The format of each set of these facing pages is designed to summarize, accurately and concisely, the relationships of a given tract or pathway. This includes, but is not limited to: 1) the location of the cells of origin for a given tract or pathway; 2) its entire course throughout the neuraxis and cerebrum; 3) the location of the decussation of these fibers, if applicable; 4) the neurotransmitters associated with the neurons comprising the tract or pathway; 5) a brief review of its blood supply; and 6) a summary of a number of deficits seen as a result of lesions at various points in the tract or pathway.

Clinical Orientation

Twelve of the systems pathways, with particular emphasis on those essential to understanding the patient with neurological problems, are also illustrated in **Clinical Orientation.** These pathway illustrations do not replace their counterparts shown in Anatomical Orientation, but are designed to complement these existing drawings. These sets of facing pages are formatted to show the pathway superimposed on MRI at representative levels of the central nervous system (CNS) (left page) and summarize the deficits seen following lesions at various CNS levels that involve the pathway (right page). These illustrations show: 1) the position of the tract/fibers in MRI at representative levels; 2) the somatotopy (if applicable) of the tract as it appears in MRI/clinical orientation; 3) the trajectory of the tract/fibers through the CNS; 4) deficits correlated with the location of lesions at various locations and levels; and 5) the laterality (R/L) of the deficit as dictated by the position of the lesion in the MRI.

Intra-axial brainstem lesions **frequently result in both sensory and motor deficits.** Recognizing this fact, both types of deficits are listed for those lesions illustrated on the MRI pathways. However, for sensory pathways, sensory deficits are listed first and motor deficits are listed last. For motor pathways, the reverse is used: motor deficits are listed first, and sensory deficits listed last. This approach emphasizes the particular pathway being described but, at the same time, acknowledges the multiplicity of deficits resulting from CNS lesions.

Additional Points

The structure of an atlas does not allow a detailed definition of each clinical term on the printed page. However, as in other chapters, the full definition of each clinical term or phrase, when used, is available from the online resources that come with this atlas; here these definitions are taken from the current edition of *Stedman's Medical Dictionary,* but they are also available from any standard medical dictionary, neurology text, or colleagues in the clinics. Researching the full definition of a clinical term or phrase is a powerful and effective learning tool.

The layout of all illustrations in this chapter clearly shows the laterality of the tract or pathway. That is, the relationship between the location of the cell of origin and the termination of the fibers making up a tract or pathway or the projections of cranial nerve nuclei. Although this is clear in the anatomical drawings, it is particularly relevant to the clinical setting, as shown in the MRI pathway illustrations. *This information is absolutely essential to understand the position of a lesion and correlate this fact with the deficits seen in the neurologically compromised patient.* For example, is the deficit on the same side as the lesion (ipsilateral), the opposite side (contralateral), or both sides (bilateral)? The concept of laterality is expressed as as "right" or commonly as R in a circle, "left" or as L in a circle, or "bilateral" in reference to the side of the deficit(s) when written on the patient's chart.

This chapter is designed to maximize the correlation between structure and function, provide a range of clinical examples for each tract or pathway, and help the user develop a knowledge base that can be easily integrated into the clinical setting.

Orientation Drawing for Pathways in Anatomical Orientation

8-1 Orientation drawing for pathways. The trajectories of pathways in the **Anatomical Orientation** are illustrated in Chapter 8 on individualized versions of a representation of the central nervous system (CNS). Although slight changes are made in each drawing, so as to more clearly diagram a specific pathway, the basic configuration of the CNS is as represented here. This allows the user to move from pathway to pathway without being required to learn a different representation or drawing for each pathway; also, laterality of the pathway, a feature essential to diagnosis, is inherently evident in each illustration. In addition, many pathways, particularly those that are essential to diagnosis, are also shown on MRI and are, therefore, shown in a **Clinical Orientation**.

The forebrain (telencephalon and diencephalon) is shown in the coronal plane, and the midbrain, pons, medulla, and spinal cord are represented through their longitudinal axes. The internal capsule is represented in the axial plane in an effort to show the rostrocaudal distribution of fibers located therein.

The reader can become familiar with the structures and regions as shown here because their locations and relationships are easily transferable to subsequent illustrations. It may be helpful to refer back to this illustration when using subsequent sections of this chapter.

Neurotransmitters

Three important facts are self-evident in the descriptions of neurotransmitters that accompany each pathway drawing. These are illustrated by noting, as an example, that glutamate is found in corticospinal fibers (see Figure 8-11). First, the **location of neuronal cell bodies** containing a specific transmitter is indicated (glutamate-containing cell bodies are found in cortical areas projecting to the spinal cord). Second, the **trajectory of fibers** containing a particular neurotransmitter is obvious from the route taken by the tract (glutaminergic corticospinal fibers are found in the internal capsule, crus cerebri, basilar pons, pyramid, and

lateral corticospinal tract). Third, the **location of terminals** containing specific neurotransmitters is indicated by the site(s) of termination of each tract (glutaminergic terminals of corticospinal fibers are located in the spinal cord gray matter). In addition, the action of most neuroactive substances is indicated as excitatory (+) or inhibitory (−). This level of neurotransmitter information, as explained here for glutaminergic corticospinal fibers, is repeated for each pathway drawing.

Clinical Correlations

The clinical correlations are designed to give the user an overview of specific deficits (i.e., **hemiplegia, resting tremor**) seen in lesions of each pathway and to provide examples of some syndromes or diseases (e.g., **Brown-Séquard syndrome, Parkinson disease**) in which these deficits are seen. Although purposefully brief, these correlations highlight examples of deficits for each pathway and provide a built-in mechanism for expanded study. For example, the words in **bold** in each correlation are clinical terms and phrases that are here taken from the current edition of *Stedman's Medical Dictionary*, but they are also available from any standard medical dictionary, neurology text, or colleagues in the clinics.

An especially useful feature of this Atlas is the fact that the full definition of all clinical terms that are indicated in **bold** (**PICA syndrome, hemiplegia, resting tremor,** etc.) is easily available when using the online resources through thePoint; instructions to access thePoint are in the inside of the front cover. Consulting these sources, especially the online resources, will significantly enhance understanding of the deficits seen in the neurologically compromised patient. Expanded information, based on the deficits mentioned in this chapter, is integrated into some of the questions for Chapter 8. Referring to such sources allows the user to glean important clinical points that correlate with the pathway under consideration, and enlarge his or her knowledge and understanding by researching the italicized words and phrases.

ABBREVIATIONS

CE	Cervical enlargement of spinal cord	IntCap, PL	Internal capsule, posterior limb
Cer	Cervical levels of spinal cord	LatSul	Lateral sulcus (Sylvian sulcus)
CinSul	Cingulate sulcus	LatVen	Lateral ventricle
CaNu	Caudate nucleus (+ Put = neostriatum)	LSE	Lumbosacral enlargement of spinal cord
CM	Centromedian (and intralaminar) nuclei	LumSac	Lumbosacral level of spinal cord
CorCl	Corpus callosum	L-VTh	Lateral and ventral thalamic nuclei excluding VPM and VPL
Dien	Diencephalon		
DMNu	Dorsomedial nucleus of thalamus	Mes	Mesencephalon
For	Fornix	Met	Metencephalon
GP	Globus pallidus (paleostriatum)	Myelen	Myelencephalon
GPl	Globus pallidus, lateral segment	Put	Putamen (+ CaNu = neostriatum)
GPm	Globus pallidus, medial segment	SThNu	Subthalamic nucleus
HyTh	Hypothalamic area	Telen	Telencephalon
IC	Internal capsule	Thor	Thoracic levels of spinal cord
IntCap, AL	Internal capsule, anterior limb	VPL	Ventral posterolateral nucleus of thalamus
IntCap, G	Internal capsule, genu	VPM	Ventral posteromedial nucleus of thalamus

8-1 Orientation Drawing for Pathways in Anatomical Orientation

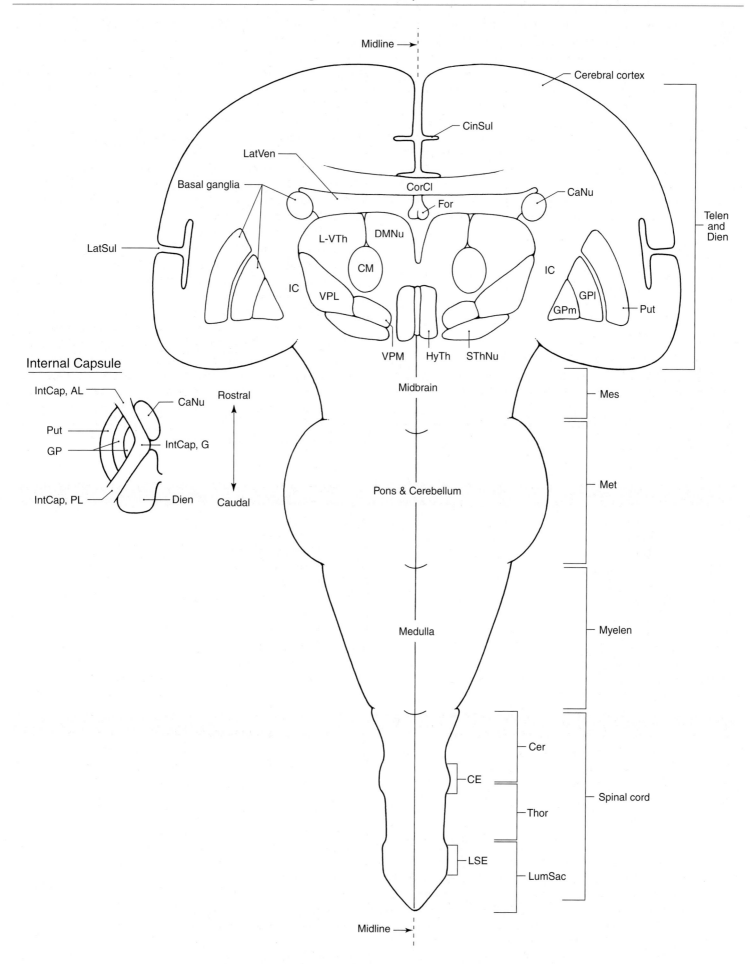

Midline →

Cerebral cortex

CinSul

LatVen

Basal ganglia

CorCl

CaNu

For

L-VTh

DMNu

CM

IC

IC

LatSul

VPL

GPl

GPm

Put

VPM

HyTh

SThNu

Telen and Dien

Internal Capsule

IntCap, AL

CaNu

Put

GP

IntCap, G

IntCap, PL

Dien

Rostral

Caudal

Midbrain

Mes

Pons & Cerebellum

Met

Medulla

Myelen

Cer

CE

Thor

Spinal cord

LSE

LumSac

Midline →

Posterior (Dorsal) Column–Medial Lemniscus System in Anatomical Orientation

8-2 The origin, course, and distribution of fibers comprising the **posterior (dorsal) column–medial lemniscus (PC–ML)** system. This illustration shows the longitudinal extent, positions in representative cross sections of brainstem and spinal cord, and somatotopy of fibers in both the posterior column (**PC**) and medial lemniscus (**ML**) portions of this system. The ML undergoes positional changes as it courses from the myelencephalon (medulla) rostrally toward the mesencephalic–diencephalic junction. In the medulla, ML and **anterolateral system (ALS)** fibers are widely separated and receive different blood supplies, whereas they are served by a common arterial source in the midbrain. As the ML makes positional changes, the somatotopy therein follows accordingly. Fibers of the postsynaptic posterior column system (shown in green) are considered in detail in Figure 8-6 on p. 200.

Neurotransmitters

Acetylcholine and the excitatory amino acids, glutamate and aspartate, are associated with some of the large-diameter, heavily myelinated fibers of the posterior horn and posterior columns.

Clinical Correlations

An ipsilateral loss of vibratory sensation, position sense, and discriminative touch (**stereoanesthesia, impaired graphesthesia,** and **tactile localization**) on one side of the body below the level of the lesion correlates with damage to the PC on the same side of the spinal cord (e.g., **Brown-Séquard syndrome**). While astereognosis, stereoagnosis, or tactile agnosia are sometimes used to describe PC damage, they are most commonly used to specify parietal lobe lesions.

The term **stereoanesthesia** is also frequently used to specify a lesion of peripheral nerves that results in an inability to perceive proprioceptive and tactile sensations. Bilateral damage (e.g., **tabes dorsalis** [tabetic neurosyphilis] or **subacute combined degeneration of the spinal cord**) produces bilateral losses. Although **ataxia** is the most common feature in patients with tabes dorsalis, they also have a loss of **muscle stretch reflexes**, severe **lancinating pain** over the body below the head (more common in the lower extremity), and bladder dysfunction. The **ataxia** that may be seen in patients with posterior column lesions (**sensory ataxia**) is due to a lack of proprioceptive input and position sense. These individuals tend to forcibly place their feet to the floor in an attempt to stimulate the missing sensory input. A patient with mild ataxia due to posterior column disease may compensate for the motor deficit by using visual cues. Patients with **subacute combined degeneration of the spinal cord** first have signs and symptoms of posterior column involvement, followed later by signs of **corticospinal tract damage** (spastic weakness of legs, increased muscle stretch reflexes [hyperreflexia], Babinski sign).

Rostral to the sensory decussation, medial lemniscus lesions result in contralateral losses that include the entire body, excluding the head. Brainstem lesions involving medial lemniscus fibers usually include adjacent structures, result in motor and additional sensory losses, and may reflect the distribution patterns of vessels (e.g., **medial medullary** or **medial pontine syndromes**). Large lesions in the forebrain may result in a complete contralateral loss of modalities carried in the posterior columns and anterolateral systems, or may produce **pain** or **paresthesia** (e.g., the **thalamic syndrome**).

ABBREVIATIONS

ALS	Anterolateral system	**NuGr**	Gracile nucleus
BP	Basilar pons	**PC**	Posterior column
CC	Crus cerebri	**PO**	Principal olivary nucleus
CTT	Central tegmental tract	**PoCGy**	Postcentral gyrus
FCu	Cuneate fasciculus	**PPGy**	Posterior paracentral gyrus
FGr	Gracile fasciculus	**PRG**	Posterior (dorsal) root ganglia
IAF	Internal arcuate fibers	**Py**	Pyramid
IC	Internal capsule	**RB**	Restiform body
ML	Medial lemniscus	**RNu**	Red nucleus
MLF	Medial longitudinal fasciculus	**SN**	Substantia nigra
NuCu	Cuneate nucleus	**VPL**	Ventral posterolateral nucleus of thalamus

---

SOMATOPY OF BODY AREAS

LE	Fibers conveying input from lower extremity	**C2**	Fibers from approximately the second cervical level
N	Fibers conveying input from neck	**S5**	Fibers from approximately the fifth sacral level
T	Fibers conveying input from trunk	**T5**	Fibers from approximately the fifth thoracic level
UE	Fibers conveying input from upper extremity		

Review of Blood Supply to PC–ML System

Structures	Arteries
PC in Spinal Cord	Penetrating branches of arterial vasocorona (see Figure 6-8)
ML in Medulla	Anterior spinal (see Figure 6-16)
ML in Pons	Overlap of paramedian and long circumferential branches of basilar (see Figure 6-23)
ML in Midbrain	Short circumferential branches of posterior cerebral, quadrigeminal, choroidal arteries (see Figure 6-30)
VPL	Thalamogeniculate branches of posterior cerebral (see Figure 6-41)
Posterior Limb of IC	Lateral striate branches of middle cerebral (see Figure 6-41)

8-2 Posterior (Dorsal) Column–Medial Lemniscus System in Anatomical Orientation

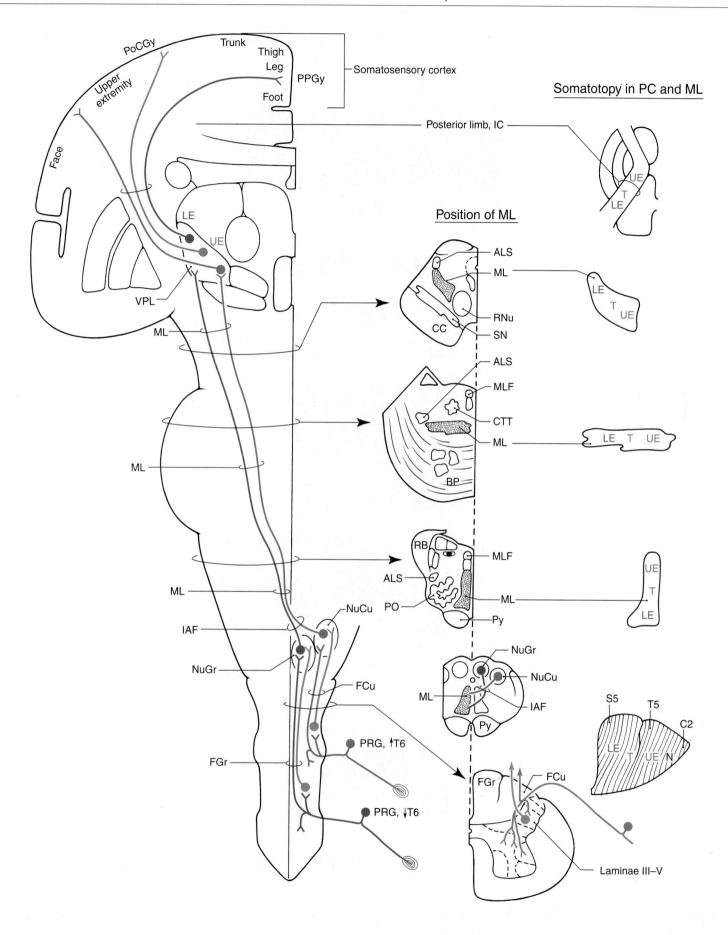

Somatotopy in PC and ML

Position of ML

Posterior Column–Medial Lemniscus System in Clinical Orientation

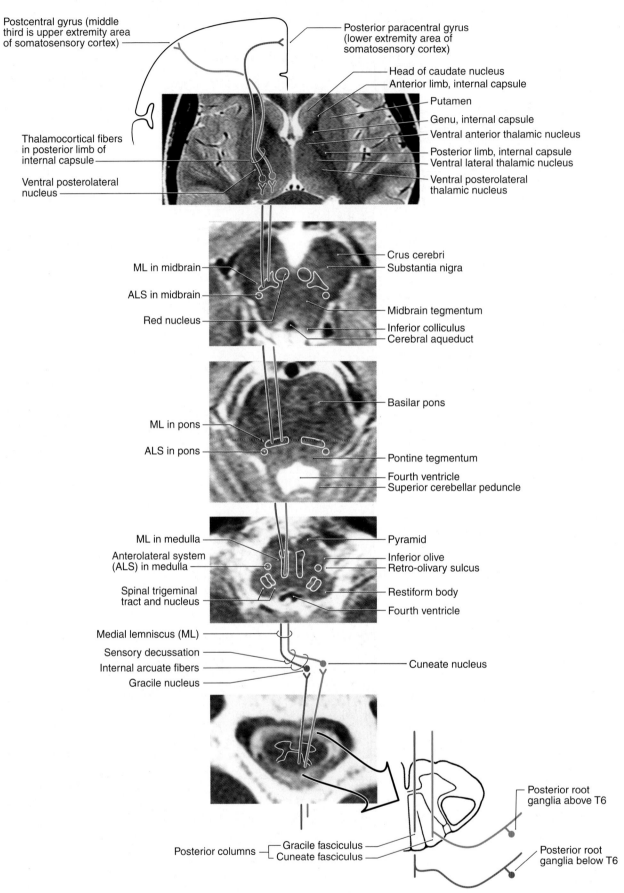

Postcentral gyrus (middle third is upper extremity area of somatosensory cortex)

Posterior paracentral gyrus (lower extremity area of somatosensory cortex)

Head of caudate nucleus
Anterior limb, internal capsule
Putamen
Genu, internal capsule
Ventral anterior thalamic nucleus
Posterior limb, internal capsule
Ventral lateral thalamic nucleus
Ventral posterolateral thalamic nucleus

Thalamocortical fibers in posterior limb of internal capsule

Ventral posterolateral nucleus

ML in midbrain
ALS in midbrain
Red nucleus

Crus cerebri
Substantia nigra

Midbrain tegmentum
Inferior colliculus
Cerebral aqueduct

ML in pons
ALS in pons

Basilar pons

Pontine tegmentum
Fourth ventricle
Superior cerebellar peduncle

ML in medulla
Anterolateral system (ALS) in medulla
Spinal trigeminal tract and nucleus

Pyramid
Inferior olive
Retro-olivary sulcus
Restiform body
Fourth ventricle

Medial lemniscus (ML)
Sensory decussation
Internal arcuate fibers
Gracile nucleus

Cuneate nucleus

Posterior root ganglia above T6

Posterior root ganglia below T6

Posterior columns — Gracile fasciculus
Cuneate fasciculus

8-3A The **posterior column–medial lemniscus (PC–ML)** system superimposed on CT (spinal cord, myelogram) and MRI (brainstem and forebrain, T2-weighted MRI) showing the location, topography, and trajectory of this pathway in a clinical orientation. The red and blue fibers correlate with those of the same color in Figure 8-2.

Posterior Column–Medial Lemniscus System in Clinical Orientation: Representative Lesions and Deficits

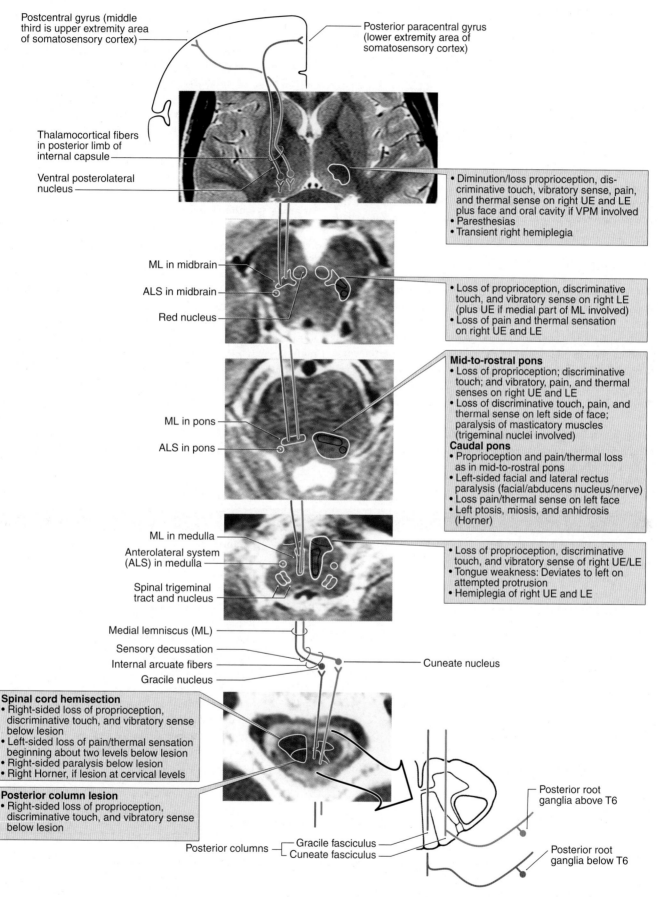

Postcentral gyrus (middle third is upper extremity area of somatosensory cortex)

Posterior paracentral gyrus (lower extremity area of somatosensory cortex)

Thalamocortical fibers in posterior limb of internal capsule

Ventral posterolateral nucleus

- Diminution/loss proprioception, discriminative touch, vibratory sense, pain, and thermal sense on right UE and LE plus face and oral cavity if VPM involved
- Paresthesias
- Transient right hemiplegia

ML in midbrain

ALS in midbrain

Red nucleus

- Loss of proprioception, discriminative touch, and vibratory sense on right LE (plus UE if medial part of ML involved)
- Loss of pain and thermal sensation on right UE and LE

Mid-to-rostral pons
- Loss of proprioception; discriminative touch; and vibratory, pain, and thermal senses on right UE and LE
- Loss of discriminative touch, pain, and thermal sense on left side of face; paralysis of masticatory muscles (trigeminal nuclei involved)

Caudal pons
- Proprioception and pain/thermal loss as in mid-to-rostral pons
- Left-sided facial and lateral rectus paralysis (facial/abducens nucleus/nerve)
- Loss pain/thermal sense on left face
- Left ptosis, miosis, and anhidrosis (Horner)

ML in pons

ALS in pons

ML in medulla

Anterolateral system (ALS) in medulla

Spinal trigeminal tract and nucleus

- Loss of proprioception, discriminative touch, and vibratory sense of right UE/LE
- Tongue weakness: Deviates to left on attempted protrusion
- Hemiplegia of right UE and LE

Medial lemniscus (ML)

Sensory decussation

Internal arcuate fibers

Gracile nucleus

Cuneate nucleus

Spinal cord hemisection
- Right-sided loss of proprioception, discriminative touch, and vibratory sense below lesion
- Left-sided loss of pain/thermal sensation beginning about two levels below lesion
- Right-sided paralysis below lesion
- Right Horner, if lesion at cervical levels

Posterior column lesion
- Right-sided loss of proprioception, discriminative touch, and vibratory sense below lesion

Posterior root ganglia above T6

Posterior columns ⎧ Gracile fasciculus ⎩ Cuneate fasciculus

Posterior root ganglia below T6

8-3B Representative lesions within the CNS that involve the **PC–ML** system and the deficits (in pink boxes) that correlate with the level and laterality of each lesion. Note that the laterality (R/L) of the deficits is determined by whether the lesion is on the left or right side of the MRI/CT; this reinforces important clinical concepts.

Anterolateral System in Anatomical Orientation

8-4 The longitudinal extent and somatotopy of fibers comprising the **anterolateral system** (**ALS**). The ALS is a composite bundle containing ascending fibers that terminate in the reticular formation (**spinoreticular fibers**), mesencephalon (**spinotectal fibers** to deep layers of the superior colliculus, **spinoperiaqueductal fibers** to the periaqueductal gray), hypothalamus (**spinohypothalamic fibers**), and sensory relay nuclei of the dorsal thalamus (**spinothalamic fibers**). Other fibers in the ALS include spino-olivary projections to the accessory olivary nuclei. Spinothalamic fibers terminate primarily in the VPL and reticulothalamic fibers terminate in some intralaminar nuclei and medial areas of the posterior thalamic complex.

Descending fibers from the PAG and nucleus raphe dorsalis enter the nucleus raphe magnus and adjacent reticular area. These latter sites, in turn, project to laminae I, II, and V of the spinal cord via raphespinal and reticulospinal fibers that participate in the modulation of pain transmission in the spinal cord.

Neurotransmitters

Glutamate (+), calcitonin gene–related peptide, and substance P (+)-containing posterior (dorsal) root ganglion cells project into laminae I, II (heavy), V (moderate), and III, IV (sparse). Some spinoreticular and spinothalamic fibers contain enkephalin (–), somatostatin (–), and cholecystokinin (+). In addition to enkephalin and somatostatin, some spinomesencephalic fibers contain vasoactive intestinal polypeptide (+). Neurons in the PAG and nucleus raphe dorsalis containing serotonin and neurotensin project into the nuclei raphe magnus and adjacent reticular formation. Cells in these latter centers that contain serotonin and enkephalin send processes to spinal cord laminae I, II, and V. Serotonergic raphespinal or enkephalinergic reticulospinal fibers may inhibit primary sensory fibers or projection neurons, conveying nociceptive (pain) information.

Clinical Correlations

A loss of pain and temperature sensations on one side of the body signifies a lesion involving the ALS; the deficit begins about two levels caudal to the lesion but on the contralateral side (e.g., **Brown-Séquard syndrome**). A bilateral loss of the same modalities, but in a dermatomal distribution, is characteristic of **syringomyelia**; the anterior white commissure is damaged by a cavitation (not ependymal lined) in the central cord area. A central cord cavitation lined by ependymal cells is a **hydromyelia**. Vascular lesions in the spinal cord (e.g., **acute central cervical cord syndrome**) may result in a bilateral and splotchy loss of pain and thermal sense below the lesion because the ALS has a dual vascular supply.

Vascular lesions in the lateral medulla (**posterior inferior cerebellar artery syndrome**) or lateral pons (**anterior inferior cerebellar artery occlusion**) result in a loss of pain and thermal sensations over the entire contralateral side of the body (ALS) as well as on the ipsilateral face (spinal trigeminal tract and nucleus), coupled with other motor and/or sensory deficits based on damage to structures these vessels serve. Note that the ALS and PC–ML systems are separated in the medulla (in different vascular territories) but are adjacent to each other in the midbrain (the same vascular territory). Consequently, medullary lesions will not result in deficits related to both pathways, whereas a lesion in the midbrain may result in a contralateral loss of pain, thermal, vibratory, and discriminative touch sensations on the body, excluding the head.

Profound loss of posterior column and anterolateral system modalities, or **intractable pain** and/or **paresthesias** (e.g., the **thalamic syndrome**), may result from vascular lesions in the posterolateral thalamus. So-called thalamic pain also may be experienced by patients who have brainstem lesions that damage fibers in the ALS and PC–ML system.

ABBREVIATIONS

ALS	Anterolateral system	Py	Pyramid
AWCom	Anterior (ventral) white commissure	RaSp	Raphespinal fibers
CC	Crus cerebri	RB	Restiform body
IC	Internal capsule	RetF	Reticular formation (of midbrain)
LE	Input from lower extremity regions	RetTh	Reticulothalamic fibers
MCP	Middle cerebellar peduncle	RNu	Red nucleus
ML	Medial lemniscus	S	Input from sacral regions
MLF	Medial longitudinal fasciculus	SC	Superior colliculus
Nu	Nuclei	SpRet	Spinoreticular fibers
NuDark	Nucleus of Darkschewitsch	SpTec	Spinotectal fibers
NuRa, d	Nucleus raphe, dorsalis	SpTh	Spinothalamic fibers (rostral midbrain and above)
NuRa, m	Nucleus raphe, magnus	T	Input from thoracic regions
PAG	Periaqueductal gray	UE	Input from upper extremity regions
PoCGy	Postcentral gyrus	VPL	Ventral posterolateral nucleus of thalamus
PPGy	Posterior paracentral gyrus	I–VIII	Laminae I–VIII of Rexed
PRG	Posterior (dorsal) root ganglion		

Review of Blood Supply to ALS

Structures	Arteries
ALS in Spinal Cord	Penetrating branches of arterial vasocorona and branches of anterior spinal (see Figures 6-8 and 6-16)
ALS in Medulla	Caudal third, vertebral; rostral two-thirds, posterior inferior cerebellar (see Figure 6-16)
ALS in Pons	Long circumferential branches of basilar (see Figure 6-23)
ALS in Midbrain	Short circumferential branches of posterior cerebral, superior cerebellar (see Figure 6-30)
VPL	Thalamogeniculate branches of posterior cerebral (see Figure 6-41)
Posterior Limb of IC	Lateral striate branches of middle cerebral (see Figure 6-41)

8-4 Anterolateral System in Anatomical Orientation

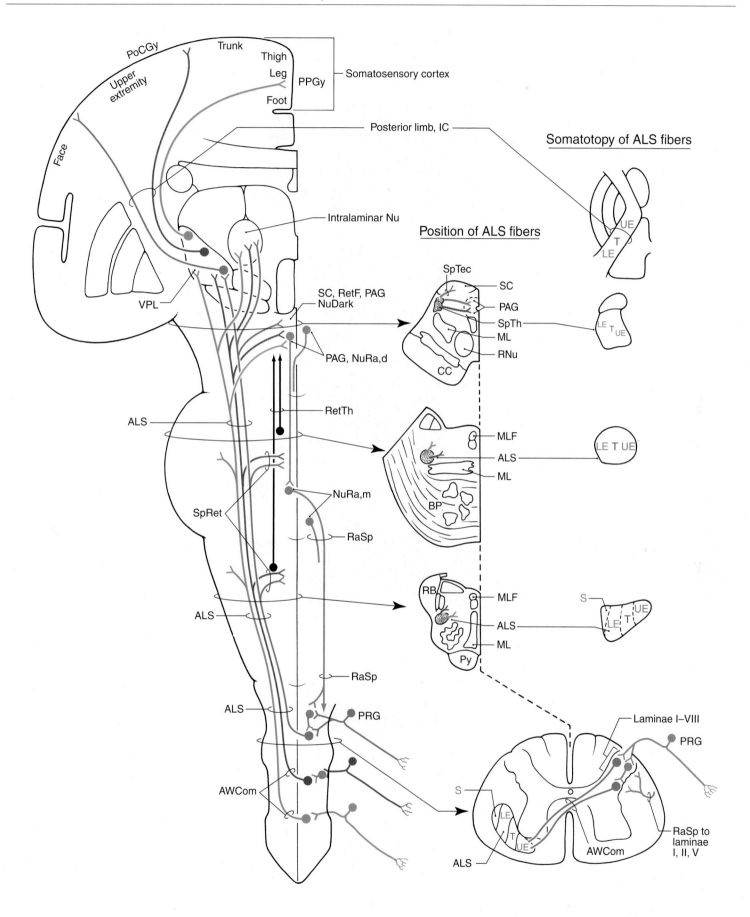

Somatotopy of ALS fibers

Position of ALS fibers

Anterolateral System in Clinical Orientation

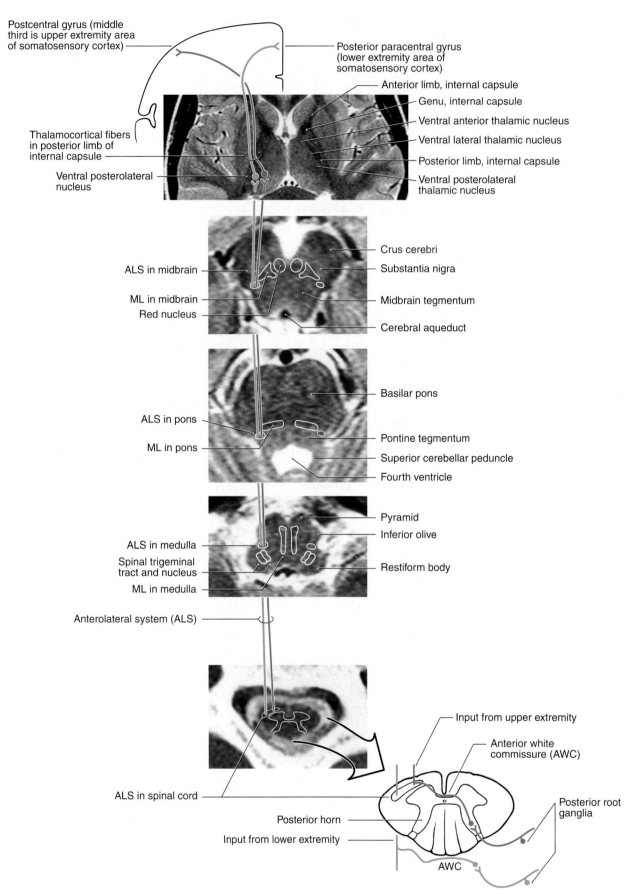

Postcentral gyrus (middle third is upper extremity area of somatosensory cortex)

Posterior paracentral gyrus (lower extremity area of somatosensory cortex)

Anterior limb, internal capsule

Genu, internal capsule

Ventral anterior thalamic nucleus

Ventral lateral thalamic nucleus

Posterior limb, internal capsule

Ventral posterolateral thalamic nucleus

Thalamocortical fibers in posterior limb of internal capsule

Ventral posterolateral nucleus

Crus cerebri

Substantia nigra

Midbrain tegmentum

Cerebral aqueduct

ALS in midbrain

ML in midbrain

Red nucleus

Basilar pons

ALS in pons

ML in pons

Pontine tegmentum

Superior cerebellar peduncle

Fourth ventricle

Pyramid

Inferior olive

ALS in medulla

Spinal trigeminal tract and nucleus

ML in medulla

Restiform body

Anterolateral system (ALS)

Input from upper extremity

Anterior white commissure (AWC)

Posterior root ganglia

ALS in spinal cord

Posterior horn

Input from lower extremity

AWC

8-5A The **anterolateral system** (**ALS**) superimposed on CT (spinal cord, myelogram) and MRI (brainstem and forebrain, T2-weighted MRI) showing the location, topography, and trajectory of this pathway in a clinical orientation. The blue and green fibers correlate with those of the same color in Figure 8-4.

Anterolateral System in Clinical Orientation: Representative Lesions and Deficits

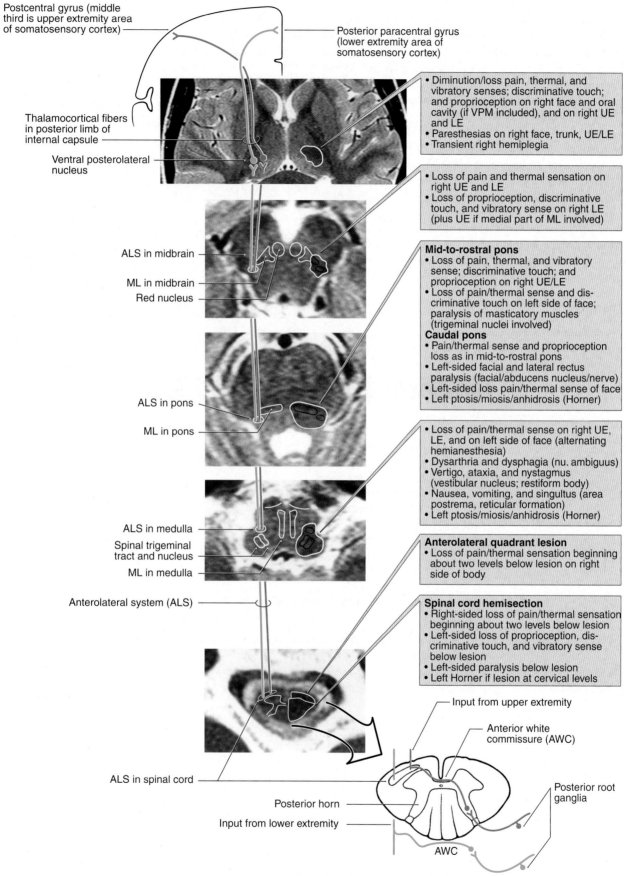

Postcentral gyrus (middle third is upper extremity area of somatosensory cortex)

Posterior paracentral gyrus (lower extremity area of somatosensory cortex)

Thalamocortical fibers in posterior limb of internal capsule

Ventral posterolateral nucleus

ALS in midbrain

ML in midbrain

Red nucleus

ALS in pons

ML in pons

ALS in medulla

Spinal trigeminal tract and nucleus

ML in medulla

Anterolateral system (ALS)

ALS in spinal cord

Posterior horn

Input from lower extremity

Input from upper extremity

Anterior white commissure (AWC)

Posterior root ganglia

AWC

- Diminution/loss pain, thermal, and vibratory senses; discriminative touch; and proprioception on right face and oral cavity (if VPM included), and on right UE and LE
- Paresthesias on right face, trunk, UE/LE
- Transient right hemiplegia

- Loss of pain and thermal sensation on right UE and LE
- Loss of proprioception, discriminative touch, and vibratory sense on right LE (plus UE if medial part of ML involved)

Mid-to-rostral pons
- Loss of pain, thermal, and vibratory sense; discriminative touch; and proprioception on right UE/LE
- Loss of pain/thermal sense and discriminative touch on left side of face; paralysis of masticatory muscles (trigeminal nuclei involved)

Caudal pons
- Pain/thermal sense and proprioception loss as in mid-to-rostral pons
- Left-sided facial and lateral rectus paralysis (facial/abducens nucleus/nerve)
- Left-sided loss pain/thermal sense of face
- Left ptosis/miosis/anhidrosis (Horner)

- Loss of pain/thermal sense on right UE, LE, and on left side of face (alternating hemianesthesia)
- Dysarthria and dysphagia (nu. ambiguus)
- Vertigo, ataxia, and nystagmus (vestibular nucleus; restiform body)
- Nausea, vomiting, and singultus (area postrema, reticular formation)
- Left ptosis/miosis/anhidrosis (Horner)

Anterolateral quadrant lesion
- Loss of pain/thermal sensation beginning about two levels below lesion on right side of body

Spinal cord hemisection
- Right-sided loss of pain/thermal sensation beginning about two levels below lesion
- Left-sided loss of proprioception, discriminative touch, and vibratory sense below lesion
- Left-sided paralysis below lesion
- Left Horner if lesion at cervical levels

8-5B Representative lesions within the CNS that involve the **ALS** and the deficits (in pink boxes) that correlate with the level and laterality of each lesion. Note that the laterality (R/L) of the deficits is determined by whether the lesion is on the left or right side of the MRI/CT; this reinforces important clinical concepts.

Postsynaptic–Posterior (Dorsal) Column System and the Spinocervicothalamic Pathway in Anatomical Orientation

8-6 The origin, course, and distribution of fibers comprising the **postsynaptic–posterior column system** (upper) and the **spinocervicothalamic pathway** (lower). Postsynaptic–posterior column fibers originate primarily from cells in lamina IV (some cells in laminae III and V–VII also contribute), ascend in the ipsilateral dorsal fasciculi, and end in their respective nuclei in the caudal medulla. Moderate-to-sparse collaterals project to a few other medullary targets.

Fibers of the spinocervical part of the spinocervicothalamic pathway also originate from cells in lamina IV (less so from III and V). The axons of these cells ascend in the posterior part of the lateral funiculus (this is sometimes called the dorsolateral funiculus) and end in a topographic fashion in the lateral cervical nucleus: lumbosacral projections terminate posterolaterally and cervical projections anteromedially. Axons arising from cells of the lateral cervical nucleus decussate in the anterior white commissure, and ascend to targets in the midbrain and thalamus. Cells of the posterior column nuclei also convey information to the contralateral thalamus via the medial lemniscus.

Neurotransmitters

Glutamate (+) and possibly substance P (+) are present in some spinocervical projections. Because some cells in laminae III–V have axons that collateralize to both the lateral cervical nucleus *and* the dorsal column nuclei, glutamate (and substance P) also may be present in some postsynaptic dorsal column fibers.

Clinical Correlations

The postsynaptic–posterior column and spinocervicothalamic pathways are not known to be major circuits in the human nervous system. However, the occurrence of these fibers may explain a well-known clinical observation. Patients who have received an **anterolateral cordotomy** (this lesion is placed just ventral to the denticulate ligament) for **intractable pain** may experience complete or partial relief, or there may be a recurrence of pain perception within days or weeks. Although the cordotomy transects fibers of the anterolateral system (the main pain pathway), this lesion spares the posterior horn, posterior columns, and spinocervical fibers. Consequently, the recurrence of pain perception (or even the partial relief of pain) in these patients may be explained by these postsynaptic–dorsal column and spinocervicothalamic projections. Through these connections, some nociceptive (pain) information may be transmitted to the ventral posterolateral nucleus and on to the sensory cortex, via circuits that bypass the anterolateral system and are spared in a cordotomy.

ABBREVIATIONS	
ALS	Anterolateral system
AWCom	Anterior (ventral) white commissure
FCu	Cuneate fasciculus
FGr	Gracile fasciculus
IAF	Internal arcuate fibers
LCerNu	Lateral cervical nucleus
ML	Medial lemniscus
NuCu	Cuneate nucleus
NuGr	Gracile nucleus
PRG	Posterior (dorsal) root ganglion

Review of Blood Supply to Posterior Horn, FGr, Fcu, and LcerNu	
Structures	**Arteries**
FGr, FCu in Spinal Cord	Penetrating branches of arterial vasocorona and some branches from central (sulcal) (see Figure 6-8)
LCerNu	Penetrating branches of arterial vasocorona and branches from central (see Figure 6-8)
NuGr NuCu	Posterior spinal (see Figure 6-16)

8-6 Postsynaptic–Posterior (Dorsal) Column System and the Spinocervicothalamic Pathway in Anatomical Orientation

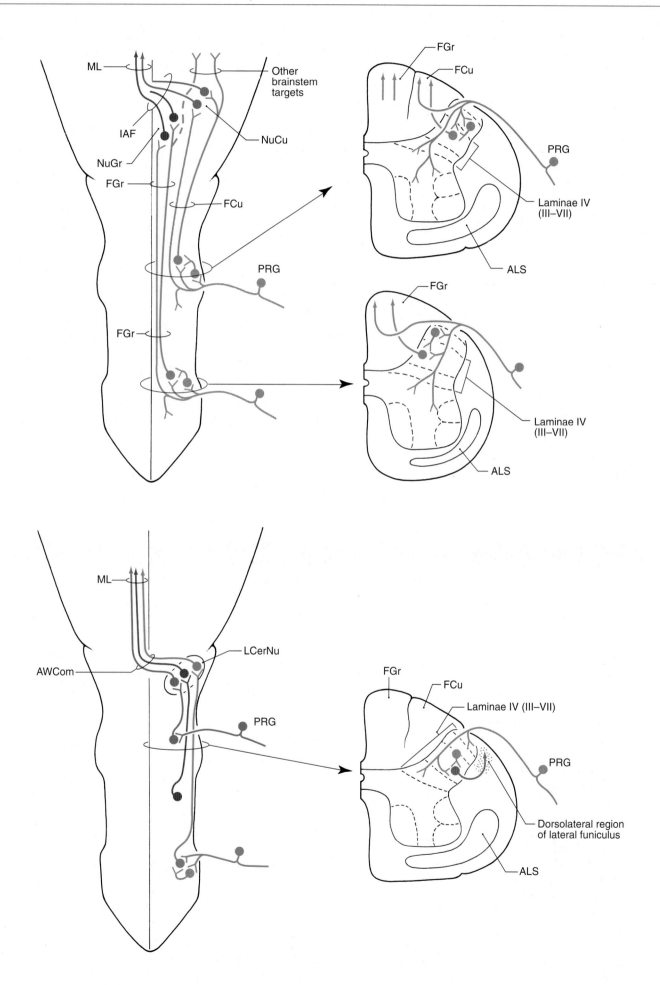

Trigeminal Pathways in Anatomical Orientation

8-7 The distribution of general sensory GSA or SA information originating on CNs V (trigeminal), VII (facial), IX (glossopharyngeal), and X (vagus). Some of these primary sensory fibers end in the principal sensory nucleus, but many form the spinal trigeminal tract and end in the spinal trigeminal nucleus.

Neurons in the **spinal trigeminal nucleus** and in ventrolateral parts of the principal sensory nucleus give rise to crossed **ventral trigeminothalamic fibers**. Collaterals of these fibers influence the hypoglossal, facial (**corneal reflex, supraorbital,** or **trigeminofacial reflex**), and trigeminal motor nuclei; mesencephalic collaterals are involved in the **jaw reflex,** or the **jaw-jerk reflex.** Collaterals also enter the dorsal motor vagal nucleus (**vomiting reflex**), the superior salivatory nucleus (**tearing/lacrimal reflex**), and the nucleus ambiguus and adjacent reticular formation (**sneezing reflex**). Uncrossed **dorsal trigeminothalamic fibers** arise from dorsomedial regions of the principal sensory nucleus.

Neurotransmitters

Substance P (+)-containing and cholecystokinin (+)-containing trigeminal ganglion cells project to the spinal trigeminal nucleus, especially its caudal part (pars caudalis). Glutamate (+) is found in many trigeminothalamic fibers arising from the principal sensory nucleus and the pars interpolaris of the spinal nucleus. It is present in fewer trigeminothalamic fibers from the pars caudalis and in almost none from the pars oralis. The locus ceruleus (noradrenergic fibers) and the raphe nuclei (serotonergic fibers) also project to the spinal nucleus. Enkephalin (–)-containing cells are present in caudal regions of the spinal nucleus, and enkephalinergic fibers are found in the nucleus ambiguus and in the hypoglossal, facial, and trigeminal motor nuclei.

Clinical Correlations

A loss of: 1) pain, temperature, and tactile sensation from the ipsilateral face, oral cavity, and teeth; 2) ipsilateral paralysis of masticatory muscles; and 3) ipsilateral loss of the corneal reflex may indicate a lesion of the trigeminal ganglion or nerve proximal to the ganglion. Damage to peripheral portions of the trigeminal nerve may be traumatic (skull fracture, especially of supraorbital and infraorbital branches), inflammatory (e.g., **herpes zoster**), or result from tumor growth (large **vestibular schwannoma** or **meningioma**). The deficit would reflect the peripheral portion of the trigeminal nerve damaged.

Trigeminal neuralgia (**tic douloureux**) is a severe burning pain restricted to the peripheral distribution of the trigeminal nerve, usually its V$_2$ (maxillary) division. This pain may be initiated by any contact to areas of the face, such as the corner of the mouth, nose, lips, or cheek (e.g., shaving, putting on make-up, chewing, or even smiling). The attacks frequently occur without warning, may happen only a few times a month to many times in a single day, and are usually seen in patients 40 years of age or older. One probable cause of trigeminal neuralgia is compression of the trigeminal root by aberrant vessels, most commonly a loop of the superior cerebellar artery (see p. 49). Other causes may include tumor, **multiple sclerosis,** and ephaptic transmission (**ephapse**) in the trigeminal ganglion. This is the most common type of neuralgia.

In the medulla, fibers of the spinal trigeminal tract and ALS are served by the posterior inferior cerebellar artery (PICA). Consequently, an **alternating** (**alternate** or **crossed**) **hemianesthesia** is one characteristic feature of the **PICA syndrome.** This is a loss of pain and thermal sensations on one side of the body and the opposite side of the face. **Pontine gliomas** may produce a paralysis of masticatory muscles (motor trigeminal damage) and some loss of tactile input (principal sensory nucleus damage), as well as other deficits based on the adjacent structures involved.

ABBREVIATIONS

ALS	Anterolateral system	OpthV	Ophthalmic division of trigeminal nerve	VPM	Ventral posteromedial nucleus of thalamus
CC	Crus cerebri				
DTTr	Dorsal (posterior) trigeminothalamic tract	PSNu	Principal (chief) sensory nucleus	VTTr	Ventral (anterior) trigeminothalamic tract
FacNu	Facial nucleus	RB	Restiform body		
GSA	General somatic afferent	RetF	Reticular formation		

Ganglia

HyNu	Hypoglossal nucleus
IC	Internal capsule
ManV	Mandibular division of trigeminal nerve
MaxV	Maxillary division of trigeminal nerve
MesNu	Mesencephalic nucleus
ML	Medial lemniscus

RNu	Red nucleus
SpTNu	Spinal trigeminal nucleus
SpTTr	Spinal trigeminal tract
TriMoNu	Trigeminal motor nucleus
TMJ	Temporomandibular joint
VPL	Ventral posterolateral nucleus of thalamus

1 Trigeminal ganglion
2 Geniculate ganglion
3 Superior of glossopharyngeal
4 Superior of vagus

Review of Blood Supply to SpTT, SpTNu, and Trigeminothalamic Tracts

Structures	Arteries
SpTTr and **SpTNu** in Medulla	Caudal third, vertebral; rostral two-thirds, posterior inferior cerebellar (see Figure 6-16)
SpTTr and **SpTNu** in Pons	Long circumferential branches of basilar (see Figure 6-23)
Trigeminothalamic Fibers in Midbrain	Short circumferential branches of posterior cerebral and superior cerebellar (see Figure 6-30)
VPM	Thalamogeniculate branches of posterior cerebral (see Figure 6-41)
Posterior Limb of IC	Lateral striate branches of middle cerebral (see Figure 6-41)

8-7 Trigeminal Pathways in Anatomical Orientation

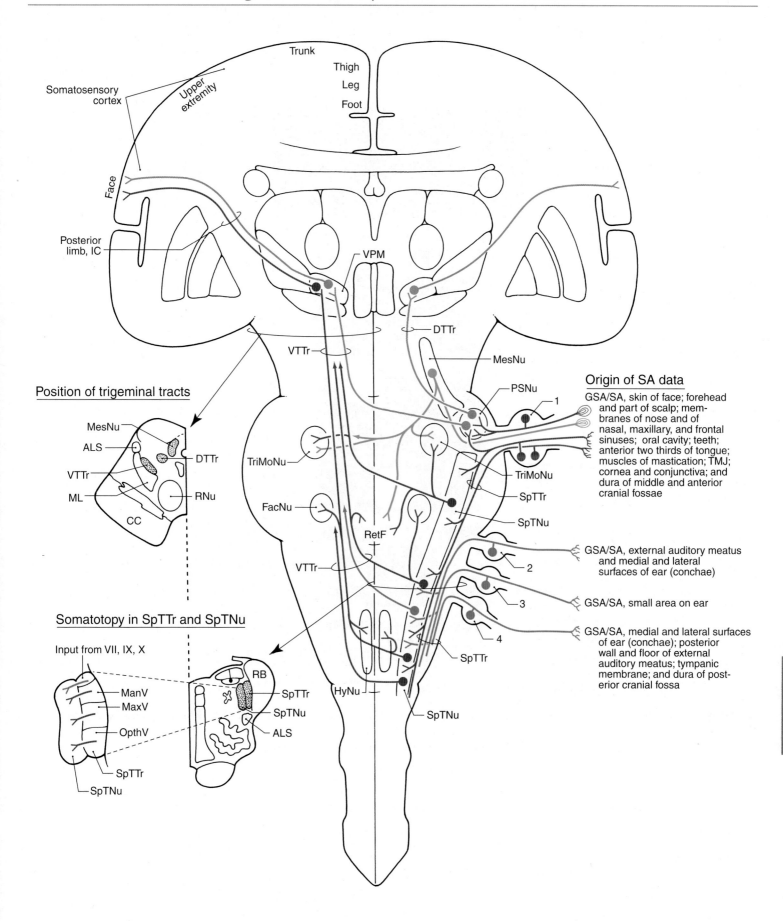

Trunk

Thigh

Leg

Foot

Somatosensory cortex

Upper extremity

Face

Posterior limb, IC

VPM

DTTr

VTTr

MesNu

Position of trigeminal tracts

MesNu

ALS

VTTr

ML

DTTr

RNu

CC

PSNu

1

TriMoNu

TriMoNu

SpTTr

SpTNu

FacNu

RetF

VTTr

Somatotopy in SpTTr and SpTNu

Input from VII, IX, X

ManV

MaxV

OpthV

SpTTr

SpTNu

RB

SpTTr

SpTNu

ALS

HyNu

SpTTr

SpTNu

Origin of SA data

GSA/SA, skin of face; forehead and part of scalp; membranes of nose and of nasal, maxillary, and frontal sinuses; oral cavity; teeth; anterior two thirds of tongue; muscles of mastication; TMJ; cornea and conjunctiva; and dura of middle and anterior cranial fossae

2

GSA/SA, external auditory meatus and medial and lateral surfaces of ear (conchae)

3

GSA/SA, small area on ear

4

GSA/SA, medial and lateral surfaces of ear (conchae); posterior wall and floor of external auditory meatus; tympanic membrane; and dura of posterior cranial fossa

Trigeminal Pathways in Clinical Orientation

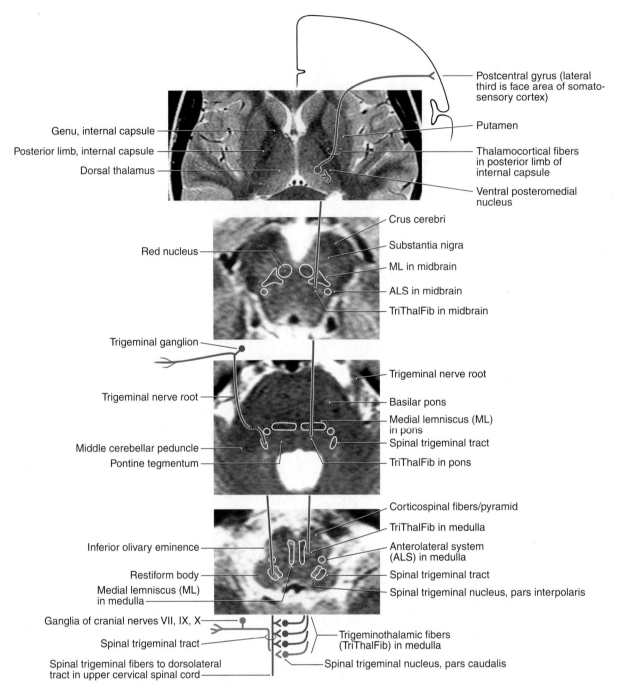

Postcentral gyrus (lateral third is face area of somato-sensory cortex)

Genu, internal capsule

Posterior limb, internal capsule

Dorsal thalamus

Putamen

Thalamocortical fibers in posterior limb of internal capsule

Ventral posteromedial nucleus

Red nucleus

Crus cerebri

Substantia nigra

ML in midbrain

ALS in midbrain

TriThalFib in midbrain

Trigeminal ganglion

Trigeminal nerve root

Trigeminal nerve root

Basilar pons

Medial lemniscus (ML) in pons

Spinal trigeminal tract

Middle cerebellar peduncle

Pontine tegmentum

TriThalFib in pons

Corticospinal fibers/pyramid

TriThalFib in medulla

Anterolateral system (ALS) in medulla

Inferior olivary eminence

Restiform body

Medial lemniscus (ML) in medulla

Spinal trigeminal tract

Spinal trigeminal nucleus, pars interpolaris

Ganglia of cranial nerves VII, IX, X

Spinal trigeminal tract

Trigeminothalamic fibers (TriThalFib) in medulla

Spinal trigeminal fibers to dorsolateral tract in upper cervical spinal cord

Spinal trigeminal nucleus, pars caudalis

8-8A   **Spinal trigeminal** and **trigeminothalamic fibers** superimposed on MRI (brainstem and forebrain, T2-weighted MRI) showing the location, topography, and trajectory of these fibers in a clinical orientation. The red and blue fibers correlate with those of the same color in Figure 8-7.

Trigeminal Pathways in Clinical Orientation: Representative Lesions and Deficits

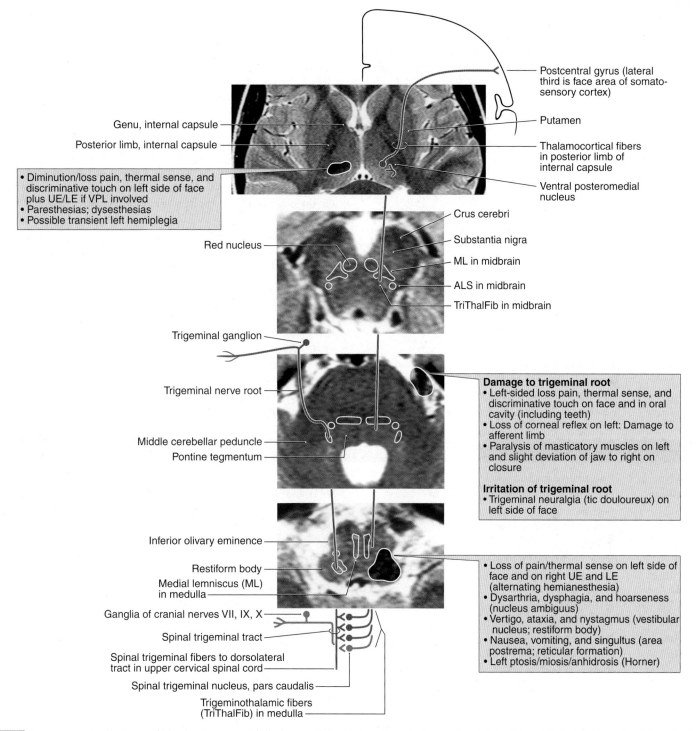

Postcentral gyrus (lateral third is face area of somatosensory cortex)

Genu, internal capsule

Posterior limb, internal capsule

Putamen

Thalamocortical fibers in posterior limb of internal capsule

Ventral posteromedial nucleus

- Diminution/loss pain, thermal sense, and discriminative touch on left side of face plus UE/LE if VPL involved
- Paresthesias; dysesthesias
- Possible transient left hemiplegia

Red nucleus

Crus cerebri

Substantia nigra

ML in midbrain

ALS in midbrain

TriThalFib in midbrain

Trigeminal ganglion

Trigeminal nerve root

Damage to trigeminal root
- Left-sided loss pain, thermal sense, and discriminative touch on face and in oral cavity (including teeth)
- Loss of corneal reflex on left: Damage to afferent limb
- Paralysis of masticatory muscles on left and slight deviation of jaw to right on closure

Irritation of trigeminal root
- Trigeminal neuralgia (tic douloureux) on left side of face

Middle cerebellar peduncle

Pontine tegmentum

Inferior olivary eminence

Restiform body

Medial lemniscus (ML) in medulla

Ganglia of cranial nerves VII, IX, X

Spinal trigeminal tract

Spinal trigeminal fibers to dorsolateral tract in upper cervical spinal cord

Spinal trigeminal nucleus, pars caudalis

Trigeminothalamic fibers (TriThalFib) in medulla

- Loss of pain/thermal sense on left side of face and on right UE and LE (alternating hemianesthesia)
- Dysarthria, dysphagia, and hoarseness (nucleus ambiguus)
- Vertigo, ataxia, and nystagmus (vestibular nucleus; restiform body)
- Nausea, vomiting, and singultus (area postrema; reticular formation)
- Left ptosis/miosis/anhidrosis (Horner)

8-8B Representative lesions of the brainstem and thalamus that involve elements of the **trigeminal system** and the deficits (in pink boxes) that correlate with the level and laterality of each lesion.

Note that the laterality (R/L) of the deficits is determined by whether the lesion is on the left or right side of the MRI; this reinforces important clinical concepts.

Solitary Pathways in Anatomical Orientation

8-9 Visceral afferent input (SVA, taste; GVA, **general visceral sensa-tion**) on CNs VII (**facial**), IX (**glossopharyngeal**), and X (**vagus**) enters the **solitary nuclei** via the **solitary tract**. Recall that the SVA and GVA functional components may be collectively grouped as VA; Visceral Afferent. What is commonly called the solitary "nucleus" is a series of small nuclei that collectively form this rostrocaudal-oriented cell column.

Solitary cells project to the salivatory, hypoglossal, and dorsal motor vagal nuclei and the nucleus ambiguus. Solitary projections to the nucleus ambiguus are the intermediate neurons in the pathway for the **gag reflex**. The afferent limb of the **gag reflex** is carried on the glos-sopharyngeal nerve, and the efferent limb originates from the nucleus ambiguus; the efferent limb travels on both CNs IX and X. Although not routinely tested, the **gag reflex** should be evaluated in patients with **dysarthria, dysphagia, or hoarseness.** Solitariospinal fibers are bilateral with a contralateral preponderance and project to the phrenic nucleus, intermediolateral cell column, and ventral horn. The VPM is the thalamic center through which visceral afferent information is relayed onto the cerebral cortex. See Figures 8-27 to 8-31 (pp. 236–238) and Table 8-1 (p. 240) for brainstem reflexes.

Neurotransmitters

Substance P (+)-containing and cholecystokinin (+)-containing cells in the geniculate ganglion (facial nerve) and the inferior ganglia of the glossopharyngeal and vagus nerves project to the solitary nucleus. Enkephalin (–), neurotensin, and GABA (+) are present in some solitary neurons that project into the adjacent dorsal motor vagal nucleus. Cholecystokinin (+), somatostatin (–), and enkephalin (–) are present in solitary neurons, cells of the parabrachial nuclei, and some thalamic neurons that project to taste and other visceral areas of the cortex.

Clinical Correlations

An ipsilateral loss of taste (**ageusia**) from the anterior two-thirds of the tongue and an ipsilateral **facial (Bell) palsy** may indicate damage to the geniculate ganglion or facial nerve proximal to the ganglion. Although a glossopharyngeal nerve lesion will result in ageusia from the posterior third of the tongue on the ipsilateral side, this loss is difficult to test. On the other hand, **glossopharyngeal neuralgia** (this may also be called **glossopharyngeal tic**) is an idiopathic pain localized to the peripheral sensory branches of the ninth nerve in the posterior pharynx, posterior tongue, and tonsillar area. Although comparatively rare, glossopha-ryngeal neuralgia may be aggravated by talking or even swallowing. Occlusion of the posterior inferior cerebellar artery (e.g., the **posterior inferior cerebellar artery** or **lateral medullary syndrome**), in addition to producing an **alternate hemianesthesia**, also results in **ageusia** from the ipsilateral side of the tongue because the posterior inferior cerebellar artery serves the solitary tract and nuclei in the medulla.

Interestingly, lesions of the olfactory nerves or tract (**anosmia,** loss of olfactory sensation; **dysosmia,** distorted olfactory sense) may affect how the patient perceives taste. Witness the fact that the nasal congestion accompanying a severe cold markedly affects the sense of taste.

ABBREVIATIONS

AmyNu	Amygdaloid nucleus (complex)	**SalNu**	Salivatory nuclei
CardResp	Cardiorespiratory portion (caudal) of solitary nucleus	**SolTr and Nu**	Solitary tract and nuclei
		SVA	Special visceral afferent
GustNu	Gustatory nucleus (rostral portion of solitary nucleus)	**Tr**	Tract
		VA	Visceral afferent
GVA	General visceral afferent	**VPM**	Ventral posteromedial nucleus of thalamus
HyNu	Hypoglossal nucleus		
HyTh	Hypothalamus		

Number Key

1 Geniculate ganglion of facial
2 Inferior ganglion of glossopharyngeal
3 Inferior ganglion of vagus
4 Dorsal motor vagal nucleus

InfVNu	Inferior (or spinal) vestibular nucleus
MVNu	Medial vestibular nucleus
NuAm	Nucleus ambiguus
PBNu	Parabrachial nuclei
RB	Restiform body

Review of Blood Supply to SolNu and SolTr

Structures	Arteries
SolNu and **Tr** in **Medulla**	Caudal medulla, anterior spinal; rostral medulla, posterior inferior cerebellar (see Figure 6-16)
Ascending Fibers in Pons	Long circumferential branches of basilar and branches of superior cerebellar (see Figure 6-23)
VPM	Thalamogeniculate branches of posterior cerebral (see Figure 6-41)
Posterior Limb of *IC*	Lateral striate branches of middle cerebral (see Figure 6-41)

8-9 Solitary Pathways in Anatomical Orientation

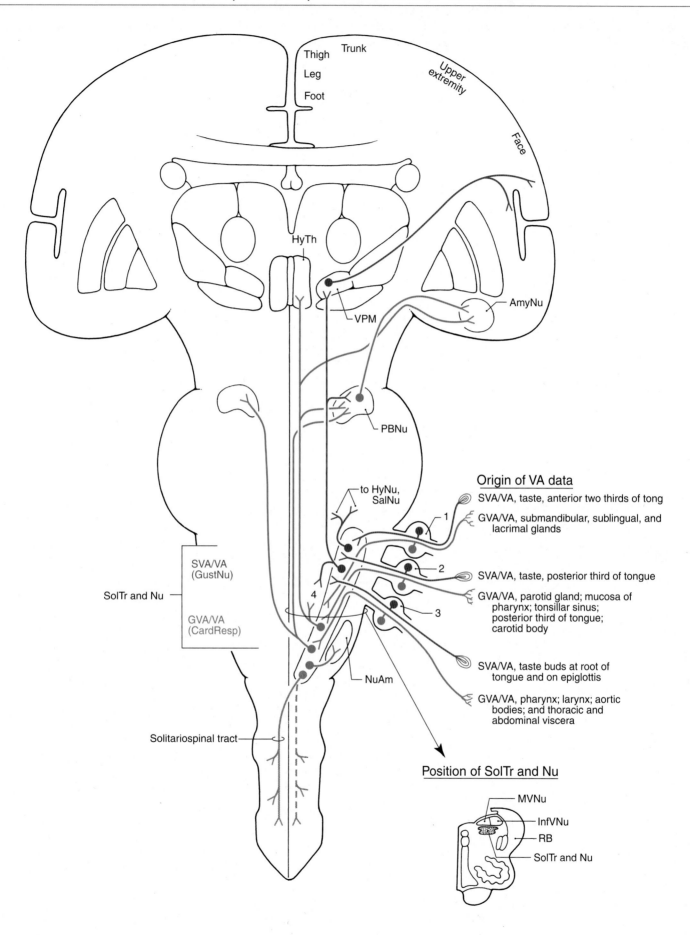

Thigh
Trunk
Leg
Foot
Upper extremity
Face

HyTh

VPM

AmyNu

PBNu

Origin of VA data

SVA/VA, taste, anterior two thirds of tong

GVA/VA, submandibular, sublingual, and lacrimal glands

to HyNu, SalNu

1

SVA/VA, taste, posterior third of tongue

SVA/VA (GustNu)

2

SolTr and Nu

GVA/VA, parotid gland; mucosa of pharynx; tonsillar sinus; posterior third of tongue; carotid body

GVA/VA (CardResp)

4

3

SVA/VA, taste buds at root of tongue and on epiglottis

NuAm

GVA/VA, pharynx; larynx; aortic bodies; and thoracic and abdominal viscera

Solitariospinal tract

Position of SolTr and Nu

MVNu

InfVNu

RB

SolTr and Nu

Blank Master Drawing for Sensory Pathways

8-10 Blank master drawing for sensory pathways. This illustration is provided for self-evaluation of sensory pathway under-standing, for the instructor to expand on sensory pathways not covered in the atlas, or both.

NOTES

8-10 Blank Master Drawing for Sensory Pathways

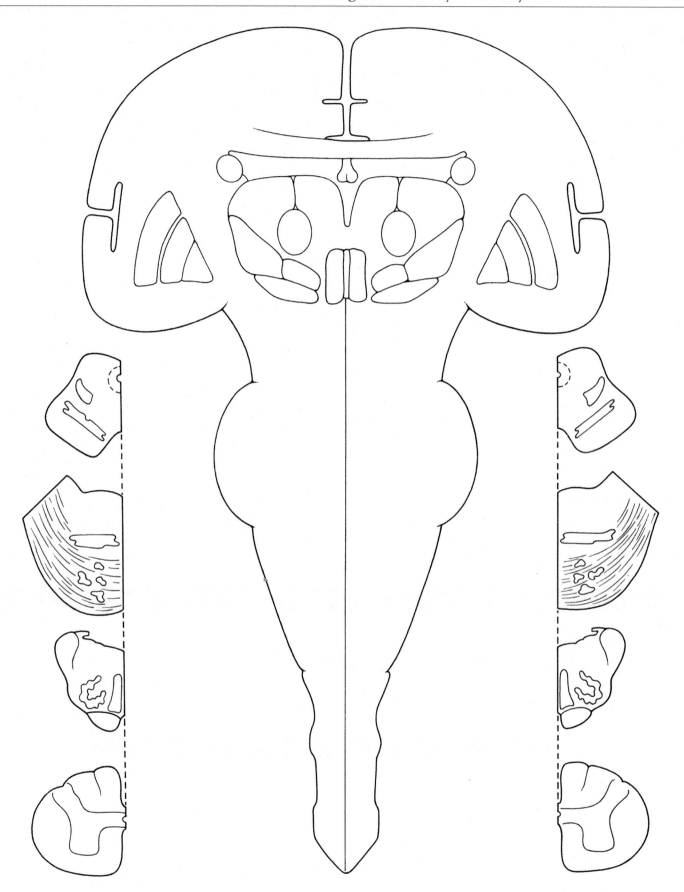

Corticospinal Tracts in Anatomical Orientation

8-11 The longitudinal extent of **corticospinal fibers** and their position and somatotopy at representative levels within the neuraxis. The somatotopy of corticospinal fibers in the **basilar pons** is less obvious than in the **internal capsule, crus cerebri, pyramid, or spinal cord**. In the **motor decussation** (pyramidal decussation), fibers originating from upper extremity areas of the cerebral cortex cross rostral to those that arise from lower extremity areas. In addition to fibers arising from the **precentral gyrus** (somatomotor area, area 4), a significant contingent also originates from the **postcentral gyrus** (areas 3, 1, 2); the former terminate primarily in laminae VI–IX, whereas the latter end mainly in laminae IV and V. Frontal area 6, and parietal areas 5 and 7 also contribute to the corticospinal tract.

Neurotransmitters

Acetylcholine, γ-aminobutyric acid (–), and substance P (+, plus other peptides) are found in small cortical neurons presumed to function as local circuit cells or in cortico-cortical connections. Glutamate (+) is present in cortical efferent fibers that project to the spinal cord. Glutaminergic corticospinal fibers and terminals are found in all spinal levels, but are especially concentrated in cervical and lumbosacral enlargements. This correlates with the fact that approximately 55% of all corticospinal fibers terminate in cervical levels of the spinal cord, approximately 20% in thoracic levels, and approximately 25% in lumbosacral levels. Some corticospinal fibers may branch and terminate at multiple spinal levels. Lower motor neurons are influenced by corticospinal fibers, either directly or indirectly, via interneurons. Acetylcholine and calcitonin gene–related peptides are present in these large motor cells and in their endings in skeletal muscle.

Clinical Correlations

Myasthenia gravis, a disease characterized by moderate to profound weakness of skeletal muscles, is caused by circulating antibodies that react with postsynaptic nicotinic acetylcholine receptors. Progressive muscle **fatigability** throughout the day is a hallmark of this disease. Ocular muscles are affected first in about 45% of patients (**diplopia, ptosis**) and ultimately in about 85% of individuals. In over 50% of patients, facial and oropharyngeal muscles are commonly affected (**facial weakness, dysphagia, dysarthria**). Weakness also may be seen in limb muscles, but almost always in combination with facial/oral weaknesses.

Injury to corticospinal fibers on one side of the cervical spinal cord (e.g., the **Brown-Séquard syndrome**) results in paralysis (**hemiplegia**) of the ipsilateral upper and lower extremities. With time, these patients may also exhibit features of an **upper motor neuron lesion** (**hyperreflexia, spasticity,** loss of superficial **abdominal reflexes,** and the **Babinski sign**). Bilateral cord damage above C4–C5 may result in quadriplegia; at C1–C2, respiratory arrest is an additional complication. Unilateral cord lesions in thoracic levels may result in paralysis of the ipsilateral lower extremity (**monoplegia**). If the thoracic spinal cord damage is bilateral both lower extremities may be paralyzed (**paraplegia**). Small lesions within the decussation of the pyramids may result in a bilateral paresis of the upper extremities (lesion in rostral portions) or a bilateral paresis of the lower extremities (lesion in caudal portions) based on the crossing patterns of fibers within the decussation. Recall that -plegia, as in **hemiplegia,** refers to a paralysis whereas **-paresis,** as in **hemiparesis,** refers to a weakness or incomplete paralysis.

Rostral to the pyramidal decussation, vascular lesions in the medulla (the **medial medullary syndrome** or **Déjèrine syndrome**), pons (the **Millard-Gubler** or **Foville syndromes**), or midbrain (the **Weber syndrome**) all produce **crossed** (**alternate** or **alternating**) hemiplegias. These present as a contralateral hemiplegia of the upper and lower extremities, coupled with an ipsilateral paralysis of the tongue (medulla), facial muscles or lateral rectus muscle (pons), and most eye movements (midbrain). Sensory deficits are frequently seen as part of these syndromes. Lesions in the internal capsule (**lacunar strokes**) produce contralateral hemiparesis sometimes coupled with various cranial nerve signs due to corticonuclear fiber involvement. Bilateral weakness, indicative of corticospinal involvement, is also present in **amyotrophic lateral sclerosis.**

ABBREVIATIONS

ACSp	Anterior corticospinal tract	CSp	Corticospinal fibers	PrCGy	Precentral gyrus
ALS	Anterolateral system	IC	Internal capsule	Py	Pyramid
APGy	Anterior paracentral gyrus	LCSp	Lateral corticospinal tract	RB	Restiform body
BP	Basilar pons	ML	Medial lemniscus	RNu	Red nucleus
CC	Crus cerebri	MLF	Medial longitudinal fasciculus	SN	Substantia nigra
CNu	Corticonuclear (corticobulbar) fibers	PO	Principal olivary nucleus		

SOMATOTOPY OF CSP FIBERS

LE	Position of fibers coursing to lower extremity regions of spinal cord	UE	Position of fibers coursing to upper extremity regions of spinal cord
T	Position of fibers coursing to thoracic regions of spinal cord		

Review of Blood Supply to Corticospinal Fibers

Structures	Arteries
Posterior Limb of IC	Lateral striate branches of middle cerebral (see Figure 6-41)
Crus Cerebri in Midbrain	Paramedian and short circumferential branches of basilar and posterior communicating (see Figure 6-30)
CSp in BP	Paramedian branches of basilar (see Figure 6-23)
Py in Medulla	Anterior spinal (see Figure 6-16)
LCSp in Spinal Cord	Penetrating branches of arterial vasocorona (LE fibers), branches of central artery (UE fibers) (see Figure 6-8)

8-11 Corticospinal Tracts in Anatomical Orientation

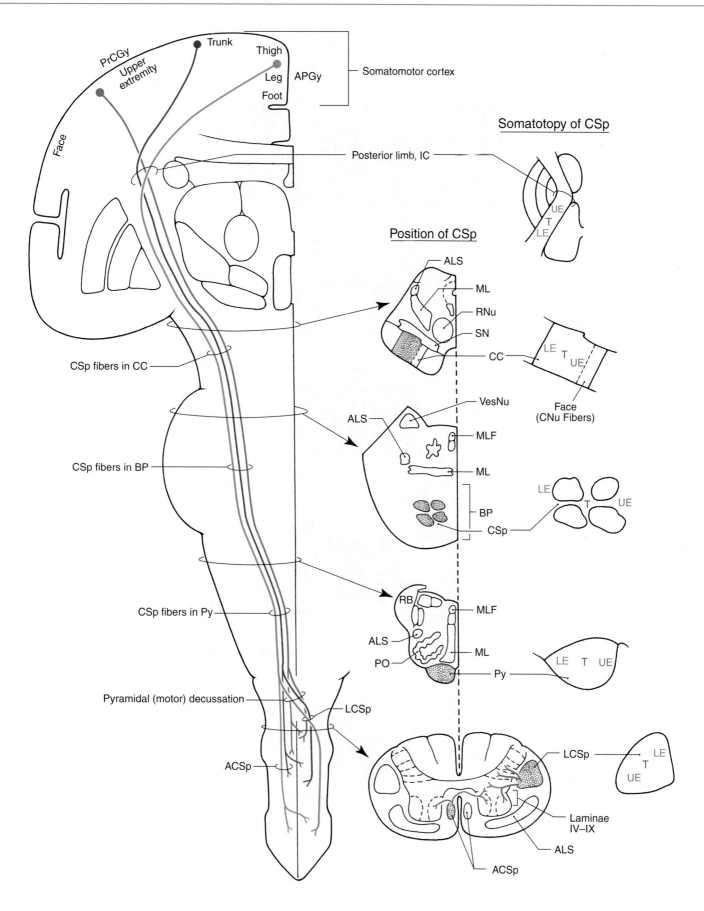

Corticospinal Tracts in Clinical Orientation

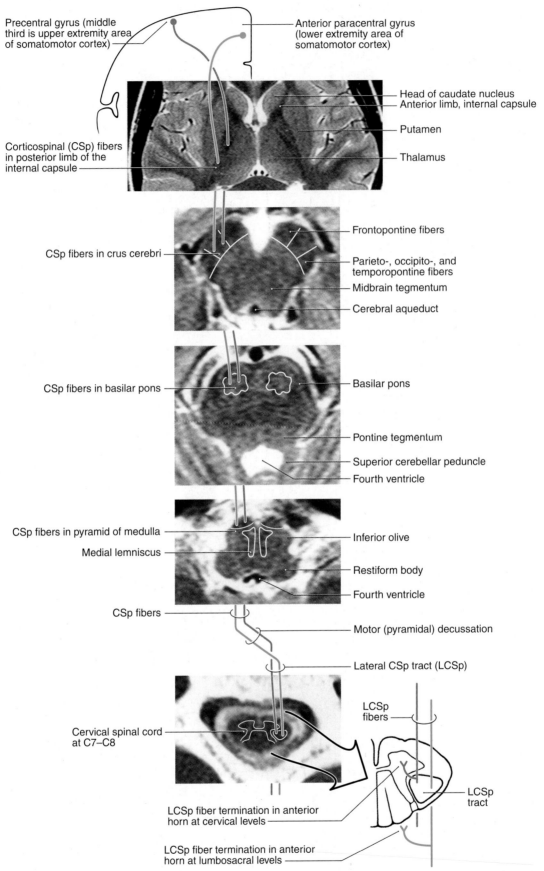

Precentral gyrus (middle third is upper extremity area of somatomotor cortex)

Anterior paracentral gyrus (lower extremity area of somatomotor cortex)

Head of caudate nucleus

Anterior limb, internal capsule

Putamen

Thalamus

Corticospinal (CSp) fibers in posterior limb of the internal capsule

Frontopontine fibers

CSp fibers in crus cerebri

Parieto-, occipito-, and temporopontine fibers

Midbrain tegmentum

Cerebral aqueduct

CSp fibers in basilar pons

Basilar pons

Pontine tegmentum

Superior cerebellar peduncle

Fourth ventricle

CSp fibers in pyramid of medulla

Medial lemniscus

Inferior olive

Restiform body

Fourth ventricle

CSp fibers

Motor (pyramidal) decussation

Lateral CSp tract (LCSp)

LCSp fibers

Cervical spinal cord at C7–C8

LCSp tract

LCSp fiber termination in anterior horn at cervical levels

LCSp fiber termination in anterior horn at lumbosacral levels

8-12A The **corticospinal system** superimposed on CT (spinal cord, myelogram) and MRI (brainstem and forebrain, T2-weighted MRI) showing the location, topography, and trajectory of this pathway in a clinical orientation. The blue and green fibers correlate with those of the same color in Figure 8-11.

Corticospinal Tracts in Clinical Orientation: Representative Lesions and Deficits

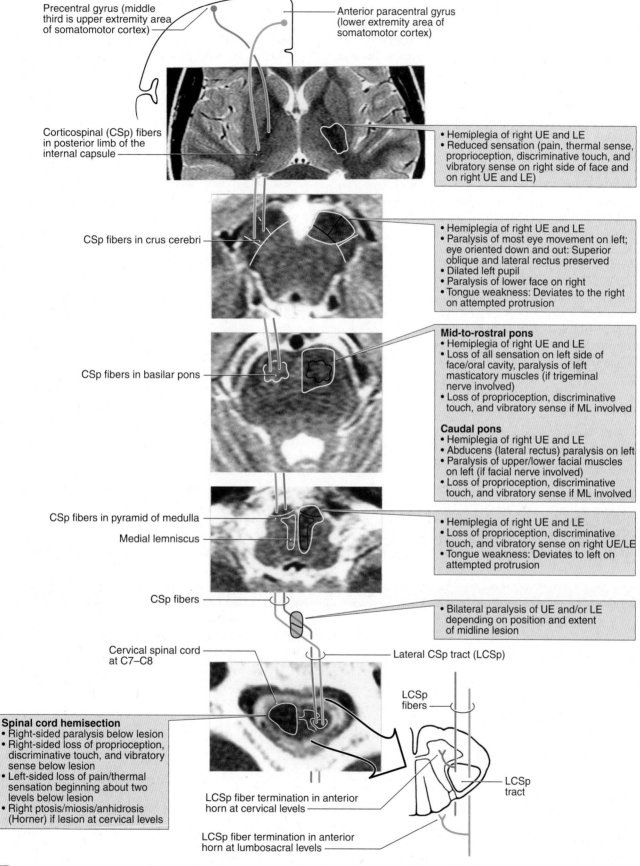

Precentral gyrus (middle third is upper extremity area of somatomotor cortex)

Anterior paracentral gyrus (lower extremity area of somatomotor cortex)

Corticospinal (CSp) fibers in posterior limb of the internal capsule

- Hemiplegia of right UE and LE
- Reduced sensation (pain, thermal sense, proprioception, discriminative touch, and vibratory sense on right side of face and on right UE and LE)

CSp fibers in crus cerebri

- Hemiplegia of right UE and LE
- Paralysis of most eye movement on left; eye oriented down and out: Superior oblique and lateral rectus preserved
- Dilated left pupil
- Paralysis of lower face on right
- Tongue weakness: Deviates to the right on attempted protrusion

CSp fibers in basilar pons

Mid-to-rostral pons
- Hemiplegia of right UE and LE
- Loss of all sensation on left side of face/oral cavity, paralysis of left masticatory muscles (if trigeminal nerve involved)
- Loss of proprioception, discriminative touch, and vibratory sense if ML involved

Caudal pons
- Hemiplegia of right UE and LE
- Abducens (lateral rectus) paralysis on left
- Paralysis of upper/lower facial muscles on left (if facial nerve involved)
- Loss of proprioception, discriminative touch, and vibratory sense if ML involved

CSp fibers in pyramid of medulla

Medial lemniscus

- Hemiplegia of right UE and LE
- Loss of proprioception, discriminative touch, and vibratory sense on right UE/LE
- Tongue weakness: Deviates to left on attempted protrusion

CSp fibers

- Bilateral paralysis of UE and/or LE depending on position and extent of midline lesion

Cervical spinal cord at C7–C8

Lateral CSp tract (LCSp)

LCSp fibers

Spinal cord hemisection
- Right-sided paralysis below lesion
- Right-sided loss of proprioception, discriminative touch, and vibratory sense below lesion
- Left-sided loss of pain/thermal sensation beginning about two levels below lesion
- Right ptosis/miosis/anhidrosis (Horner) if lesion at cervical levels

LCSp tract

LCSp fiber termination in anterior horn at cervical levels

LCSp fiber termination in anterior horn at lumbosacral levels

8-12B Representative lesions within the CNS that involve the **corticospinal system** and the deficits (in pink boxes) that correlate with the level and laterality of each lesion. Note that the laterality (R/L) of the deficits is determined by whether the lesion is on the left or right side of the MRI/CT; this reinforces important clinical concepts.

Corticonuclear Fibers in Anatomical Orientation

8-13 The origin, course, and distribution of **corticonuclear fibers** to brainstem motor nuclei. These fibers influence—either directly or through neurons in the immediately adjacent reticular formation—the **motor nuclei of oculomotor, trochlear, trigeminal, abducens, facial, glossopharyngeal** and **vagus** (both via **nucleus ambiguus**), **accessory,** and **hypoglossal** nerves.

Corticonuclear fibers arise in the frontal eye fields (areas 6 and 8 in caudal portions of the middle frontal gyrus), the precentral gyrus (somatomotor cortex, area 4), and some originate from the postcentral gyrus (areas 3, 1, and 2). Fibers from area 4 occupy the genu of the internal capsule, but those from the frontal eye fields (areas 8 and 6) may traverse caudal portions of the anterior limb, and some (from areas 3, 1, and 2) may occupy the most rostral portions of the posterior limb. Fibers that arise in areas 8 and 6 terminate in the **rostral interstitial nucleus of the medial longitudinal fasciculus (vertical gaze center)** and the **paramedian pontine reticular formation (horizontal gaze center)**; these areas, in turn, project respectively to the third, fourth, and sixth nuclei. Fibers from area 4 terminate in, or adjacent to, cranial nerve motor nuclei excluding those of III, IV, and VI.

Although not illustrated here, the superior colliculus receives cortical input from area 8 and from the parietal eye field (area 7) and also projects to the riMLF and PPRF. In addition, note that descending cortical fibers (many arising in areas 3, 1, and 2) project to sensory relay nuclei of some cranial nerves and to other sensory relay nuclei in the brainstem.

Neurotransmitters

Glutamate (+) is found in many corticofugal axons that directly innervate cranial nerve motor nuclei and in those fibers that terminate near, but not in, the various motor nuclei (indirect).

Clinical Correlations

Lesions involving the motor cortex (e.g., **cerebral artery occlusion**) or the internal capsule (e.g., **lacunar strokes** or occlusion of **lenticulostriate branches of M₁**) give rise to a contralateral **hemiplegia** of the upper and lower extremities (corticospinal fiber involvement) coupled with certain cranial nerve signs. Strictly cortical lesions may produce a transient **gaze palsy** in which the eyes deviate toward the lesioned side and away from the side of the hemiplegia. In addition to a **contralateral hemiplegia,** common cranial nerve findings in capsular lesions may include: 1) **deviation of the tongue** toward the side of the weakness and away from the side of the lesion when protruded; and 2) **paralysis of facial muscles** on the contralateral lower half of the face (**central facial palsy**). This reflects the fact that corticonuclear fibers to genioglossus motor neurons and to facial motor neurons serving the lower face are primarily crossed. Interruption of corticonuclear fibers to the nucleus ambiguus may result in **weakness of palatal muscles** contralateral to the lesion; the **uvula will deviate** toward the ipsilateral (lesioned) side on attempted phonation. In addition, a lesion involving corticonuclear fibers to the accessory nucleus may result in drooping of the ipsilateral shoulder (or an inability to elevate the shoulder against resistance) due to trapezius weakness, and difficulty in turning the head (against resistance) to the contralateral side due to weakness of the sternocleidomastoid muscle. In contrast to the **crossed** (**alternating**) **hemiplegia** characteristic of brainstem lesions, hemisphere lesions result in spinal and cranial nerve deficits that are generally, but not exclusively, contralateral to the cerebral injury.

Brainstem lesions, especially in the midbrain or pons, may result in the following: 1) **vertical gaze palsies** (midbrain); 2) the **Parinaud syndrome**—paralysis of upward gaze (tumors in area of pineal); 3) **internuclear ophthalmoplegia** (lesion in the MLF between motor nuclei of III and VI); 4) **horizontal gaze palsies** (lesion in abducens nucleus + PPRF); or 5) the **one-and-a-half syndrome** (see also Figure 3-8 and Table 3-2, pp. 53–54). In the latter case, the lesion is adjacent to the midline and involves mainly the abducens nucleus, internuclear fibers from the ipsilateral abducens that are crossing to enter the contralateral MLF, and internuclear fibers from the contralateral abducens nucleus that cross to enter the MLF on the ipsilateral (lesioned) side. The result is a loss of ipsilateral abduction (lateral rectus) and adduction (medial rectus, the "one") and a contralateral loss of adduction (medial rectus, the "half"); the only remaining horizontal movement is contralateral abduction via the intact abducens motor neurons.

ABBREVIATIONS

AbdNu	Abducens nucleus	**OcNu**	Oculomotor nucleus
AccNu	Accessory nucleus	**PPRF**	Paramedian pontine reticular formation
EWpgNu	Edinger-Westphal nucleus	**riMLF**	Rostral interstitial nucleus of the medial longitudinal fasciculus
FacNu	Facial nucleus		
HyNu	Hypoglossal nucleus	**TriMoNu**	Trigeminal motor nucleus
IC	Internal capsule	**TroNu**	Trochlear nucleus
NuAm	Nucleus ambiguus		

Review of Blood Supply to Cranial Nerve Motor Nuclei

Structures	Arteries
OcNu and **EWpgNu**	Paramedian branches of basilar bifurcation and medial branches of posterior cerebral and posterior communicating (see Figure 6-30)
TriMoNu	Long circumferential branches of basilar (see Figure 6-23)
AbdNu and **FacNu**	Long circumferential branches of basilar (see Figure 6-23)
NuAm	Posterior inferior cerebellar (see Figure 6-16)
HyNu	Anterior spinal (see Figure 6-16)

8-13 Corticonuclear Fibers in Anatomical Orientation

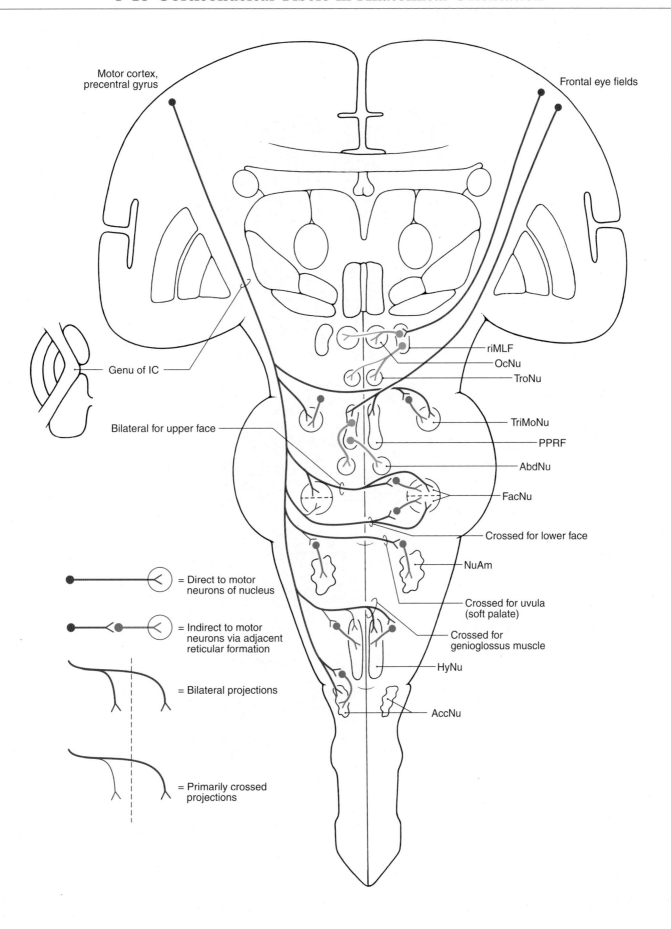

Motor cortex, precentral gyrus

Frontal eye fields

Genu of IC

Bilateral for upper face

riMLF

OcNu

TroNu

TriMoNu

PPRF

AbdNu

FacNu

Crossed for lower face

NuAm

Crossed for uvula (soft palate)

Crossed for genioglossus muscle

HyNu

AccNu

= Direct to motor neurons of nucleus

= Indirect to motor neurons via adjacent reticular formation

= Bilateral projections

= Primarily crossed projections

Corticonuclear Fibers in Clinical Orientation

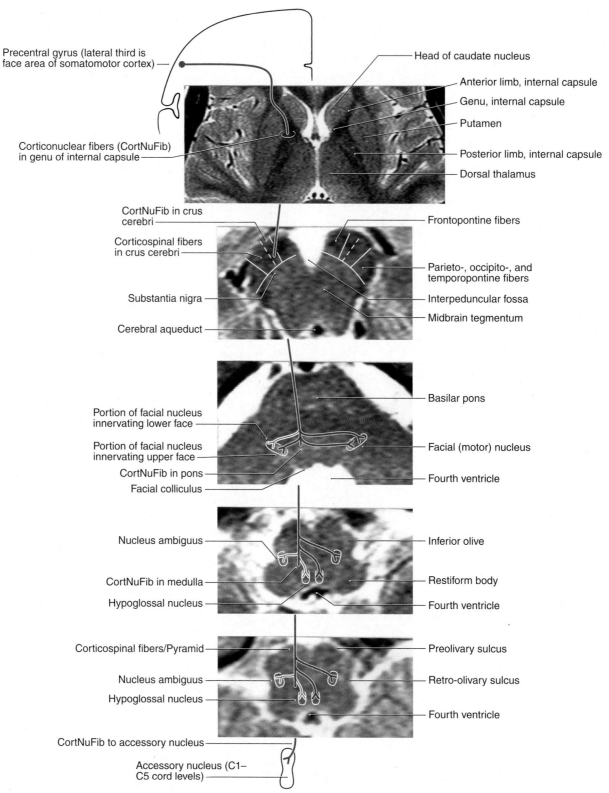

Precentral gyrus (lateral third is face area of somatomotor cortex)

Corticonuclear fibers (CortNuFib) in genu of internal capsule

Head of caudate nucleus

Anterior limb, internal capsule

Genu, internal capsule

Putamen

Posterior limb, internal capsule

Dorsal thalamus

CortNuFib in crus cerebri

Corticospinal fibers in crus cerebri

Substantia nigra

Cerebral aqueduct

Frontopontine fibers

Parieto-, occipito-, and temporopontine fibers

Interpeduncular fossa

Midbrain tegmentum

Portion of facial nucleus innervating lower face

Portion of facial nucleus innervating upper face

CortNuFib in pons

Facial colliculus

Basilar pons

Facial (motor) nucleus

Fourth ventricle

Nucleus ambiguus

CortNuFib in medulla

Hypoglossal nucleus

Inferior olive

Restiform body

Fourth ventricle

Corticospinal fibers/Pyramid

Nucleus ambiguus

Hypoglossal nucleus

CortNuFib to accessory nucleus

Accessory nucleus (C1– C5 cord levels)

Preolivary sulcus

Retro-olivary sulcus

Fourth ventricle

8-14A Fibers comprising the **corticonuclear system** superimposed on MRI (brainstem and forebrain, T2-weighted MRI) showing their location, topography, and trajectory in a clinical orientation. The main projection is indicated by the larger diameter branches. The red fibers correlate with those of the same color in Figure 8-13.

Corticonuclear Fibers in Clinical Orientation:
Representative Lesions and Deficits

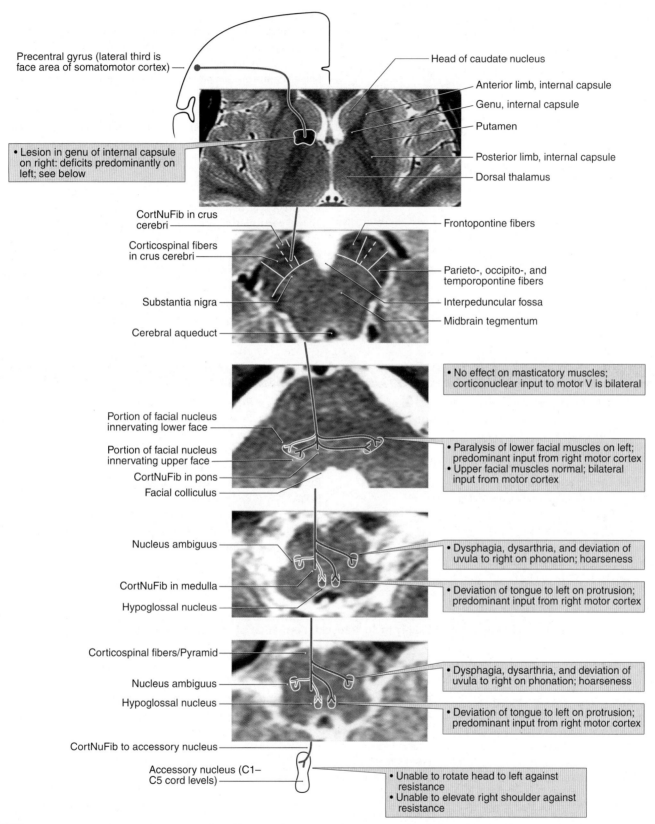

Precentral gyrus (lateral third is face area of somatomotor cortex)

Head of caudate nucleus

Anterior limb, internal capsule

Genu, internal capsule

Putamen

Posterior limb, internal capsule

Dorsal thalamus

- Lesion in genu of internal capsule on right: deficits predominantly on left; see below

CortNuFib in crus cerebri

Corticospinal fibers in crus cerebri

Frontopontine fibers

Parieto-, occipito-, and temporopontine fibers

Substantia nigra

Interpeduncular fossa

Midbrain tegmentum

Cerebral aqueduct

- No effect on masticatory muscles; corticonuclear input to motor V is bilateral

Portion of facial nucleus innervating lower face

Portion of facial nucleus innervating upper face

CortNuFib in pons

Facial colliculus

- Paralysis of lower facial muscles on left; predominant input from right motor cortex
- Upper facial muscles normal; bilateral input from motor cortex

Nucleus ambiguus

- Dysphagia, dysarthria, and deviation of uvula to right on phonation; hoarseness

CortNuFib in medulla

Hypoglossal nucleus

- Deviation of tongue to left on protrusion; predominant input from right motor cortex

Corticospinal fibers/Pyramid

Nucleus ambiguus

- Dysphagia, dysarthria, and deviation of uvula to right on phonation; hoarseness

Hypoglossal nucleus

- Deviation of tongue to left on protrusion; predominant input from right motor cortex

CortNuFib to accessory nucleus

Accessory nucleus (C1–C5 cord levels)

- Unable to rotate head to left against resistance
- Unable to elevate right shoulder against resistance

8-14B Representative lesion of corticonuclear fibers in the genu of the internal capsule that results in deficits (in pink boxes) related to the motor function of certain cranial nerves. Note that the laterality (R/L) of the deficits is determined by the location of the lesion in the genu on the right; this reinforces important clinical concepts.

Tectospinal and Reticulospinal Tracts in Anatomical Orientation

8-15 The origin, course, and position in representative cross sections of brainstem and spinal cord, and the general distribution of **tectospinal** and **reticulospinal tracts**. Tectospinal fibers originate from deeper layers of the superior colliculus, cross in the posterior (dorsal) tegmental decussation, and distribute to cervical cord levels. Several regions of cerebral cortex (e.g., frontal, parietal, temporal) project to the tectum, but the most highly organized corticotectal projections arise from the visual cortex. **Pontoreticulospinal fibers (medial reticulospinal)** tend to be uncrossed, whereas those from the medulla (**bulboreticulospinal** or **lateral reticulospinal**) are bilateral, but with a pronounced ipsilateral preponderance. Corticoreticular fibers are bilateral with a slight contralateral preponderance and originate from several cortical areas.

Neurotransmitters

Corticotectal projections, especially those from the visual cortex, use glutamate (+). This substance is also present in most corticoreticular fibers. Some neurons of the gigantocellular reticular nucleus that send their axons to the spinal cord, as reticulospinal projections, contain enkephalin (–) and substance P (+). Enkephalinergic reticulospinal fibers may be part of the descending system that modulates pain transmission at the spinal level. Many reticulospinal fibers influence the activity of lower motor neurons.

Clinical Correlations

Isolated lesions of only tectospinal and reticulospinal fibers are essentially never seen. **Tectospinal fibers** project to upper cervical levels where they influence reflex movement of the head and neck. Such movements may be diminished or slowed in patients with damage to these fibers. **Pontoreticulospinal (medial reticulospinal) fibers** are excitatory to extensor motor neurons and to neurons innervating axial musculature; some of these fibers also may inhibit flexor motor neurons. In contrast, some **bulboreticulospinal (lateral reticulospinal) fibers** are primarily inhibitory to extensor motor neurons and neurons innervating muscles of the neck and back; these fibers also may excite flexor motor neurons via interneurons.

Reticulospinal (and vestibulospinal) fibers contribute to the **spasticity** that develops in patients having lesions of corticospinal fibers. These fibers, particularly reticulospinal fibers, also contribute to the tonic extension of the arms and legs seen in **decerebrate rigidity** when spinal motor neurons are released from descending cortical control. The sudden increase in extensor rigidity, seen in decerebrate patients when a noxious stimulus is applied to, for example, the skin between the toes, is mediated via spinoreticular fibers (traveling in the ALS) that end on reticulospinal neurons whose axons descend to increase the level of excitation to extensor motor neurons.

ABBREVIATIONS

ALS	Anterolateral system	PO	Principal olivary nucleus
ATegDec	Anterior tegmental decussation (rubrospinal fibers)	PTegDec	Posterior tegmental decussation (tectospinal fibers)
BP	Basilar pons	Py	Pyramid
CC	Crus cerebri	RB	Restiform body
CRet	Corticoreticular fibers	RetNu	Reticular nuclei
CTec	Corticotectal fibers	RetSp	Reticulospinal tract(s)
GigRetNu	Gigantocellular reticular nucleus	RNu	Red nucleus
LCSp	Lateral corticospinal tract	RuSp	Rubrospinal tract
ML	Medial lemniscus	SC	Superior colliculus
MLF	Medial longitudinal fasciculus	SN	Substantia nigra
MVNu	Medial vestibular nucleus	SpVNu	Spinal (or inferior) vestibular nucleus
OcNu	Oculomotor nucleus	TecSp	Tectospinal tract

Review of Blood Supply to SC, Reticular Formation of Pons and Medulla, and TecSp and RetSp Tracts	
Structures	**Arteries**
SC	Long circumferential branches (quadrigeminal branch) of posterior cerebral plus some from superior cerebellar and posterior choroidal (see Figure 6-30)
Pontine Reticular Formation	Long circumferential branches of basilar plus branches of superior cerebellar in rostral pons (see Figure 6-23)
Medullary Recticular Formation	Branches of vertebral plus paramedian branches of basilar at medulla–pons junction (see Figure 6-16)
TecSp and RetSp	Branches of central artery (TecSp and Medullary RetSp); tracts penetrating branches of arterial vasocorona (Pontine RetSp) (see Figures 6-16 and 6-8)

8-15 Tectospinal and Reticulospinal Tracts in Anatomical Orientation

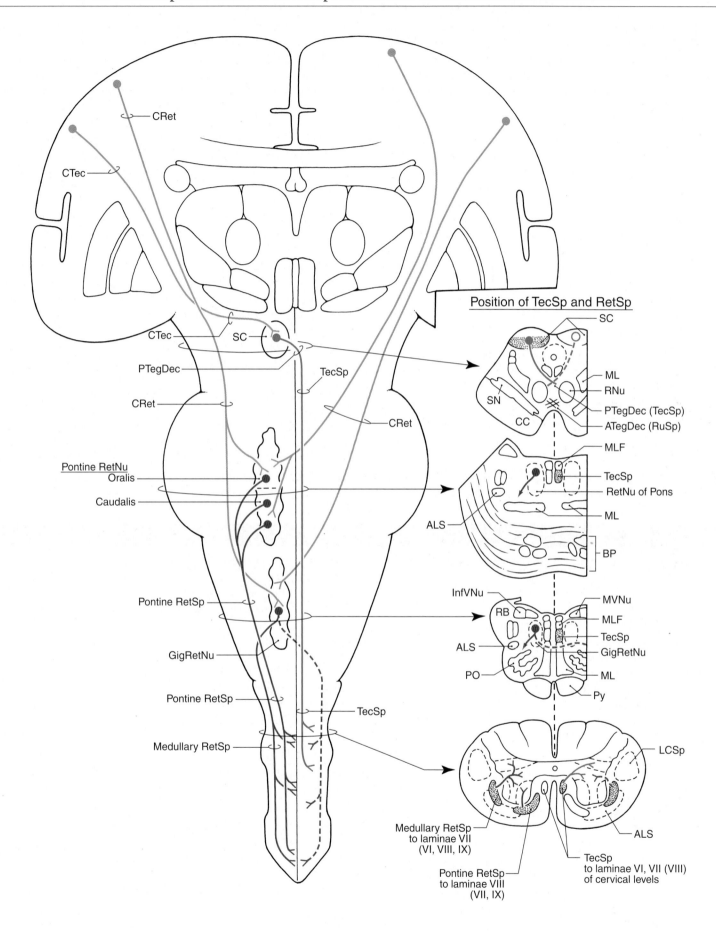

Position of TecSp and RetSp

CRet
CTec
CTec
SC
PTegDec
CRet
TecSp
CRet
Pontine RetNu
Oralis
Caudalis
Pontine RetSp
GigRetNu
Pontine RetSp
TecSp
Medullary RetSp

SC
ML
RNu
SN
CC
PTegDec (TecSp)
ATegDec (RuSp)

MLF
TecSp
RetNu of Pons
ALS
ML
BP

InfVNu
RB
ALS
PO
MVNu
MLF
TecSp
GigRetNu
ML
Py

LCSp
Medullary RetSp
to laminae VII
(VI, VIII, IX)
Pontine RetSp
to laminae VIII
(VII, IX)
TecSp
to laminae VI, VII (VIII)
of cervical levels
ALS

Rubrospinal and Vestibulospinal Tracts in Anatomical Orientation

8-16 The origin, course, and position in representative cross sections of brainstem and spinal cord, and the general distribution of **rubrospinal** and **vestibulospinal tracts**. **Rubrospinal fibers** cross in the anterior (ventral) tegmental decussation and distribute to all spinal levels, although projections to cervical levels clearly predominate. Cells in dorsomedial regions of the red nucleus receive input from upper extremity areas of the motor cortex and project to cervical levels, but those in ventrolateral areas of the nucleus receive some fibers from lower extremity areas of the motor cortex and may project in sparse numbers to lumbosacral levels. The red nucleus also projects, via the central tegmental tract, to the ipsilateral inferior olivary complex (rubro-olivary fibers).

Medial and lateral vestibular nuclei give rise to the **medial and lateral vestibulospinal tracts,** respectively. The former tract is primarily ipsilateral, projects to upper spinal levels, and is considered a component of the medial longitudinal fasciculus in the spinal cord. The latter tract is ipsilateral and somatotopically organized; fibers to lumbosacral levels originate from dorsal and caudal regions of the lateral nucleus, whereas those to cervical levels arise from its rostral and more ventral areas.

Neurotransmitters

Glutamate (+) is present in corticorubral fibers. Some lateral vestibulospinal fibers contain aspartate (+), whereas glycine (–) is present in a portion of the medial vestibulospinal projection. There are numerous γ-aminobutyric acid (–)-containing fibers in the vestibular complex; these represent the endings of cerebellar corticovestibular fibers.

Clinical Correlations

Isolated injury to rubrospinal and vestibulospinal fibers is really not seen in humans. Deficits in fine distal limb movements seen in monkeys following experimental rubrospinal lesions may be present in humans. However, these deficits are overshadowed by the **hemiplegia** associated with injury to the adjacent corticospinal fibers. The **rubral tremor** (Holmes tremor) and the **cerebellar ataxia**/tremor (all predominately contralateral), as seen in patients with the **Claude syndrome** (a lesion of the medial midbrain), is related to damage to the red nucleus and the adjacent cerebellothalamic fibers, respectively. These patients also may have a **paucity of most eye movement** on the ipsilateral side and a **dilated pupil** (**oculomotor palsy** and **mydriasis**) due to concurrent damage to exiting rootlets of the oculomotor nerve. The sudden increase in extensor rigidity, seen in **decerebrate** patients when a noxious stimulus is applied to, for example, the skin between the toes, is mediated via spinoreticular fibers (traveling in the ALS) that end on reticulospinal neurons whose axons descend to excite extensor motor neurons.

Medial vestibulospinal fibers primarily inhibit motor neurons innervating extensors and neurons serving muscles of the back and neck. **Lateral vestibulospinal fibers** may inhibit some flexor motor neurons, but they mainly facilitate spinal reflexes via their excitatory influence on spinal motor neurons innervating extensors. Vestibulospinal and reticulospinal (see Figure 8-17 on pp. 222–223) fibers contribute to the **spasticity** seen in patients with damage to corticospinal fibers or to the tonic extension of the extremities in patients with **decerebrate rigidity**. In the case of decerebrate rigidity, the descending influences on spinal flexor motor neurons (corticospinal, rubrospinal) are removed; the descending brainstem influence on spinal extensor motor neurons predominates; this is augmented by excitatory spinoreticular input (via ALS) to some of the centers giving rise to reticulospinal fibers (see also Figure 8-15 on pp. 218–219). See Figure 8-17 for lesions that influence the activity of rubrospinal and reticulospinal fibers.

ABBREVIATIONS

ATegDec	Anterior tegmental decussation (rubrospinal fibers)	MVesSp	Medial vestibulospinal tract
CC	Crus cerebri	MVNu	Medial vestibular nucleus
CorRu	Corticorubral fibers	OcNu	Oculomotor nucleus
FacNu	Facial nucleus	PTegDec	Posterior tegmental decussation (tectospinal fibers)
InfVNu	Inferior (or spinal) vestibular nucleus	Py	Pyramid
LCSp	Lateral corticospinal tract	RNu	Red nucleus
LRNu	Lateral reticular nucleus	RuSp	Rubrospinal tract
LVNu	Lateral vestibular nucleus	SC	Superior colliculus
LVesSp	Lateral vestibulospinal tract	SVNu	Superior vestibular nucleus
ML	Medial lemniscus	TecSp	Tectospinal tract
MLF	Medial longitudinal fasciculus	VesSp	Vestibulospinal tracts

Review of Blood Supply to RNu, Vestibular Nuclei, MFL and RuSp, and Vestibulospinal Tracts

Structures	Arteries
RNu	Medial branches of posterior cerebral and posterior communicating plus some from short circumferential branches of posterior cerebral (see Figure 6-30)
Vestibular Nuclei	Posterior inferior cerebellar in medulla (see Figure 6-16) and long circumferential branches in pons (see Figure 6-23)
MLF	Long circumferential branches of basilar in pons (see Figure 6-23) and anterior spinal in medulla (see Figure 6-16)
MVesSp	Branches of central artery (see Figures 6-8 and 6-16)
LVesSp and RuSp	Penetrating branches of arterial vasocorona plus terminal branches of central artery (see Figure 6-8)

8-16 Rubrospinal and Vestibulospinal Tracts in Anatomical Orientation

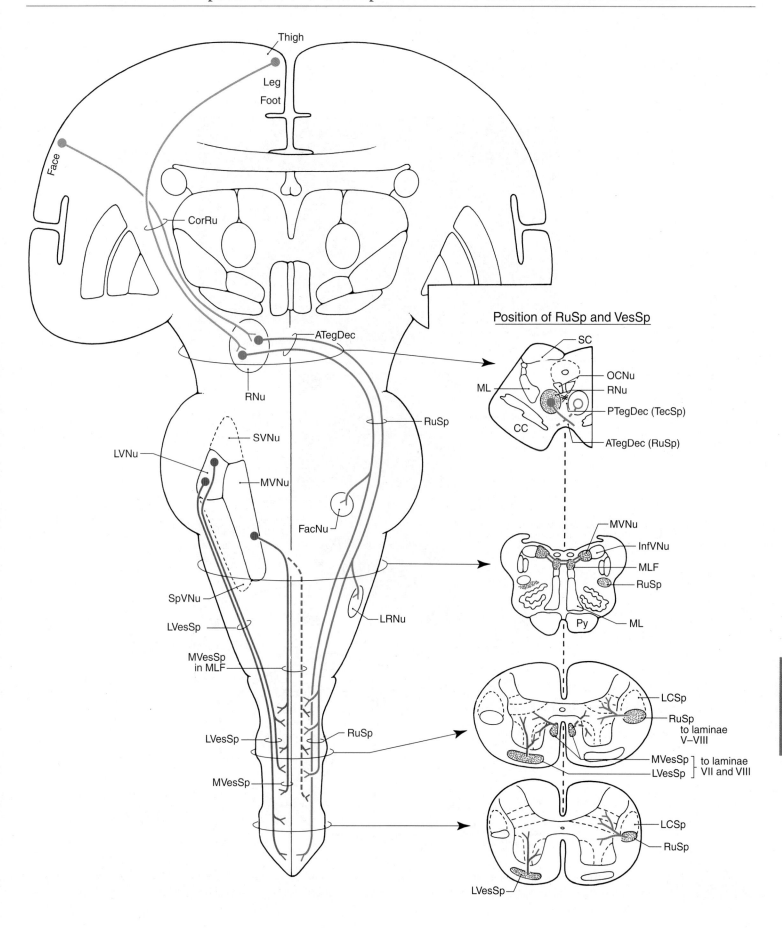

Position of RuSp and VesSp

Rubrospinal, Reticulospinal, and Vestibulospinal Fibers: Clinical Orientation

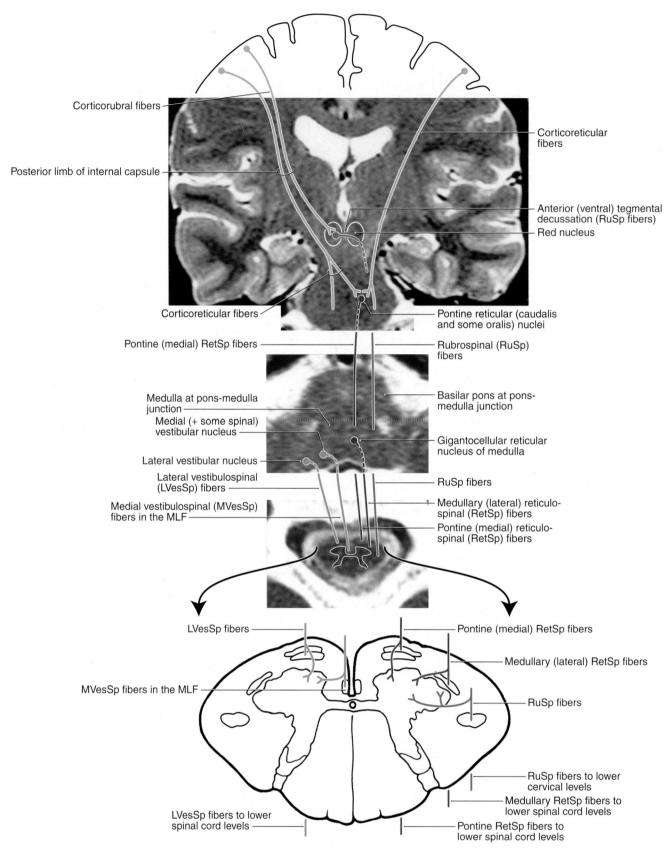

Corticorubral fibers

Posterior limb of internal capsule

Corticoreticular fibers

Corticoreticular fibers

Anterior (ventral) tegmental decussation (RuSp fibers)

Red nucleus

Pontine reticular (caudalis and some oralis) nuclei

Pontine (medial) RetSp fibers

Rubrospinal (RuSp) fibers

Medulla at pons-medulla junction

Medial (+ some spinal) vestibular nucleus

Lateral vestibular nucleus

Lateral vestibulospinal (LVesSp) fibers

Medial vestibulospinal (MVesSp) fibers in the MLF

Basilar pons at pons-medulla junction

Gigantocellular reticular nucleus of medulla

RuSp fibers

Medullary (lateral) reticulo-spinal (RetSp) fibers

Pontine (medial) reticulo-spinal (RetSp) fibers

LVesSp fibers

MVesSp fibers in the MLF

Pontine (medial) RetSp fibers

Medullary (lateral) RetSp fibers

RuSp fibers

RuSp fibers to lower cervical levels

Medullary RetSp fibers to lower spinal cord levels

LVesSp fibers to lower spinal cord levels

Pontine RetSp fibers to lower spinal cord levels

8-17A **Rubrospinal, reticulospinal,** and **vestibulospinal fibers** superimposed on CT (spinal cord, myelogram) and MRI (brainstem and forebrain, T2-weighted MRI) showing their origin, location, and trajectory in clinical orientation.

Rubrospinal, Reticulospinal, and Vestibulospinal Fibers:
Clinical Orientation—Lesions Affecting Their Influence on Spinal Motor Neurons

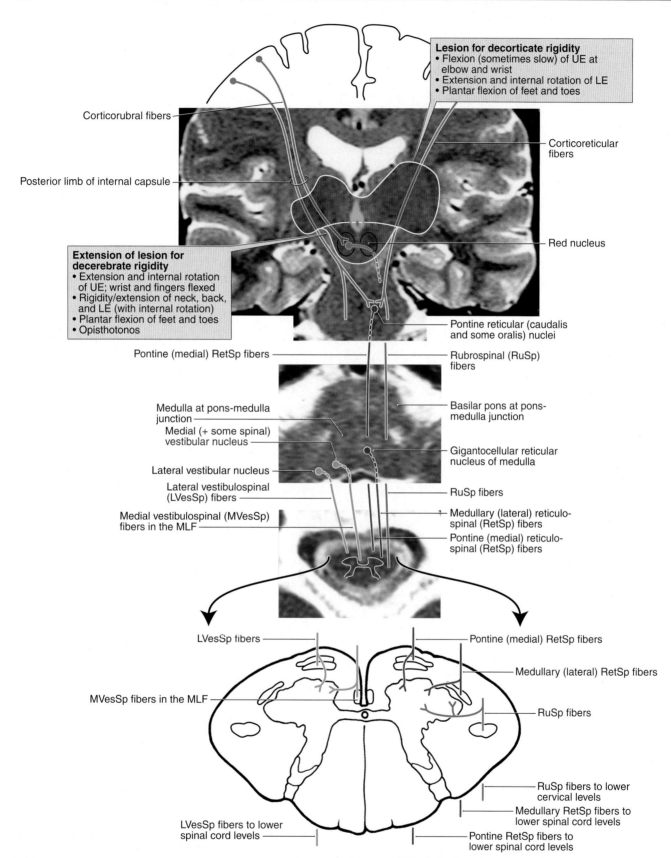

Lesion for decorticate rigidity
- Flexion (sometimes slow) of UE at elbow and wrist
- Extension and internal rotation of LE
- Plantar flexion of feet and toes

Corticorubral fibers

Posterior limb of internal capsule

Extension of lesion for decerebrate rigidity
- Extension and internal rotation of UE; wrist and fingers flexed
- Rigidity/extension of neck, back, and LE (with internal rotation)
- Plantar flexion of feet and toes
- Opisthotonos

Pontine (medial) RetSp fibers

Medulla at pons-medulla junction

Medial (+ some spinal) vestibular nucleus

Lateral vestibular nucleus

Lateral vestibulospinal (LVesSp) fibers

Medial vestibulospinal (MVesSp) fibers in the MLF

Corticoreticular fibers

Red nucleus

Pontine reticular (caudalis and some oralis) nuclei

Rubrospinal (RuSp) fibers

Basilar pons at pons-medulla junction

Gigantocellular reticular nucleus of medulla

RuSp fibers

Medullary (lateral) reticulo-spinal (RetSp) fibers

Pontine (medial) reticulo-spinal (RetSp) fibers

LVesSp fibers

MVesSp fibers in the MLF

Pontine (medial) RetSp fibers

Medullary (lateral) RetSp fibers

RuSp fibers

RuSp fibers to lower cervical levels

Medullary RetSp fibers to lower spinal cord levels

LVesSp fibers to lower spinal cord levels

Pontine RetSp fibers to lower spinal cord levels

8-17B Representative lesions in the forebrain that are **supratentorial** (located above the tentorial notch) and then extend downward through the notch and become **infratentorial**. These lesions alter the activity of **rubrospinal, vestibulospinal,** and **reticulospinal fibers** that results in the characteristic deficit (in pink boxes) seen in these patients. In a large supratentorial lesion (**decorticate**), all brainstem nuclei (including the red nucleus) are intact. When the lesion becomes infratentorial, the red nucleus influence is removed, the extensor rigidity predominates and the patient becomes **decerebrate**. This extensor posturing is, exacerbated by incoming signals from the anterolateral system; the **decerebrate posturing** is increased during stimulation. See Chapter 9 for additional information on herniation syndromes.

Blank Master Drawing for Motor Pathways

8-18 Blank master drawing for motor pathways. This illustration is provided for self-evaluation of motor pathways understanding, for the instructor to expand on motor pathways not covered in this atlas, or both.

NOTES

8-18 Blank Master Drawing for Motor Pathways

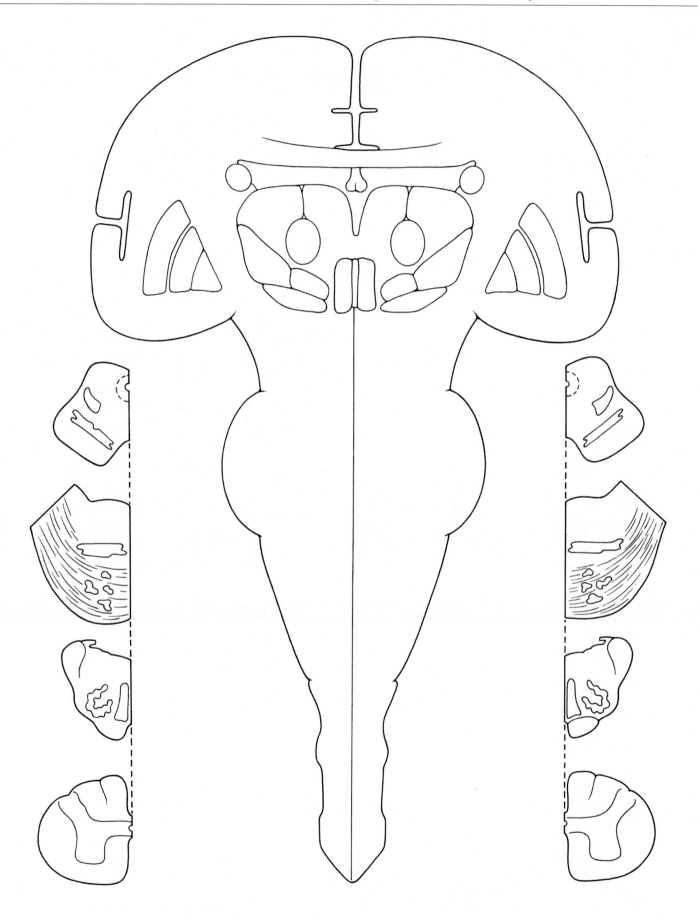

Cranial Nerve Efferents (III, IV, VI, XI–AccNu, XII) in Anatomical Orientation

8-19 The origin and peripheral distribution of GSE or SE fibers from the **oculomotor, trochlear, abducens, accessory,** and **hypoglossal nuclei.** Edinger-Westphal cells adjacent to the oculomotor nucleus are organized into the **Edinger-Westphal centrally projecting nucleus (EWcpNu)** and the **Edinger-Westphal preganglionic nucleus (EWpgNu).** Neurons of the **EWcpNu** project to the spinal cord and a variety of brainstem nuclei (such as parabrachial, inferior olivary, dorsal raphe) that are involved in stress and food/drink intake behaviors. Neurons of the **EWpgNu** are the origin of the VE preganglionic parasympathetic input to the ciliary ganglion traveling on the third nerve; this is part of the **pupillary light reflex** pathway. **Internuclear abducens neurons** (in green) project, via the MLF, to contralateral oculomotor neurons that innervate the medial rectus muscle (**internuclear ophthalmoplegia** pathway).

The **trapezius** and **sternocleidomastoid muscles** originate from cervical somites located caudal to the last pharyngeal arch; they are designated here as SE. In addition, the motor neurons innervating these same muscles are found in cervical cord levels C1 to about C6.

Neurotransmitters

Acetylcholine (and probably calcitonin gene–related peptide, CGRP) is found in the motor neurons of cranial nerve nuclei and in their peripheral endings. This substance is also found in cells of the Edinger-Westphal preganglionic nucleus and the ciliary ganglion.

Clinical Correlations

Myasthenia gravis (MG) is a disease caused by autoantibodies that may directly block **nicotinic acetylcholine receptors** or damage the postsynaptic membrane (via complement-mediated lysis) thereby reducing the number of viable receptor sites. Ocular movement disorders (**diplopia, ptosis**) are the initial deficits observed in approximately 50% of patients and are present in approximately 85% of all MG patients. Movements of the neck and tongue also may be impaired, with the latter contributing to **dysphagia** and **dysarthria.**

The patient who presents with: 1) **ptosis;** 2) lateral and downward deviation of the eye; and 3) **diplopia** (except on ipsilateral lateral gaze) may have a lesion of third nerve (e.g., as in the **Weber syndrome** or in a **carotid cavernous aneurysm**). In addition, the pupil may be unaffected (**pupillary sparing**) or **dilated** and fixed. Lesions in the midbrain that involve the root of the third nerve and the crus cerebri give rise to a **superior crossed (alternating) hemiplegia.** This is an ipsilateral paralysis of most eye movement and a dilated pupil on the ipsilateral side and a contralateral hemiplegia of the extremities.

Damage to the MLF (e.g., **multiple sclerosis** or small vessel occlusion) between the sixth and third nuclei results in **internuclear ophthalmoplegia;** on attempted lateral gaze, the opposite medial rectus muscle will not adduct. A lesion of the fourth nerve (frequently caused by trauma) produces **diplopia** on downward and inward gaze (tilting the head may give some relief), and the eye is slightly elevated when the patient looks straight ahead.

Diabetes mellitus, trauma, or **pontine gliomas** are some causes of sixth nerve dysfunction. In these patients, the affected eye is slightly adducted, and **diplopia** is pronounced on attempted gaze to the lesioned side. Damage in the caudal and medial pons may involve the fibers of the sixth nerve and the adjacent corticospinal fibers in the basilar pons, giving rise to a **middle crossed (alternating) hemiplegia.** The deficits are an ipsilateral paralysis of the lateral rectus muscle and a contralateral hemiplegia of the extremities. The eleventh nerve may be damaged centrally (e.g., **syringobulbia** or **amyotrophic lateral sclerosis**) or at the jugular foramen with resultant paralysis of the ipsilateral sternocleidomastoid and upper parts of the trapezius muscle.

Central injury to the twelfth nucleus or fibers (e.g., the **medial medullary syndrome** or in **syringobulbia**) or to its peripheral parts (e.g., **polyneuropathy,** trauma, or tumor) results in deviation of the tongue toward the lesioned side on attempted protrusion. A lesion in the medial aspects of the medulla will give rise to an **inferior crossed (alternating) hemiplegia.** This is characterized by a paralysis of the ipsilateral side of the tongue (twelfth root damage) and contralateral hemiplegia of the extremities (damage to corticospinal fibers in the pyramid).

ABBREVIATIONS

AbdNr	Abducens nerve	**OcNu**	Oculomotor nucleus
AbdNu	Abducens nucleus	**PO**	Principal olivary nucleus
AccNr	Accessory nerve	**Py**	Pyramid
AccNu	Accessory nucleus	**RNu**	Red nucleus
BP	Basilar pons	**SC**	Superior colliculus
CC	Crus cerebri	**SCP, Dec**	Superior cerebellar peduncle, decussation
EWpgNu	Edinger-Westphal preganglionic nucleus	**TroDec**	Trochlear decussation
FacCol	Facial colliculus	**TroNr**	Trochlear nerve
HyNr	Hypoglossal nerve	**TroNu**	Trochlear nucleus
HyNu	Hypoglossal nucleus		
ML	Medial lemniscus		**Ganglion**
MLF	Medial longitudinal fasciculus	1 Ciliary	
OcNr	Oculomotor nerve		

Review of Blood Supply to OcNu, TroNu, AbdNu, and HyNu and the Internal Course of Their Fibers	
Structures	**Arteries**
OcNu and Fibers	Medial branches of posterior cerebral and posterior communicating (see Figure 6-30)
TroNu	Paramedian branches of basilar bifurcation (see Figure 6-30)
AbdNu	Long circumferential branches of basilar (see Figure 6-23)
Abducens Fibers in **BP**	Paramedian branches of basilar (see Figure 6-23)
HyNu and Fibers	Anterior spinal (see Figure 6-16)

8-19 Cranial Nerve Efferents (III, IV, VI, XI—AccNu, and XII) in Anatomical Orientation

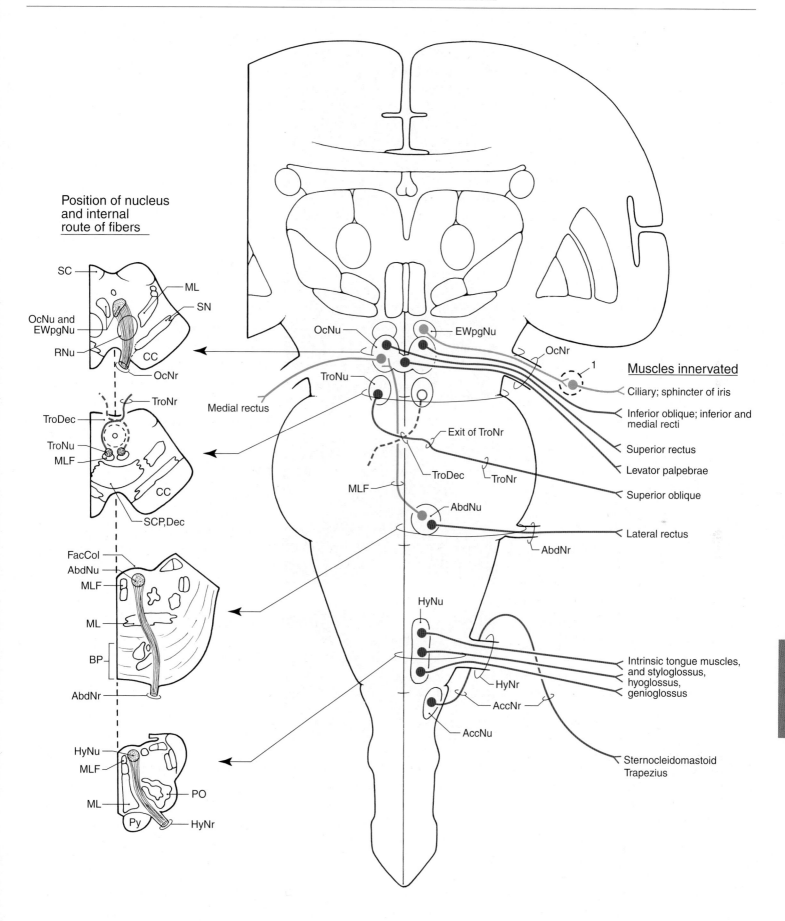

Position of nucleus and internal route of fibers

SC
ML
OcNu and EWpgNu
SN
RNu
CC
OcNr

TroNr
TroDec
TroNu
MLF
CC
SCP,Dec

FacCol
AbdNu
MLF
ML
BP
AbdNr

HyNu
MLF
ML
Py
PO
HyNr

OcNu
EWpgNu
OcNr
1

Muscles innervated

Ciliary; sphincter of iris

Inferior oblique; inferior and medial recti

Superior rectus

Levator palpebrae

Superior oblique

Lateral rectus

Intrinsic tongue muscles, and styloglossus, hyoglossus, genioglossus

Sternocleidomastoid Trapezius

TroNu
Medial rectus
Exit of TroNr
TroDec
TroNr
MLF
AbdNu
AbdNr

HyNu
HyNr
AccNr
AccNu

Cranial Nerve Efferents (III, IV, VI, and XII) in Clinical Orientation

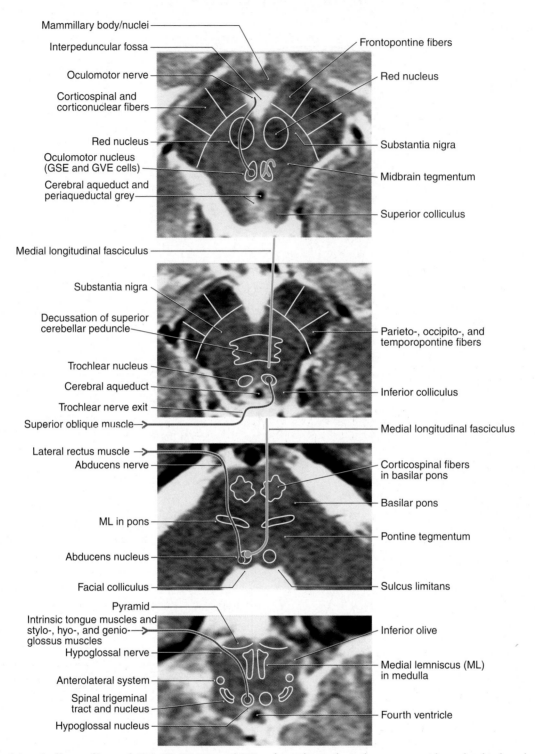

Mammillary body/nuclei

Interpeduncular fossa

Oculomotor nerve

Corticospinal and corticonuclear fibers

Red nucleus

Oculomotor nucleus (GSE and GVE cells)

Cerebral aqueduct and periaqueductal grey

Frontopontine fibers

Red nucleus

Substantia nigra

Midbrain tegmentum

Superior colliculus

Medial longitudinal fasciculus

Substantia nigra

Decussation of superior cerebellar peduncle

Trochlear nucleus

Cerebral aqueduct

Trochlear nerve exit

Superior oblique muscle →

Parieto-, occipito-, and temporopontine fibers

Inferior colliculus

Medial longitudinal fasciculus

Lateral rectus muscle →

Abducens nerve

ML in pons

Abducens nucleus

Facial colliculus

Corticospinal fibers in basilar pons

Basilar pons

Pontine tegmentum

Sulcus limitans

Pyramid

Intrinsic tongue muscles and stylo-, hyo-, and genio- → glossus muscles

Hypoglossal nerve

Anterolateral system

Spinal trigeminal tract and nucleus

Hypoglossal nucleus

Inferior olive

Medial lemniscus (ML) in medulla

Fourth ventricle

8-20A The nuclei and **efferent fibers of CNs III, IV, VI, and XII** superimposed on MRI (brainstem, T2-weighted MRI) shown in a clinical orientation. Also shown is the internuclear pathway from the sixth nucleus on one side to the third nucleus on the contralateral side. The red and green fibers correlate with those of the same color in Figure 8-19.

Cranial Nerve Efferents (III, IV, VI, and XII) in Clinical Orientation: Representative Lesions and Deficits

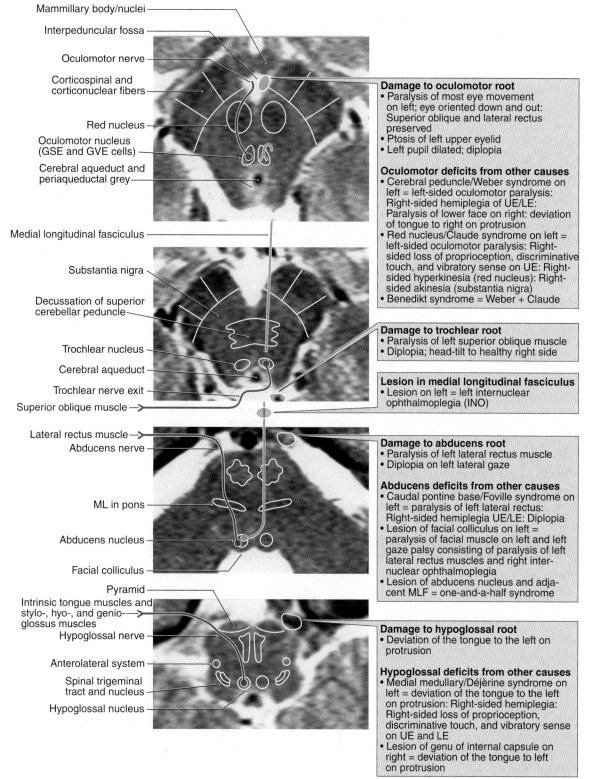

Mammillary body/nuclei

Interpeduncular fossa

Oculomotor nerve

Corticospinal and corticonuclear fibers

Red nucleus

Oculomotor nucleus (GSE and GVE cells)

Cerebral aqueduct and periaqueductal grey

Medial longitudinal fasciculus

Substantia nigra

Decussation of superior cerebellar peduncle

Trochlear nucleus

Cerebral aqueduct

Trochlear nerve exit

Superior oblique muscle →

Lateral rectus muscle →
Abducens nerve

ML in pons

Abducens nucleus

Facial colliculus

Pyramid

Intrinsic tongue muscles and stylo-, hyo-, and genio-glossus muscles →

Hypoglossal nerve

Anterolateral system

Spinal trigeminal tract and nucleus

Hypoglossal nucleus

Damage to oculomotor root
- Paralysis of most eye movement on left; eye oriented down and out: Superior oblique and lateral rectus preserved
- Ptosis of left upper eyelid
- Left pupil dilated; diplopia

Oculomotor deficits from other causes
- Cerebral peduncle/Weber syndrome on left = left-sided oculomotor paralysis: Right-sided hemiplegia of UE/LE: Paralysis of lower face on right: deviation of tongue to right on protrusion
- Red nucleus/Claude syndrome on left = left-sided oculomotor paralysis: Right-sided loss of proprioception, discriminative touch, and vibratory sense on UE: Right-sided hyperkinesia (red nucleus): Right-sided akinesia (substantia nigra)
- Benedikt syndrome = Weber + Claude

Damage to trochlear root
- Paralysis of left superior oblique muscle
- Diplopia; head-tilt to healthy right side

Lesion in medial longitudinal fasciculus
- Lesion on left = left internuclear ophthalmoplegia (INO)

Damage to abducens root
- Paralysis of left lateral rectus muscle
- Diplopia on left lateral gaze

Abducens deficits from other causes
- Caudal pontine base/Foville syndrome on left = paralysis of left lateral rectus: Right-sided hemiplegia UE/LE: Diplopia
- Lesion of facial colliculus on left = paralysis of facial muscle on left and left gaze palsy consisting of paralysis of left lateral rectus muscles and right internuclear ophthalmoplegia
- Lesion of abducens nucleus and adjacent MLF = one-and-a-half syndrome

Damage to hypoglossal root
- Deviation of the tongue to the left on protrusion

Hypoglossal deficits from other causes
- Medial medullary/Déjèrine syndrome on left = deviation of the tongue to the left on protrusion: Right-sided hemiplegia: Right-sided loss of proprioception, discriminative touch, and vibratory sense on UE and LE
- Lesion of genu of internal capsule on right = deviation of the tongue to left on protrusion

8-20B Representative lesions of the roots of CNs III, IV, VI, and XII and the deficits (in pink boxes) that correlate with each lesion. Also shown is a lesion of the medial longitudinal fasciculus. Additional examples of the causes of deficits related to these particular cranial nerves are also indicated. Note that lesions of these cranial nerve roots result in motor deficits on the side of the lesion.

Cranial Nerve Efferents (V, VII, IX, and X) in Anatomical Orientation

8-21 The origin and peripheral distribution of fibers arising from the **motor nuclei** of the **trigeminal, facial,** and **glossopharyngeal** and **vagus** (via the **nucleus ambiguus**) **nerves.** Also shown is the origin of GVE or VE preganglionic parasympathetic fibers from the **superior** (to facial nerve) and **inferior** (to glossopharyngeal nerve) **salivatory nuclei** and from the **dorsal motor vagal nucleus.** The functional component for cranial nerve motor nuclei innervating muscles arising from pharyngeal arches may be classified as SE neurons (see Figures 6-1 and 6-2 on pp. 96–97). Muscles innervated by the trigeminal nerve (V) come from the first arch, those served by the facial nerve (VII) from the second arch; the stylopharyngeal muscle originates from the third arch and is innervated by the glossopharyngeal nerve (IX), and the muscles derived from the fourth arch are served by the vagus nerve (X).

Neurotransmitters

The transmitter found in the cells of cranial nerve motor nuclei, and in their peripheral endings, is acetylcholine; calcitonin gene–related peptide (CGRP) is also colocalized in these motor neurons. This substance is also present in preganglionic and postganglionic parasympathetic neurons.

Clinical Correlations

Patients with **myasthenia gravis** frequently have oropharyngeal symptoms and complications that result in **dysarthria,** and **dysphagia.** These individuals have difficulty chewing and swallowing, their jaw may hang open, and the mobility of facial muscles is decreased. **Impaired hearing** (weakness of tensor tympani) and **hyperacusis** (increased hearing sensitivity caused by weakness of the stapedius muscle) also may be present.

Symptoms of: 1) a loss of pain, temperature, and touch on the ipsilateral face and in the oral and nasal cavities; 2) **paralysis** of ipsilateral masticatory muscles (jaw deviates to the lesioned side when closed); and 3) loss of the afferent limb of the **corneal reflex** may specify damage to the fifth nerve (e.g., **meningioma, trauma**). If especially large, a **vestibular schwannoma** may compress the trigeminal nerve root and result in a hemifacial sensory loss that may include the oral cavity. **Trigeminal neuralgia (tic douloureux)** is an intense, sudden, intermittent pain in the area of the cheek, oral cavity, or adjacent parts of the nose (distribution of V_2 or V_3, see also Figure 8-7 on p. 202). One cause is an aberrant loop of the **superior cerebellar artery** impinging on the trigeminal root (see Figure 3-4, p. 49).

Tumors (e.g., **chordoma** or **vestibular schwannoma**), **trauma,** or **meningitis** may damage the seventh nerve, resulting in: 1) an ipsilateral **facial palsy** (or **Bell palsy**); 2) loss of taste from the ipsilateral two-thirds of the tongue; and 3) decreased secretion from the ipsilateral lacrimal, nasal, and sublingual and submandibular glands. Injury distal to the chorda tympani produces only an ipsilateral **facial palsy.** A paralysis of the muscles on one side of the face with no paralysis of the extremities is a **facial hemiplegia,** whereas intermittent and involuntary contraction of the facial muscles is called **hemifacial spasm.** One cause of hemifacial spasm is compression of the facial root by an aberrant loop from the **anterior inferior cerebellar artery.** These patients also may have **vertigo, tinnitus,** or **hearing loss** suggesting involvement of the adjacent vestibulocochlear nerve.

Because of their common origin from NuAm, adjacent exit from the medulla, and passage through the jugular foramen, the ninth and tenth nerves may be damaged together (e.g., **amyotrophic lateral sclerosis** or in **syringobulbia**). The results are **dysarthria, dysphagia, dyspnea,** loss of taste from the ipsilateral caudal tongue, and loss of the **gag reflex.** Damage to structures at, or traversing, the jugular foramen results in combinations of deficits called **jugular foramen syndromes.** Internal to the foramen, the deficits may reflect injury to CNs IX, X (described above), and XI (ipsilateral trapezius and sternocleidomastoid weakness), the **Vernet syndrome,** while a lesion immediately external to the foramen may compromise CNs IX to XI plus XII (**Collet-Sicard syndrome**). In this latter case, along with the other deficits, the tongue will deviate to the side of the lesion on protrusion. Bilateral lesions of the tenth nerve may be life-threatening because of the resultant total paralysis (and closure) of the muscles in the vocal folds (vocalis muscle).

ABBREVIATIONS

AbdNu	Abducens nucleus	**SpTNu**	Spinal trigeminal nucleus
ALS	Anterolateral system	**SpTTr**	Spinal trigeminal tract
BP	Basilar pons	**SSNu**	Superior salivatory nucleus
DVagNu	Dorsal motor nucleus of vagus	**TecSp**	Tectospinal tract
FacNr	Facial nerve	**TriMoNu**	Trigeminal motor nucleus
FacNu	Facial nucleus	**TriNr**	Trigeminal nerve
GlNr	Glossopharyngeal nerve	**VagNr**	Vagus nerve
HyNu	Hypoglossal nucleus		
ISNu	Inferior salivatory nucleus		**Ganglia**
MesNu	Mesencephalic nucleus	1	Pterygopalatine
ML	Medial lemniscus	2	Submandibular
MLF	Medial longitudinal fasciculus	3	Otic
NuAm	Nucleus ambiguus	4	Terminal and/or intramural
PSNu	Principal (chief) sensory nucleus		

Review of Blood Supply to TriMoNu, FacNu, DMNu, and NuAm and the Internal Course of Their Fibers

Structures	Arteries
TriMoNu and Trigeminal Root	Long circumferential branches of basilar (see Figure 6-23)
FacNu and Internal Genu	Long circumferential branches of basilar (see Figure 6-23)
DMNu and **NuAm**	Branches of vertebral and posterior inferior cerebellar (see Figure 6-16)

8-21 Cranial Nerve Efferents (V, VII, IX, and X) in Anatomical Orientation

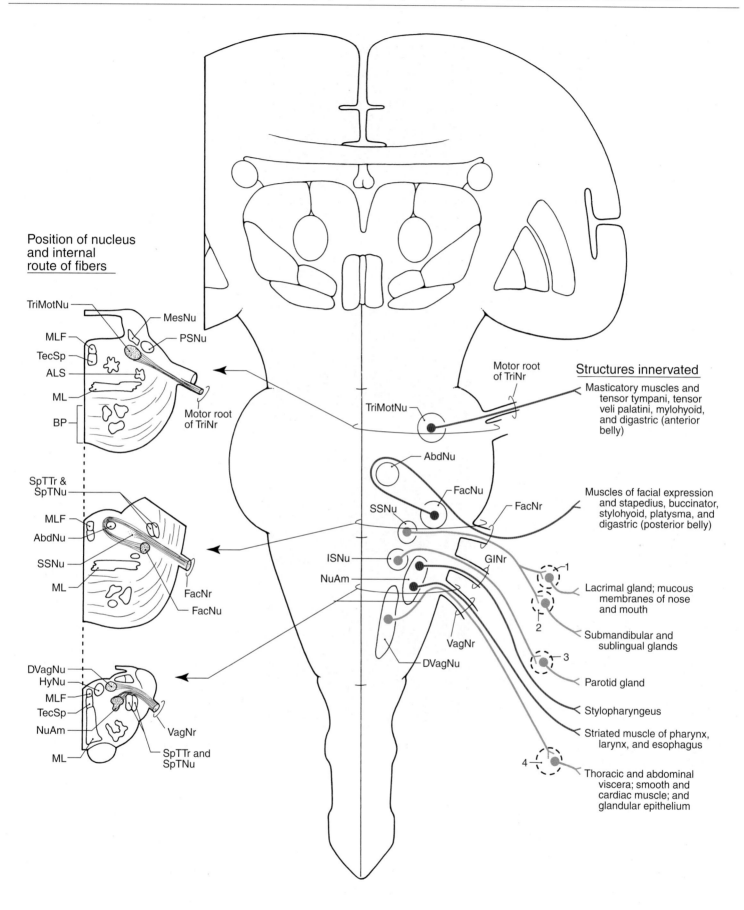

Position of nucleus
and internal
route of fibers

TriMotNu
MesNu
MLF
PSNu
TecSp
ALS
ML
BP
Motor root
of TriNr

SpTTr &
SpTNu
MLF
AbdNu
SSNu
ML
FacNr
FacNu

DVagNu
HyNu
MLF
TecSp
NuAm
VagNr
ML
SpTTr and
SpTNu

Motor root
of TriNr

TriMotNu

AbdNu
FacNu
SSNu
FacNr
ISNu
GlNr
NuAm
VagNr
DVagNu

Structures innervated

Masticatory muscles and
tensor tympani, tensor
veli palatini, mylohyoid,
and digastric (anterior
belly)

Muscles of facial expression
and stapedius, buccinator,
stylohyoid, platysma, and
digastric (posterior belly)

1

Lacrimal gland; mucous
membranes of nose
and mouth

2

Submandibular and
sublingual glands

3

Parotid gland

Stylopharyngeus

Striated muscle of pharynx,
larynx, and esophagus

4

Thoracic and abdominal
viscera; smooth and
cardiac muscle; and
glandular epithelium

Cranial Nerve Efferents (V, VII, IX, and X) in Clinical Orientation

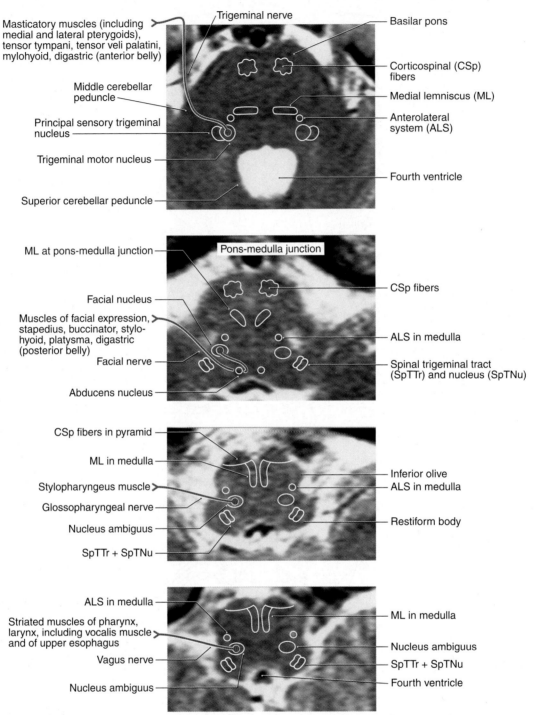

Masticatory muscles (including medial and lateral pterygoids), tensor tympani, tensor veli palatini, mylohyoid, digastric (anterior belly)

Trigeminal nerve

Basilar pons

Corticospinal (CSp) fibers

Middle cerebellar peduncle

Medial lemniscus (ML)

Principal sensory trigeminal nucleus

Anterolateral system (ALS)

Trigeminal motor nucleus

Fourth ventricle

Superior cerebellar peduncle

ML at pons-medulla junction

Pons-medulla junction

CSp fibers

Facial nucleus

Muscles of facial expression, stapedius, buccinator, stylo-hyoid, platysma, digastric (posterior belly)

ALS in medulla

Facial nerve

Spinal trigeminal tract (SpTTr) and nucleus (SpTNu)

Abducens nucleus

CSp fibers in pyramid

ML in medulla

Inferior olive

Stylopharyngeus muscle

ALS in medulla

Glossopharyngeal nerve

Nucleus ambiguus

Restiform body

SpTTr + SpTNu

ALS in medulla

ML in medulla

Striated muscles of pharynx, larynx, including vocalis muscle and of upper esophagus

Nucleus ambiguus

Vagus nerve

SpTTr + SpTNu

Nucleus ambiguus

Fourth ventricle

8-22A The **nuclei and efferent fibers of CNs V, VII, IX, and X** superimposed on MRI (brainstem, T2-weighted MRI) shown in clinical orientation. The red fibers correlate with those of the same color in Figure 8-21.

Cranial Nerve Efferents (V, VII, IX, and X) in Clinical Orientation: Representative Lesions and Deficits

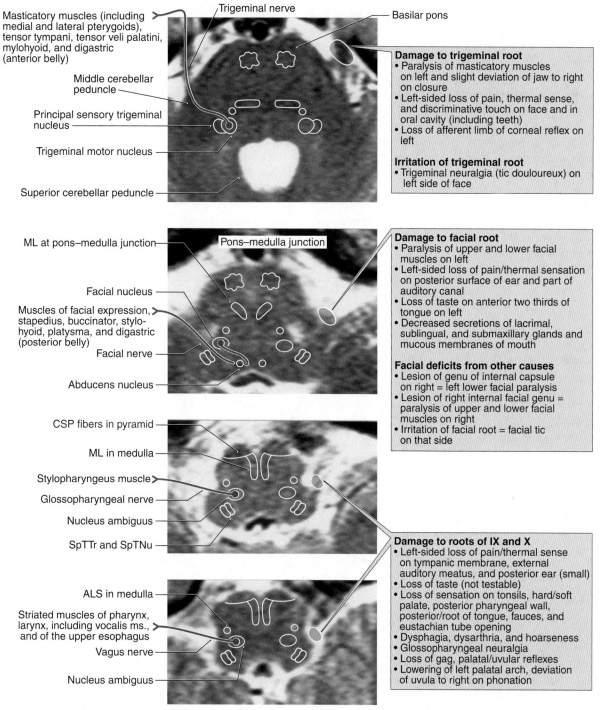

Masticatory muscles (including medial and lateral pterygoids), tensor tympani, tensor veli palatini, mylohyoid, and digastric (anterior belly)

Trigeminal nerve

Basilar pons

Middle cerebellar peduncle

Principal sensory trigeminal nucleus

Trigeminal motor nucleus

Superior cerebellar peduncle

Damage to trigeminal root
• Paralysis of masticatory muscles on left and slight deviation of jaw to right on closure
• Left-sided loss of pain, thermal sense, and discriminative touch on face and in oral cavity (including teeth)
• Loss of afferent limb of corneal reflex on left

Irritation of trigeminal root
• Trigeminal neuralgia (tic douloureux) on left side of face

ML at pons–medulla junction

Pons–medulla junction

Facial nucleus

Muscles of facial expression, stapedius, buccinator, stylohyoid, platysma, and digastric (posterior belly)

Facial nerve

Abducens nucleus

Damage to facial root
• Paralysis of upper and lower facial muscles on left
• Left-sided loss of pain/thermal sensation on posterior surface of ear and part of auditory canal
• Loss of taste on anterior two thirds of tongue on left
• Decreased secretions of lacrimal, sublingual, and submaxillary glands and mucous membranes of mouth

Facial deficits from other causes
• Lesion of genu of internal capsule on right = left lower facial paralysis
• Lesion of right internal facial genu = paralysis of upper and lower facial muscles on right
• Irritation of facial root = facial tic on that side

CSP fibers in pyramid

ML in medulla

Stylopharyngeus muscle

Glossopharyngeal nerve

Nucleus ambiguus

SpTTr and SpTNu

ALS in medulla

Striated muscles of pharynx, larynx, including vocalis ms., and of the upper esophagus

Vagus nerve

Nucleus ambiguus

Damage to roots of IX and X
• Left-sided loss of pain/thermal sense on tympanic membrane, external auditory meatus, and posterior ear (small)
• Loss of taste (not testable)
• Loss of sensation on tonsils, hard/soft palate, posterior pharyngeal wall, posterior/root of tongue, fauces, and eustachian tube opening
• Dysphagia, dysarthria, and hoarseness
• Glossopharyngeal neuralgia
• Loss of gag, palatal/uvular reflexes
• Lowering of left palatal arch, deviation of uvula to right on phonation

8-22B Representative lesions of the roots of CNs V, VII, IX, and X and the deficits (in pink boxes) that correlate with each lesion. Also indicated are deficits related to the fifth and seventh cranial nerves that may originate from other causes. Note that lesions of these cranial nerve roots result in motor deficits on the side of the lesion.

Spinal and Cranial Nerve Reflexes

Examining **reflexes** is an essential part of any **neurological examination** because it provides information critical to the diagnosis of the neurologically compromised patient. All reflexes have an **afferent limb** (usually a **primary sensory fiber** with a cell body in a ganglion) and an **efferent limb** (usually a fiber innervating skeletal muscle) originating from a motor nucleus. The afferent fiber may synapse directly on the efferent neuron, in which case it is a **monosynaptic reflex,** or there may be one, or more, interneurons insinuated between the afferent and efferent limbs; these are **polysynaptic reflexes.** In many reflexes, the influence on the motor neuron may be both monosynaptic and polysynaptic. In the case of cranial nerves, polysynaptic reflexes may also be mediated through the immediately adjacent reticular formation of the brainstem.

The **primary sensory fiber** is regarded as the **first-order neuron** in a pathway. Although the first-order neuron may participate in a reflex, it also contributes information to ascending pathways. The primary sensory fiber may synapse directly on a tract cell, or may communicate through interneurons. In either case, this **tract cell** is regarded as the **second order neuron** in the pathway.

Spinal reflexes may rely on **sensory/afferent** information that arises from the body, enters the spinal cord, influences lower motor neurons, and results in an appropriate response. The same principle applies to **cranial nerve reflexes.** The **afferent input** enters the brainstem on a cranial nerve and may influence motor neurons, and the **efferent outflow** exits the brainstem on the same, or another, cranial nerve. Because of these structural/functional features, the reflex pathways are placed at this location in Chapter 8, following "Sensory and Motor Pathways and Cranial Nerves." The circuits for the more routinely tested reflexes are described; this is not intended as an all-inclusive list.

Particularly brisk or hyperactive reflexes, commonly demonstrated in muscle stretch reflexes, are specified as **hyperreflexia.** Decreased or hypoactive reflexes are described as **hyporeflexia.** A complete absence of reflex activity is **areflexia.** These deviations from normal may be seen in spinal reflexes as well as in cranial nerve reflexes. The aberrations from normal reflex activity may indicate peripheral nerve disease or injury/disease of the brainstem, spinal cord, or forebrain.

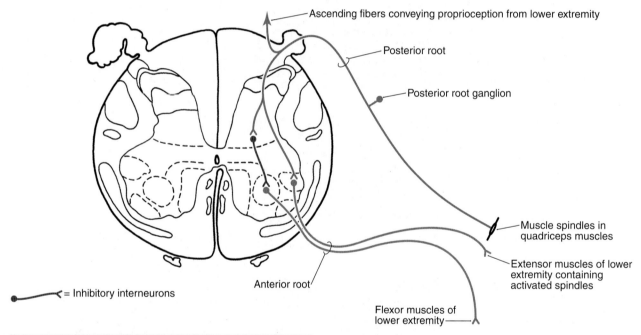

Ascending fibers conveying proprioception from lower extremity

Posterior root

Posterior root ganglion

Muscle spindles in quadriceps muscles

Extensor muscles of lower extremity containing activated spindles

Flexor muscles of lower extremity

Anterior root

= Inhibitory interneurons

8-23 The **muscle stretch reflex** (also called a **stretch** or **myotatic reflex**) is sometimes incorrectly called a tendon reflex or deep tendon reflex (these are clear misnomers); the receptor for this reflex is the **muscle spindle** (within the muscle itself, hence **muscle stretch reflex**). The afferent limb is activated by tapping the tendon of a muscle and momentarily stretching **muscle spindles (primary or secondary)** within the muscle. These action potentials are propagated on **A-alpha (13–20 mm in diameter, 80–120 m/s conduction velocity)** or **A-beta (6–12 mm, 35–75 m/s) fibers.** Their cell bodies are in **posterior root ganglia;** these fibers **monosynaptically** excite motor neurons innervating the muscle from which the afferent volley arose, and the muscle contracts,

precipitating the reflex. Collaterals of the afferent axons synapse on interneurons that, in turn, inhibit motor neurons innervating antagonistic muscles.

Muscle stretch reflexes test the functional integrity of different spinal levels. Examples of these **reflexes,** and their corresponding levels are: triceps **(C7–C8),** biceps **(C5–C6), brachioradialis (C5–C6), Achilles/ankle jerk (S1), patellar/knee jerk (L2–L4),** and the **finger flexor (C7–C8).** Concurrent with the reflex, the central processes send ascending collaterals that relay information to the **nuclei gracilis** or **cuneatus,** depending on the level of the input, and the sensation is perceived. The **patellar reflex** is shown here.

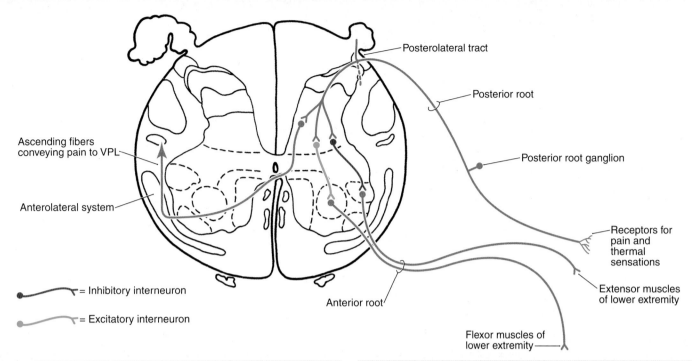

- Posterolateral tract
- Posterior root
- Posterior root ganglion
- Receptors for pain and thermal sensations
- Extensor muscles of lower extremity

Ascending fibers conveying pain to VPL

Anterolateral system

Anterior root

Flexor muscles of lower extremity

= Inhibitory interneuron

= Excitatory interneuron

8-24 The **nociceptive reflex** (also called a **withdrawal reflex** or **flexor reflex**) is activated by tissue damage; action potentials are propagated on **A-delta** (1–5 mm in diameter, 5–30 m/s conduction velocity) and **C** (0.2–5.0 mm, 0.5–2 m/s) fibers. These afferent fibers have cell bodies in the **posterior root ganglion** and they terminate on **inhibitory** and/or **excitatory** spinal interneurons. When a patient steps on a nail, flexor motor neurons of the lower extremity are excited, extensor motor neurons of the LE are inhibited, and the extremity is pulled away from the noxious stimulus. The same arrangement of circuits applies when the hand encounters a noxious stimulus and the upper extremity is withdrawn. Concurrent with this reflex, the recognition of pain is achieved via second order neurons that ascend in the ALS of the spinal cord.

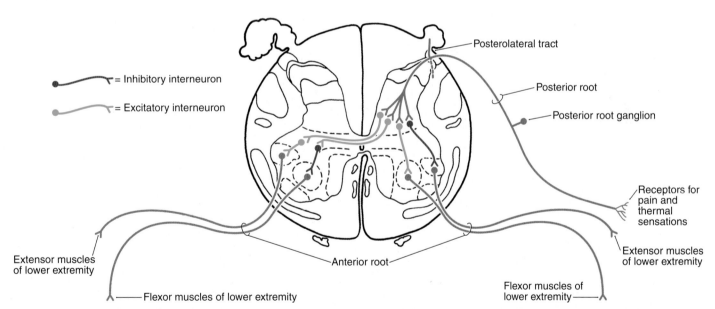

= Inhibitory interneuron

= Excitatory interneuron

- Posterolateral tract
- Posterior root
- Posterior root ganglion
- Receptors for pain and thermal sensations
- Extensor muscles of lower extremity

Extensor muscles of lower extremity

Anterior root

Flexor muscles of lower extremity

Flexor muscles of lower extremity

8-25 The **crossed extension reflex** affects extremities on both sides of the body. The afferent fibers, their input to spinal interneurons, and their respective action (excitatory/inhibitory) on flexor and extensor spinal motor neurons **on the side of the noxious stimulus is the same as in the nociceptive reflex** (see Figure 8-24). The stimulus occurs and the extremity on that side is withdrawn. In an effort to maintain stability, **when an injured foot is withdrawn on the side of the stimulus, the opposite LE is extended.** Consequently, on the side opposite the stimulus, flexor motor neurons are **inhibited** and extensor motor neurons are **excited** and the relative posture of the patient is maintained. This reflex also gives rise to ascending information that reaches a conscious level of perception.

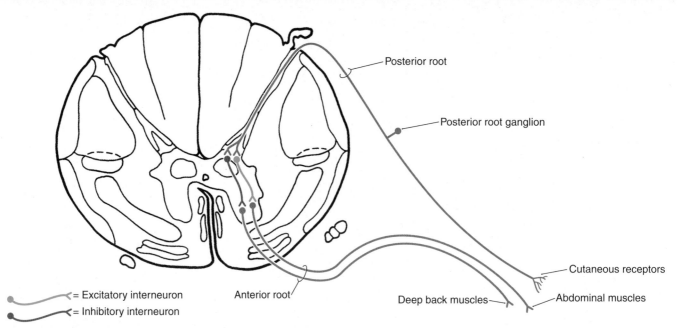

8-26 The **abdominal reflex** is a cutaneous reflex; the afferent limb arises from receptors on **A-delta and C fibers**. It is mediated through **lower thoracic spinal levels (T8–T11)** and is activated by lightly stroking the abdomen about 4–5 cm lateral to, and parallel with, the midline. The afferent fibers enter the **posterior root** and synapse on interneurons. Some of these are excitatory interneurons that, in turn, excite lower motor neurons that innervate the abdominal musculature; the muscles of the abdomen contract and the trunk flexes slightly. Other interneurons inhibit the alpha motor neurons that are innervating deep back muscles; inactivation of these motor neurons decreases the tension in the deep back muscles and increases the efficacy of the abdominal reflex. These deep back muscles extend the trunk. A normal response is occurring when the abdominal muscles contract and the umbilicus rotates slightly to the stimulated side. The sensations created by stroking the abdominal wall will also enter ascending spinal cord pathways and are consciously perceived.

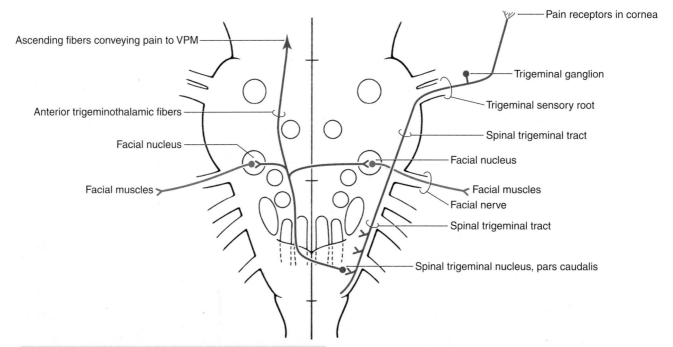

8-27 The **corneal reflex** (also called the **lid reflex**) has its afferent limb in the **trigeminal nerve (CN V)** and its efferent limb in the **facial nerve (CN VII)**. An irritating stimulus to the cornea activates C fibers, the cell bodies of which are in the **trigeminal ganglion**. These axons enter the brainstem on the trigeminal nerve, descend in the **spinal trigeminal tract**, and terminate in the **spinal trigeminal nucleus, pars caudalis**. Pars caudalis neurons project to the contralateral **ventral posteromedial thalamic nucleus** and, en route, send collaterals to the **facial motor nucleus** bilaterally; the facial response is generally more active on the side of the stimulation. Axons of the motor neurons in the **facial nucleus** exit in the **facial nerve** to eventually exit the skull via the **stylomastoid foramen**. Axons in the **zygomatic branch of the facial nerve** innervate the **orbicularis oculi muscle** and the eyelids close in response to a noxious stimulus of the cornea. The noxious information being relayed via ascending fibers eventually reaches conscious perception via anterior trigeminothalamic fibers.

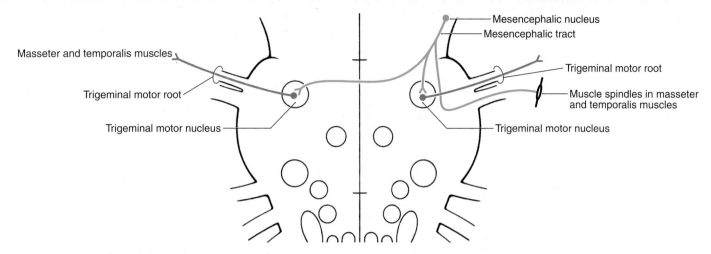

8-28 The **jaw jerk reflex** (also called the **jaw jerk** or **mandibular reflex**) is a cranial nerve version of a spinal **muscle stretch reflex**; this reflex is mediated through the **trigeminal nerve (CN V)**. The axons of the afferent limb synapse on the motor neurons that innervate skeletal muscles (it is a **monosynaptic reflex**). A gentle tap on the chin stretches **muscle spindles** in the **temporalis and masseter muscles**, initiating action potentials on **A-alpha (primary muscle spindles)** and **A-beta (secondary muscle spindles)** fibers. These fibers enter the brain on the **sensory root of** the **trigeminal nerve,** and have their primary afferent cell bodies in the **mesencephalic nucleus**. Collaterals of these afferent fibers project directly, and bilaterally, to the **trigeminal motor nucleus**; axons of these motor cells exit via **the motor root of the trigeminal nerve** to innervate the **temporalis and masseter muscles,** resulting in jaw closure in response to the tap on the chin. This information also reaches a conscious level: the patient perceives the tap on the chin. The jaw-jerk reflex is often increased/brisk (**hyperreflexia**) in patients with amyotrophic lateral sclerosis.

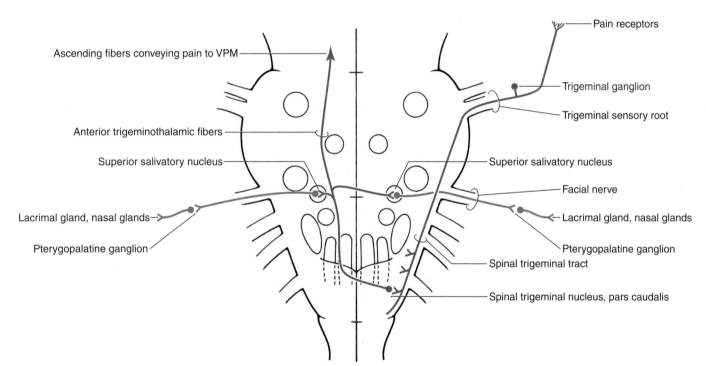

8-29 There are a variety of reflexes in which sensory input results in a visceral motor response. Examples are the **lacrimal (tearing)** and the **salivatory reflexes.** The lacrimal reflex is used here as an example of a **somato-visceral reflex**. The afferent limb is activated by stimulation of **C fibers** and **A-delta receptors/fibers** in the cornea and sclera. This afferent message enters the brainstem on the **trigeminal nerve** (cell bodies in the **trigeminal ganglion**), descends within the **spinal trigeminal tract,** and synapses in the **spinal trigeminal nucleus, pars caudalis**. Collaterals of ascending **trigeminothalamic fibers** (en route to the ventral posteromedial thalamic nucleus) synapse in the **superior salivatory nucleus (SSN)** either directly (shown here) or through interneurons. Parasympathtic preganglionic fibers from the SSN exit on the **facial nerve,** travel to the **pterygopalatine ganglion,** where they synapse, and the postganglionic fibers course to the **lacrimal gland** and to **mucous membranes of the nose.** A nocuous stimulus to the cornea results in tearing and increased nasal secretions and the discomfort is perceived through ascending fibers that eventually influence the sensory cortex.

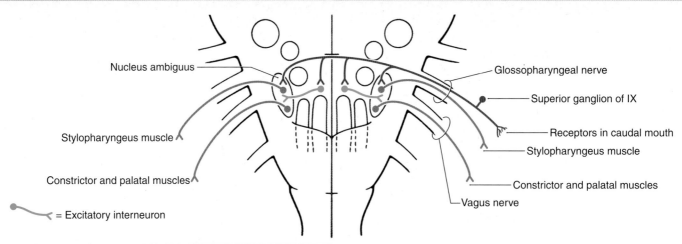

8-30 The **gag reflex** (also called the **faucial reflex**) is mediated through the **glossopharyngeal (CN IX)** and the **vagus (CN X) nerves.** The afferent limb is activated by cutaneous stimulation of **A-delta** and probably **C fibers** on the caudal base of the tongue and/or caudal roof of the mouth (soft palate). This space between the mouth and pharynx is the **fauces,** hence the term **faucial reflex.** The afferent limb is via CN IX with its cell bodies in the superior ganglion of CN IX; the central terminations are in the **nucleus ambiguus,** either directly or through interneurons (both shown here). The efferent limb from the **nucleus ambiguus** travels on CNs IX and X to the **stylopharyngeus muscle** (via IX), to the **pharyngeal constricter muscles,** and to **muscles that move the palate** (via X). In response to irritation in the caudal oral cavity, the pharynx constricts and elevates in an attempt to extrude the offending object, and the discomfort is perceived through pathways to the cerebral cortex.

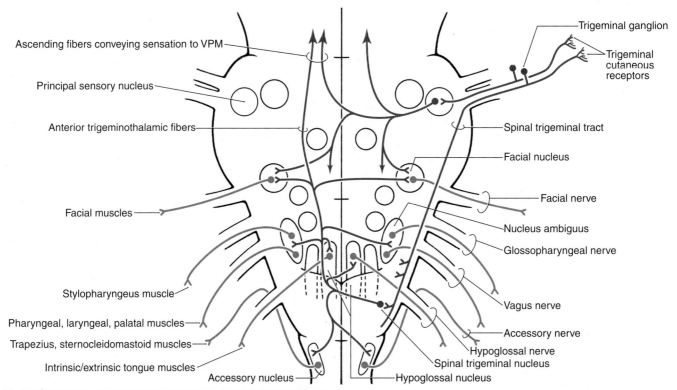

8-31 There are a variety of reflexes seen in infants mediated by CNs V, VII, IX, or XI and XII. Examples of these are the **snout, sucking,** and **rooting reflexes;** they usually disappear by about 1 year of age. These are commonly referred to as "primitive reflexes." However, these reflexes may reappear in patients with dementia, or in individuals with degenerative diseases, or dysfunction, of the frontal lobe.

The afferent limb for these reflexes is via CN V and is activated by touching around (snout, rooting), or in (sucking), the mouth opening. These afferent fibers enter the brainstem via CN V and have cell bodies in the **trigeminal ganglion.** They terminate in the **spinal trigeminal nucleus** (information relayed on **A-delta fibers** from **free nerve endings**) and in the **principal sensory nucleus** (information relayed on **A-beta fibers** from endings such as **Meissner corpuscles** and **Merkel cell complexes**).

Secondary trigeminal fibers, en route to the **ventral posteromedial nucleus** of the thalamus from both the **spinal trigeminal** and **principal sensory nuclei,** send collaterals to the **facial nucleus,** the **nucleus ambiguus,** the **accessory nucleus,** and the **hypoglossal nucleus,** either directly, or via interneurons located in the reticular formation (only the direct are shown here). In response to stimulation around, or in, the mouth opening, the infant's **facial muscles respond** (via the facial nucleus), the **head orients** toward or away from the source of the stimulus (accessory nucleus), the **laryngeal and pharyngeal muscles contract** during **sucking** (nucleus ambiguus), and the **tongue moves** in and out of the mouth or protrudes toward the stimulus (hypoglossal nucleus). These reflexes are absolutely essential to survival (orienting toward nutrition, sucking, tongue and facial muscle responses).

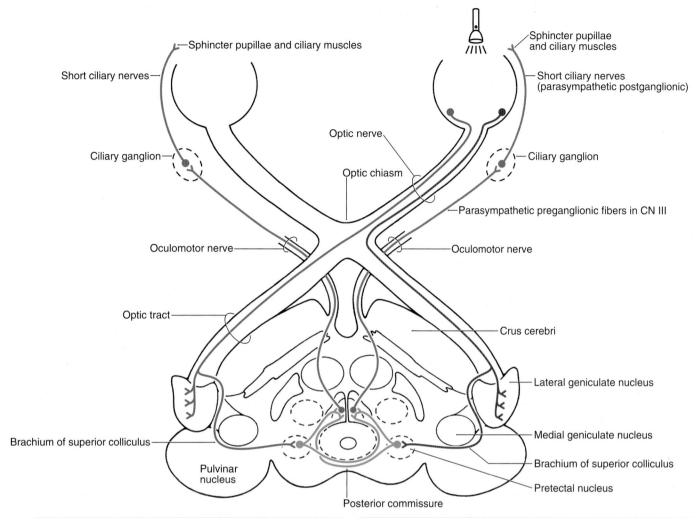

Sphincter pupillae and ciliary muscles

Short ciliary nerves

Ciliary ganglion

Optic nerve

Optic chiasm

Oculomotor nerve

Optic tract

Brachium of superior colliculus

Pulvinar nucleus

Posterior commissure

Sphincter pupillae and ciliary muscles

Short ciliary nerves (parasympathetic postganglionic)

Ciliary ganglion

Parasympathetic preganglionic fibers in CN III

Oculomotor nerve

Crus cerebri

Lateral geniculate nucleus

Medial geniculate nucleus

Brachium of superior colliculus

Pretectal nucleus

8-32 The **pupillary light reflex** (also called the **pupillary reflex** or **light reflex**) has its afferent limb in the **optic nerve** (CN II) and its efferent limb in the **oculomotor nerve** (CN III). Light shined in the eye results in the neural activity conveyed on fibers of the **optic nerve, optic chiasm** (where some cross), **optic tract,** and the **brachium of the superior colliculus,** which synapse bilaterally in the **pretectal area/nucleus.**

The **Edinger-Westphal complex** consists of two portions both of which are immediately adjacent to the oculomotor nucleus (see Figure 6-28 on p. 148). The **Edinger-Westphal centrally projecting nucleus** (EWcpNu) projects to a number of central targets such as the spinal cord, posterior column, parabrachial, trigeminal, and facial nuclei, but not to the ciliary ganglion. The **Edinger-Westphal preganglionic nucleus** (EWpgNu) preferentially projects to the **ciliary ganglion;** these EWpgNu cells are the parasympathetic preganglionic neurons of the third cranial nerve. After receipt of retinal input via the above pathway, both pretectal areas project bilaterally to the EWpgNu. In turn, the EWpgNu sends **parasympathetic preganglionic fibers** on the ipsilateral oculomotor nerve to the **ciliary ganglion,** which in turn sends **postganglionic fibers,** as **short ciliary nerves,** to the **sphincter pupillae muscle** of the iris. In the normal patient, light shined in one eye will result in a pupillary reflex in that eye (**direct response**) and in the opposite eye (**consensual response**).

Example One: In the case of a patient with previously diagnosed **retinitis pigmentosa** and absolutely no perception of light in that eye, when a light is shined in the blind eye, the patient has a direct and consensual **pupillary light reflex.** The explanation of this response is that there is a small population (<1%) of **melanopsin-containing ganglion cells** in the retina that are characterized by large cell bodies and expansive dentritic fields. These cells are intrinsically sensitive to light, do not rely on input from rods or cones, and project to central targets such as the suprachiasmatic nucleus and the EWpgNu. Melanopsin ganglion cells do not appear to participate in form recognition (vision, actually seeing/recognizing things in visual space). Their presence not only explains the pupillary reflex in a blind eye, but is the likely explanation of the fact that patients blind in both eyes may have reasonably normal circadian rhythms.

Example Two: In the case of a patient with a lesion of the optic nerve and a light is shined in the eye on the lesioned side, this patient perceives no light in that eye, **both the direct and consensual pupillary responses are absent,** and the **afferent limb of the reflex is interrupted.** In this example, there is no input to either pretectal area from the eye on the side with the optic nerve lesion.

Example Three: In the case of a patient with a lesion of one optic nerve and a light is shined in the eye opposite the side of the lesion (the good eye), this patient perceives the light in this eye, and there is **both a direct and consensual response.** In this example, the **afferent limb to both pretectal nuclei is intact,** and there is a response in the blind eye because its efferent limb is intact.

Example Four: In the case of a patient with a lesion of the oculomotor nerve on one side and a light is shined in the eye on the side of the lesion, the patient perceives the light (the **afferent limb is intact**) but there is no direct response in that eye; the **efferent limb is interrupted** by the lesion. There is a **consensual response in the opposite eye** in this situation. If the light is shined in the eye on the side opposite the oculomotor root lesion, the light is perceived, and there is a direct response but no consensual response.

Table 8-1 Flow Diagrams of Additional Common Reflexes

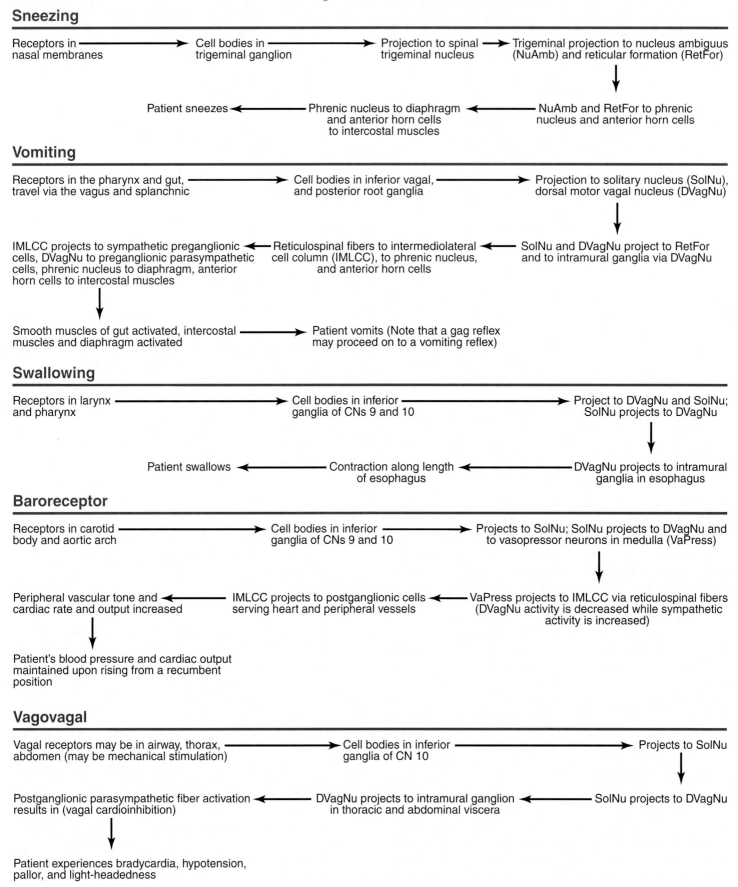

Sneezing

Receptors in nasal membranes → Cell bodies in trigeminal ganglion → Projection to spinal trigeminal nucleus → Trigeminal projection to nucleus ambiguus (NuAmb) and reticular formation (RetFor)

Patient sneezes ← Phrenic nucleus to diaphragm and anterior horn cells to intercostal muscles ← NuAmb and RetFor to phrenic nucleus and anterior horn cells

Vomiting

Receptors in the pharynx and gut, travel via the vagus and splanchnic → Cell bodies in inferior vagal, and posterior root ganglia → Projection to solitary nucleus (SolNu), dorsal motor vagal nucleus (DVagNu)

IMLCC projects to sympathetic preganglionic cells, DVagNu to preganglionic parasympathetic cells, phrenic nucleus to diaphragm, anterior horn cells to intercostal muscles ← Reticulospinal fibers to intermediolateral cell column (IMLCC), to phrenic nucleus, and anterior horn cells ← SolNu and DVagNu project to RetFor and to intramural ganglia via DVagNu

Smooth muscles of gut activated, intercostal muscles and diaphragm activated → Patient vomits (Note that a gag reflex may proceed on to a vomiting reflex)

Swallowing

Receptors in larynx and pharynx → Cell bodies in inferior ganglia of CNs 9 and 10 → Project to DVagNu and SolNu; SolNu projects to DVagNu

Patient swallows ← Contraction along length of esophagus ← DVagNu projects to intramural ganglia in esophagus

Baroreceptor

Receptors in carotid body and aortic arch → Cell bodies in inferior ganglia of CNs 9 and 10 → Projects to SolNu; SolNu projects to DVagNu and to vasopressor neurons in medulla (VaPress)

Peripheral vascular tone and cardiac rate and output increased ← IMLCC projects to postganglionic cells serving heart and peripheral vessels ← VaPress projects to IMLCC via reticulospinal fibers (DVagNu activity is decreased while sympathetic activity is increased)

Patient's blood pressure and cardiac output maintained upon rising from a recumbent position

Vagovagal

Vagal receptors may be in airway, thorax, abdomen (may be mechanical stimulation) → Cell bodies in inferior ganglia of CN 10 → Projects to SolNu

Postganglionic parasympathetic fiber activation results in (vagal cardioinhibition) ← DVagNu projects to intramural ganglion in thoracic and abdominal viscera ← SolNu projects to DVagNu

Patient experiences bradycardia, hypotension, pallor, and light-headedness

* All of these reflexes are mediated through the brainstem. As is the case with brainstem reflexes, the pathways may involve several centers, or nuclei, within the brainstem; only the basic pathways are diagrammed here.

Blank Drawing for the Spinal Cord and Brainstem

8-33 Blank master drawings for spinal cord and cranial nerve/ brainstem reflexes. These illustrations are provided for self-evaluation of the understanding of circuits related to reflexes, for the instructor to expand on reflexes not covered in this atlas, or for both activities. For a wider variety of review possibilities, a cervical spinal cord level and brainstem diagram is given here.

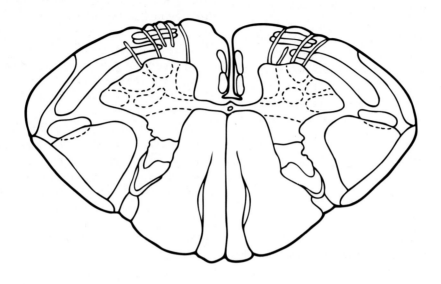

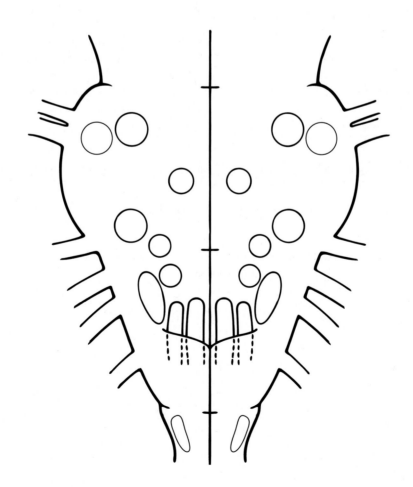

Spinocerebellar Tracts in Anatomical Orientation

8-34 The origin, course, and distribution pattern of fibers to the cerebellar cortex and nuclei from the spinal cord (**posterior [dorsal]** and **anterior [ventral] spinocerebellar tracts, rostral spinocerebellar fibers**) and from the accessory (lateral) cuneate nucleus (**cuneocerebellar fibers**). Also illustrated is the somatotopy of those fibers that enter the cerebellum via the restiform body, the larger portion of the inferior cerebellar peduncle, or in relationship to the superior cerebellar peduncle. After these fibers enter the cerebellum, collaterals are given off to the cerebellar nuclei while the parent axons of spinocerebellar and cuneocerebellar fibers pass on to the cortex, where they end as mossy fibers in the granule cell layer. Although not shown here, there are ascending spinal projections to the medial and dorsal accessory nuclei of the inferior olivary complex (spino-olivary fibers). The accessory olivary nuclei (as well as the principal olivary nucleus) project to the cerebellar cortex and send collaterals into the nuclei (see Figure 8-35 on p. 244).

Neurotransmitters

Glutamate (+) is found in some spinocerebellar fibers, in their mossy fiber terminals in the cerebellar cortex, and in their collateral branches that innervate the cerebellar nuclei.

Clinical Correlations

Lesions, or tumors, that selectively damage only spinocerebellar fibers are rarely, if ever, seen in humans. The **ataxia** one might expect to see in patients with a spinal cord hemisection (e.g., the **Brown-Séquard syndrome**) is masked by the **hemiplegia** of the ipsilateral UE and LE resulting from the concomitant damage to lateral corticospinal (and other) fibers. There are also genetic defects that affect these tracts.

Friedreich ataxia (hereditary spinal ataxia) is an autosomal recessive disorder, the symptoms of which usually appear between 8 and 15 years of age. There is degeneration of anterior and posterior spinocerebellar tracts plus the posterior columns and corticospinal tracts. Degenerative changes are also seen in cerebellar Purkinje cells, in posterior root ganglion cells, in neurons of the Clarke column, and in some nuclei of the pons and medulla. These patients have **ataxia** (early onset), **dysarthria, muscle weakness/paralysis** (particularly in the LEs), and skeletal defects. The axial and appendicular **ataxia** seen in these patients correlates partially with the spinocerebellar degeneration and also partially with proprioceptive losses via the degeneration of posterior column fibers.

ABBREVIATIONS			
ACNu	Accessory (lateral) cuneate nucleus	PSCT	Posterior (dorsal) spinocerebellar tract
ALS	Anterolateral system	PSNu	Principal (chief) sensory nucleus of trigeminal nerve
AMV	Anterior medullary velum	Py	Pyramid
ASCT	Anterior (ventral) spinocerebellar tract	RB	Restiform body
Cbl	Cerebellum	RSCF	Rostral spinocerebellar fibers
CblNu	Cerebellar nuclei	RuSp	Rubrospinal tract
CCblF	Cuneocerebellar fibers	S	Sacral representation
DNuC	Dorsal nucleus of Clarke	SBC	Spinal border cells
FNL	Flocculonodular lobe	SCP	Superior cerebellar peduncle
IZ	Intermediate zone	SpTNu	Spinal trigeminal nucleus
L	Lumbar representation	SpTTr	Spinal trigeminal tract
MesNu	Mesencephalic nucleus	T	Thoracic representation
ML	Medial lemniscus	TriMoNu	Trigeminal motor nucleus
PRG	Posterior (dorsal) root ganglion	VesNu	Vestibular nuclei

Review of Blood Supply to Spinal Cord Gray Matter, Spinocerebellar Tracts, RB, and SCP	
Structures	**Arteries**
Spinal Cord Gray	Branches of central artery (see Figure 6-8)
PSCT and **ASCT** in Cord	Penetrating branches of arterial vasocorona (see Figure 6-8)
RB	Posterior inferior cerebellar (see Figure 6-16)
SCP	Long circumferential branches of basilar and superior cerebellar (see Figure 6-23)
Cerebellum	Posterior and anterior inferior cerebellar and superior cerebellar

8-34 Spinocerebellar Tracts in Anatomical Orientation

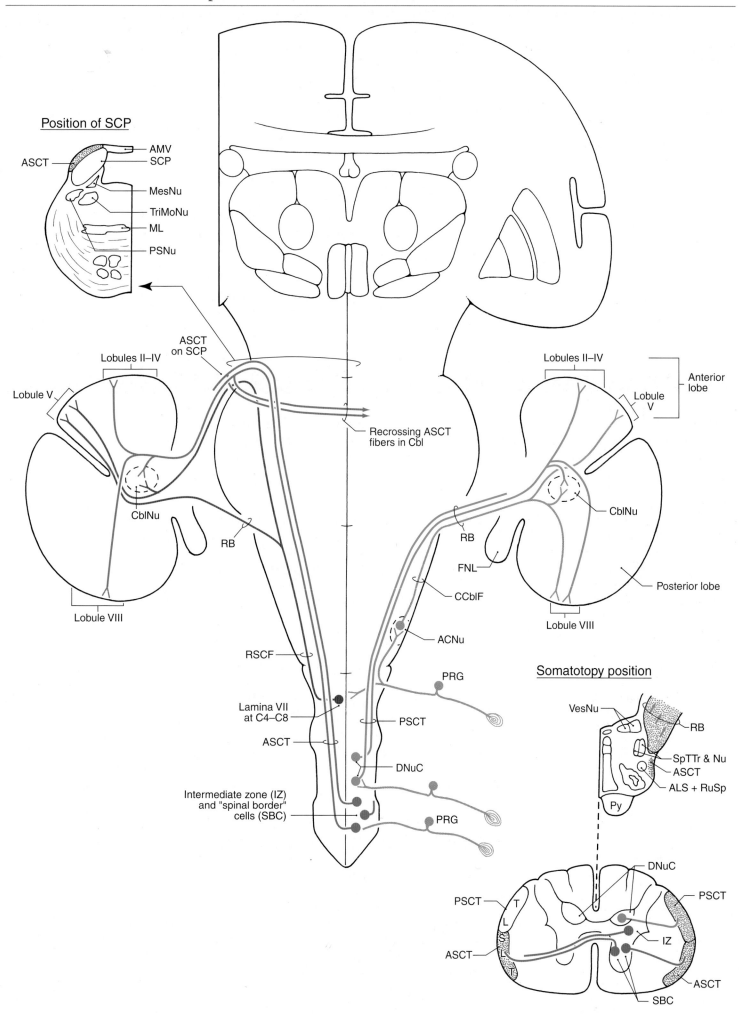

Position of SCP

AMV
SCP
ASCT
MesNu
TriMoNu
ML
PSNu

ASCT on SCP

Lobules II–IV
Lobule V

Lobules II–IV
Lobule V
Anterior lobe

Recrossing ASCT fibers in Cbl

CblNu
RB

CblNu
RB
FNL

Posterior lobe

CCblF

Lobule VIII

Lobule VIII

ACNu

RSCF

Somatotopy position

PRG

Lamina VII at C4–C8

PSCT

VesNu
RB

ASCT

SpTTr & Nu
ASCT
ALS + RuSp

DNuC

Py

Intermediate zone (IZ) and "spinal border" cells (SBC)

PRG

DNuC

PSCT

PSCT

T
L

ASCT

IZ

S
L

ASCT

SBC

Pontocerebellar, Reticulocerebellar, Olivocerebellar, Ceruleocerebellar, Hypothalamocerebellar, and Raphecerebellar Fibers in Anatomical Orientation

8-35 Afferent fibers to the cerebellum from selected brainstem areas and the organization of corticopontine fibers in the internal capsule and crus cerebri as shown here. **Pontocerebellar axons** are mainly crossed, **reticulocerebellar fibers** may be bilateral (from RetTegNu) or mainly uncrossed (from **LRNu and PRNu**), and **olivocerebellar fibers (OCblF)** are exclusively crossed. **Raphecerebellar, hypothalamocerebellar,** and **ceruleocerebellar fibers** are, to varying degrees, bilateral projections. Although all afferent fibers to the cerebellum give rise to collaterals to the cerebellar nuclei, those from pontocerebellar axons are relatively small, having comparatively small diameters. Olivocerebellar axons end as **climbing fibers**, reticulocerebellar and pontocerebellar fibers as **mossy fibers**, and hypothalamocerebellar and ceruleocerebellar axons end in all cortical layers. These latter fibers have been called **multilayered fibers** in the literature because they branch in all layers of the cerebellar cortex.

Neurotransmitters

Glutamate (+) is found in corticopontine projections and in most pontocerebellar fibers. Aspartate (+) and corticotropin (+)-releasing factor are present in many olivocerebellar fibers. Ceruleocerebellar fibers contain noradrenalin, histamine is found in hypothalamocerebellar fibers, and some reticulocerebellar fibers contain enkephalin. Serotonergic fibers to the cerebellum arise from neurons found in medial areas of the reticular formation (open gray cell in Figure 8-35 on the facing page) and, most likely, from some cells in the adjacent raphe nuclei.

Clinical Correlations

Common symptoms seen in patients with lesions involving nuclei and tracts that project to the cerebellum are **ataxia** (of trunk or limbs), an **ataxic gait, dysarthria, dysphagia,** and disorders of eye movement such as **nystagmus.** These deficits are seen in some hereditary diseases (e.g., **olivopontocerebellar degeneration, ataxia telangiectasia,** or **hereditary cerebellar ataxia**), in tumors (**brainstem gliomas**), in vascular diseases (**lateral pontine syndrome**), or in other conditions, such as **alcoholic cerebellar degeneration** or pontine hemorrhages (see Figures 8-36 and 8-38A, B on pp. 246 and 250–251 for more information on cerebellar lesions).

ABBREVIATIONS

AntLb	Anterior limb of internal capsule		PostLb	Posterior limb of internal capsule
CblNu	Cerebellar nuclei		PonNu	Pontine nuclei
CerCblF	Ceruleocerebellar fibers		PO	Principal olivary nucleus
CPonF	Cerebropontine fibers		PPon	Parietopontine fibers
CSp	Corticospinal fibers		PRNu	Paramedian reticular nuclei
DAO	Dorsal accessory olivary nucleus		Py	Pyramid
FPon	Frontopontine fibers		RB	Restiform body
Hyth	Hypothalamus		RCblF	Reticulocerebellar fibers
HythCblF	Hypothalamocerebellar fibers		RetLenLb	Retrolenticular limb of internal capsule
IC	Internal capsule		RNu	Red nucleus
IO	Inferior olive		RetTegNu	Reticulotegmental nucleus
LoCer	Nucleus (locus) ceruleus		SCP	Superior cerebellar peduncle
LRNu	Lateral reticular nucleus		SubLenLb	Sublenticular limb of internal capsule
MAO	Medial accessory olivary nucleus		SN	Substantia nigra
MCP	Middle cerebellar peduncle		TPon	Temporopontine fibers
ML	Medial lemniscus			
NuRa	Raphe nuclei			**Number Key**
OCblF	Olivocerebellar fibers			
OPon	Occipitopontine fibers		1	Nucleus raphe, pontis
PCblF	Pontocerebellar fibers		2	Nucleus raphe, magnus
			3	Raphecerebellar fibers

Review of Blood Supply to Precerebellar Relay Nuclei in Pons and Medulla, MCP, and RB	
Structures	**Arteries**
Pontine Tegmentum	Long circumferential branches of basilar plus some from superior cerebellar (see Figure 6-23)
Basilar Pons	Paramedian and short circumferential branches of basilar (see Figure 6-23)
Medulla **RetF** and **IO**	Branches of vertebral and posterior inferior cerebellar (see Figure 6-16)
MCP	Long circumferential branches of basilar and branches of anterior inferior and superior cerebellar (see Figure 6-23)
RB	Posterior inferior cerebellar (see Figure 6-16)

8-35 Pontocerebellar, Reticulocerebellar, Olivocerebellar, Ceruleocerebellar, Hypothalamocerebellar, and Raphecerebellar Fibers in Anatomical Orientation

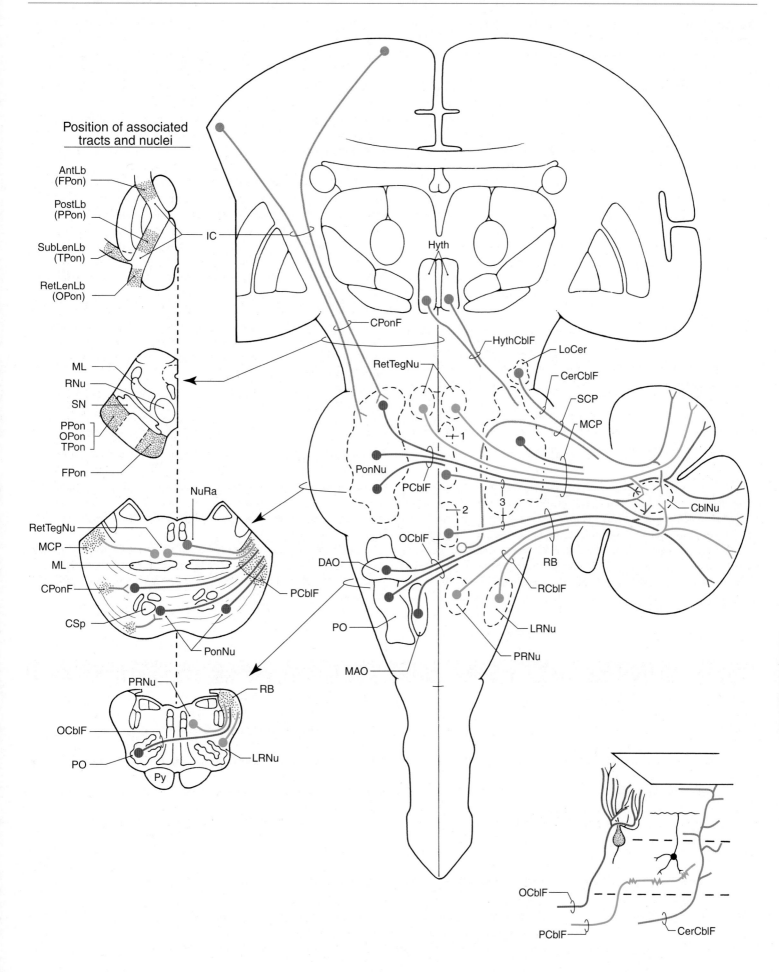

Position of associated
tracts and nuclei

AntLb
(FPon)

PostLb
(PPon)

SubLenLb
(TPon)

RetLenLb
(OPon)

IC

ML
RNu
SN
PPon
OPon
TPon
FPon

NuRa

RetTegNu
MCP
ML
CPonF
CSp
PonNu

PRNu
OCblF
PO
Py
RB
LRNu

Hyth
CPonF
RetTegNu
HythCblF
LoCer
CerCblF
SCP
MCP
1
PonNu
PCblF
3
CblNu
2
OCblF
RB
DAO
RCblF
PO
LRNu
MAO
PRNu

Cerebellar Corticonuclear, Nucleocortical, and Corticovestibular Fibers in Anatomical Orientation

8-36 **Cerebellar corticonuclear fibers** arise from all regions of the cortex and terminate in an orderly (mediolateral and rostrocaudal) sequence in the ipsilateral cerebellar nuclei. **Corticonuclear fibers** from the vermal cortex terminate in the fastigial nucleus, those from the intermediate cortex in the emboliform and globose nuclei, and those from the lateral cortex in the dentate nucleus. Also, cerebellar corticonuclear fibers from the anterior lobe typically terminate in more rostrally in these nuclei whereas those from the posterior lobe terminate more caudally. **Cerebellar corticovestibular fibers** originate primarily from the vermis and flocculonodular lobe, exit the cerebellum via the **juxtarestiform body,** and end in the ipsilateral vestibular nuclei. Corticonuclear and corticovestibular fibers arise from Purkinje cells.

Nucleocortical processes originate from cerebellar nuclear neurons and pass to the overlying cortex in a pattern that reciprocates the corticonuclear projection; they end as mossy fibers. Some nucleocortical fibers are collaterals of cerebellar efferent axons. The cerebellar cortex may influence the activity of lower motor neurons through many combinations of circuits, for example, the **cerebellovestibular–vestibulospinal** route.

Neurotransmitters

γ-Aminobutyric acid (GABA) (–) is found in Purkinje cells and is the principal transmitter substance present in cerebellar corticonuclear and corticovestibular projections. However, taurine (–) and motilin (–) are also found in some Purkinje cells. GABA-ergic terminals are numerous in the cerebellar nuclei and vestibular complex. Some of the glutamate-containing mossy fibers in the cerebellar cortex represent the endings of nucleocortical fibers that originate from cells in the cerebellar nuclei.

Clinical Correlations

Numerous disease entities can result in cerebellar dysfunction, including viral infections (**echovirus**), **hereditary diseases** (see Figure 8-35), **trauma, tumors (glioma, medulloblastoma),** occlusion of cerebellar arteries (**cerebellar stroke**), **arteriovenous malformations,** developmental errors (e.g., the **Dandy-Walker syndrome** or the **Arnold-Chiari deformity**), or the intake of alcohol or toxins. Damage to only the cortex results in transient deficits unless the lesion is quite large or causes an increase in intracranial pressure. However, lesions involving both the cortex and nuclei, or only the nuclei, may result in long-term deficits.

Lesions involving midline structures (vermal cortex, fastigial nuclei) and/or the flocculonodular lobe result in **truncal ataxia** (**titubation** or **tremor**), **nystagmus,** and head tilting. These patients also may have a **wide-based (cerebellar) gait,** are unable to **walk in tandem (heel to toe),** and may be unable to walk on their heels or on their toes. Generally, midline lesions result in bilateral motor deficits affecting axial and proximal limb musculature.

Damage to the intermediate and lateral cortices and the globose, emboliform, and dentate nuclei results in various combinations of the following: **dysarthria, dysmetria (hypometria, hypermetria), dysdiadochokinesia, tremor (static, kinetic, intention), rebound phenomenon,** unsteady and **wide-based (cerebellar) gait,** and **nystagmus.** A commonly observed deficit in patients with cerebellar lesions is an **intention tremor,** which is best seen in the **finger-nose test;** as the finger approaches the nose the tremor intensifies. The **finger-to-finger test** is also used to assess cerebellar function. The **heel-to-shin test** (sliding one heel down the opposite shin) will show **dysmetria** in that lower extremity. If the heel-to-shin test is normal in a patient with his or her eyes open, the cerebellum is intact. If this test is repeated in the same patient with eyes closed and is abnormal, this would suggest a lesion in the posterior column–medial lemniscus system.

Cerebellar damage in intermittent and lateral areas (nuclei or cortex plus nuclei) causes movement disorders on the same side of the body as the lesion; the patient may tend to fall toward the side of the lesion. This is explained by the cerebellar nuclei projecting to contralateral VL of thalamus, VL projects to ipsilateral motor cortex, motor cortex projects (corticospinal fibers) to the contralateral spinal cord. Other circuits (cerebellorubral–rubrospinal) and feedback loops (cerebello-olivary–olivocerebellar) follow similar routes. The motor expression of unilateral cerebellar damage is toward the lesioned side because of these doubly crossed pathways.

Lesions of cerebellar efferent fibers, after they cross the midline in the decussation of the superior cerebellar peduncle, will give rise to motor deficits on the contralateral side of the body (excluding the head). This is seen in midbrain lesions such as the **Claude syndrome.**

ABBREVIATIONS

CorNu	Corticonuclear fibers	MLF	Medial longitudinal fasciculus
CorVes	Corticovestibular fibers	MVesSp	Medial vestibulospinal tract
Flo	Flocculus	MVNu	Medial vestibular nucleus
IC	Intermediate cortex	NL, par	Lateral cerebellar nucleus, parvocellular region
InfVesNu	Inferior (spinal) vestibular nucleus	NM, par	Medial cerebellar nucleus, parvocellular region
JRB	Juxtarestiform body	NuCor	Nucleocortical fibers
LC	Lateral cortex	SVNu	Superior vestibular nucleus
LVesSp	Lateral vestibulospinal tract	VC	Vermal cortex
LVNu	Lateral vestibular nucleus		

Review of Blood Supply to Cerebellum and Vestibular Nuclei

Structures	Arteries
Cerebellar Cortex	Branches of posterior and anterior inferior cerebellar and superior cerebellar
Cerebellar Nuclei	Anterior inferior cerebellar and superior cerebellar
Vestibular Nuclei	Posterior inferior cerebellar in medulla, long circumferential branches of basilar in pons

8-36 Cerebellar Corticonuclear, Nucleocortical, and Corticovestibular Fibers in Anatomical Orientation

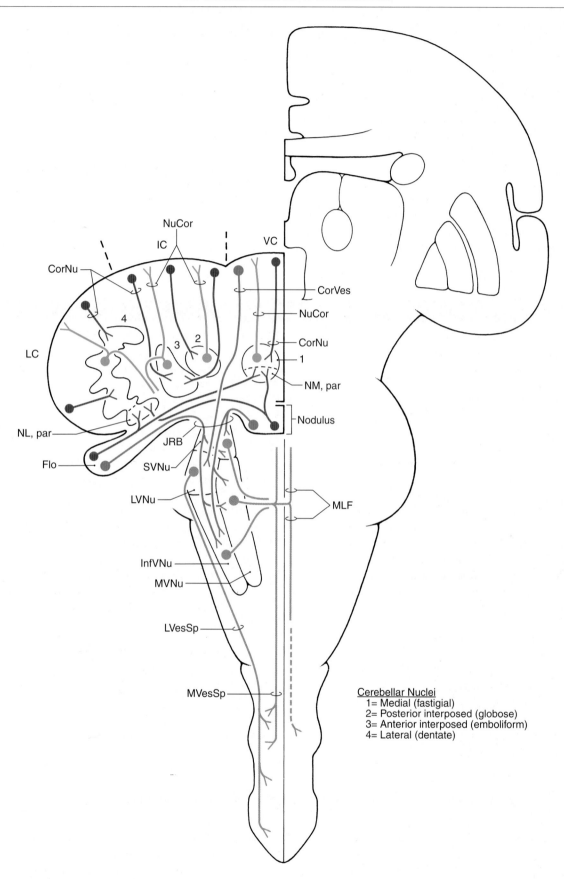

Cerebellar Nuclei
1= Medial (fastigial)
2= Posterior interposed (globose)
3= Anterior interposed (emboliform)
4= Lateral (dentate)

Cerebellar Efferent Fibers in Anatomical Orientation

8-37 The origin, course, topography, and general distribution of fibers arising in the cerebellar nuclei. **Cerebellofugal fibers** (**cerebellar efferent fibers** commonly called **cerebellothalamic fibers**) project to several thalamic areas (VL and VA), to intralaminar relay nuclei in addition to the centromedian, and a number of midbrain, pontine, and medullary targets. Most of the latter nuclei project back to the cerebellum (e.g., **reticulocerebellar, pontocerebellar**), some in a highly organized manner. For example, **cerebello-olivary fibers** from the dentate nucleus (DNu) project to the principal olivary nucleus (PO), and neurons of the PO send their axons back to the lateral cerebellar cortex, with collaterals going to the DNu.

The cerebellar nuclei can influence motor activity through, as examples, the following routes: (1) **cerebellorubral-rubrospinal;** (2) **cerebelloreticular-reticulospinal;** (3) **cerebellothalamic-thalamocortical-corticospinal;** and (4) others. In addition, some direct cerebellospinal fibers arise in the fastigial nucleus as well as in the interposed nuclei.

Neurotransmitters

Many cells in the cerebellar nuclei contain glutamate (+), aspartate (+), or γ-aminobutyric acid (–). Glutamate and aspartate are found in cerebellorubral and cerebellothalamic fibers, whereas some GABA-containing cells give rise to cerebellopontine and cerebello-olivary fibers. Some cerebelloreticular projections also may contain GABA.

Clinical Correlations

Lesions of the cerebellar nuclei result in a range of motor deficits depending on the location of the injury. Many of these are described in Figures 8-36 and 8-38B on pp. 246 and 251, respectively.

ABBREVIATIONS

ALS	Anterolateral system	NuDark	Nucleus of Darkschewitsch
AMV	Anterior medullary velum	OcNu	Oculomotor nucleus
BP	Basilar pons	PO	Principal olivary nucleus
CblOl	Cerebello-olivary fibers	PonNu	Pontine nuclei
CblTh	Cerebellothalamic fibers	RetForm	Reticular formation
CblRu	Cerebellorubral fibers	RNu	Red nucleus
CC	Crus cerebri	RuSp	Rubrospinal tract
CeGy	Central gray (periaqueductal gray)	SC	Superior colliculus
CM	Centromedian nucleus of thalamus	SCP	Superior cerebellar peduncle
CSp	Corticospinal fibers	SCP, Dec	Superior cerebellar peduncle, decussation
DAO	Dorsal accessory olivary nucleus	SN	Substantia nigra
DNu	Dentate nucleus (lateral cerebellar nucleus)	SVNu	Superior vestibular nucleus
ENu	Emboliform nucleus (anterior interposed cerebellar nucleus)	ThCor	Thalamocortical fibers
		ThFas	Thalamic fasciculus
EWpgNu	Edinger-Westphal preganglionic nucleus	TriMoNu	Trigeminal motor nucleus
FNu	Fastigial nucleus (medial cerebellar nucleus)	VL	Ventral lateral nucleus of thalamus
GNu	Globose nucleus (posterior interposed cerebellar nucleus)	VPL	Ventral posterolateral nucleus of thalamus
		VSCT	Ventral spinocerebellar tract
IC	Inferior colliculus	ZI	Zona incerta
InfVNu	Inferior (spinal) vestibular nucleus		
INu	Interstitial nucleus		
LRNu	Lateral reticular nucleus		
LVNu	Lateral vestibular nucleus		
MAO	Medial accessory olivary nucleus		
ML	Medial lemniscus		
MLF	Medial longitudinal fasciculus		
MVNu	Medial vestibular nucleus		

Number Key

1 Ascending projections to superior colliculus, and possibly ventral lateral and ventromedial thalamic nuclei
2 Descending crossed fibers from superior cerebellar peduncle
3 Uncinate fasciculus (of Russell)
4 Juxtarestiform body to vestibular nuclei
5 Reticular formation

Review of Blood Supply to Cerebellar Nuclei and Their Principal Efferent Pathways	
Structures	**Arteries**
Cerebellar Nuclei	Anterior inferior cerebellar and superior cerebellar
SCP	Long circumferential branches of basilar and superior cerebellar (see Figure 6-23)
Midbrain Tegmentum (**RNu,** **CblTh, CblRu, OcNu**)	Paramedian branches of basilar bifurcation, short circumferential branches of posterior cerebral, branches of superior cerebellar (see Figure 6-30)
VPL, CM, VL, VA	Thalamogeniculate branches of posterior cerebral, thalamoperforating branches of the posteromedial group of posterior cerebral (see Figure 6-41)
IC	Lateral striate branches of middle cerebral (see Figure 6-41)

8-37 Cerebellar Efferent Fibers in Anatomical Orientation

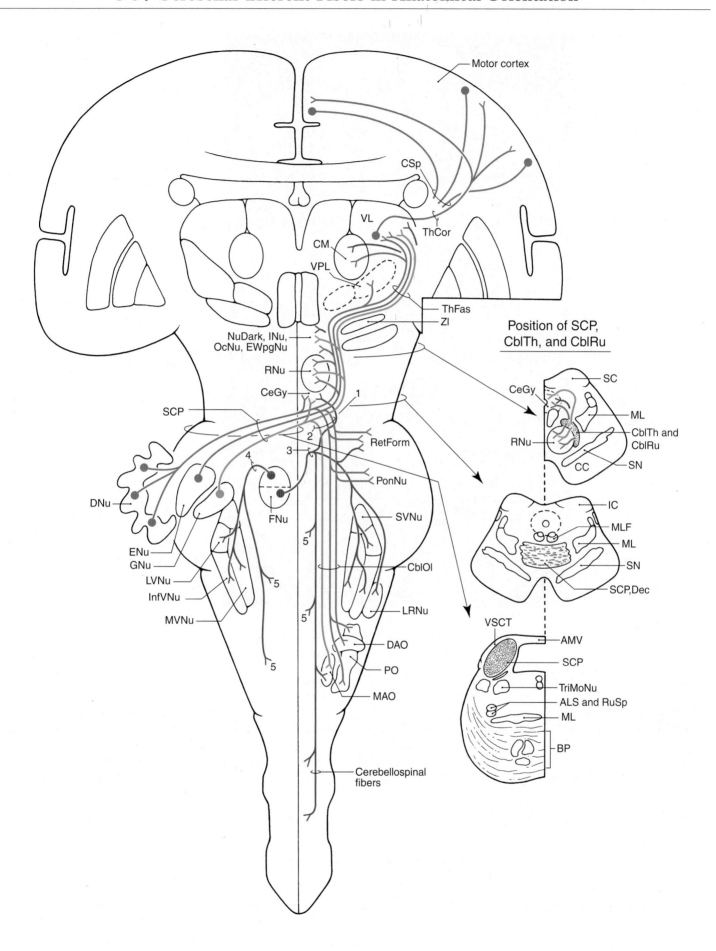

Motor cortex

CSp

VL

CM

VPL

ThCor

ThFas
ZI

NuDark, INu, OcNu, EWpgNu

RNu

CeGy

SCP

1

2

3

4

RetForm

PonNu

SVNu

DNu

FNu

ENu

GNu

LVNu

InfVNu

MVNu

5

5

5

5

CblOl

LRNu

DAO

PO

MAO

Cerebellospinal fibers

Position of SCP, CblTh, and CblRu

CeGy

RNu

SC

ML

CblTh and CblRu

SN

CC

IC

MLF

ML

SN

SCP,Dec

VSCT

AMV

SCP

TriMoNu

ALS and RuSp

ML

BP

Cerebellar Efferent Fibers in Clinical Orientation

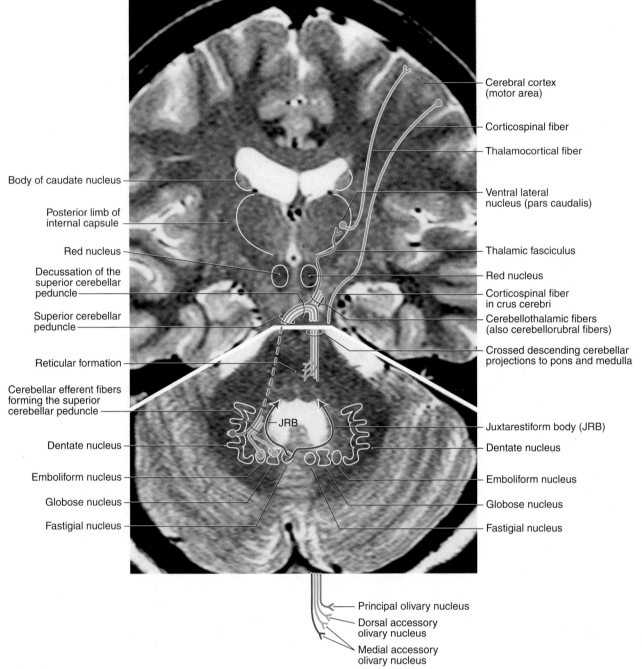

8-38A **Efferent fibers of the cerebellar nuclei** superimposed on MRI (brainstem and forebrain, T2-weighted images) showing their origin, location, and trajectory in a clinical orientation. The blue, gray, and green fibers are shown arising in the right **cerebellar nuclei,** crossing in the **decussation of the superior cerebellar peduncle,** and after decussating, they either descend or ascend to various brainstem and thalamic targets. The red fibers originating in the fastigial nucleus project bilaterally to various nuclei of the brainstem and, in much lesser numbers, to select thalamic nuclei. The blue, gray, green, and red fibers correlate with those of the same color in Figure 8-37.

Cerebellar Efferent Fibers in Clinical Orientation: Representative Lesions and Deficits

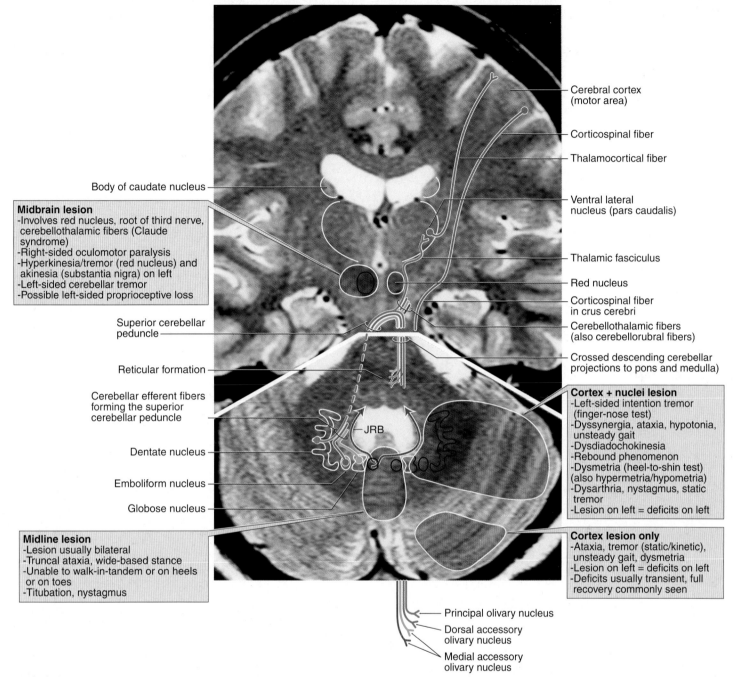

Cerebral cortex (motor area)

Corticospinal fiber

Thalamocortical fiber

Ventral lateral nucleus (pars caudalis)

Thalamic fasciculus

Red nucleus

Corticospinal fiber in crus cerebri

Cerebellothalamic fibers (also cerebellorubral fibers)

Crossed descending cerebellar projections to pons and medulla)

Body of caudate nucleus

Midbrain lesion
-Involves red nucleus, root of third nerve, cerebellothalamic fibers (Claude syndrome)
-Right-sided oculomotor paralysis
-Hyperkinesia/tremor (red nucleus) and akinesia (substantia nigra) on left
-Left-sided cerebellar tremor
-Possible left-sided proprioceptive loss

Superior cerebellar peduncle

Reticular formation

Cerebellar efferent fibers forming the superior cerebellar peduncle

JRB

Dentate nucleus

Emboliform nucleus

Globose nucleus

Cortex + nuclei lesion
-Left-sided intention tremor (finger-nose test)
-Dyssynergia, ataxia, hypotonia, unsteady gait
-Dysdiadochokinesia
-Rebound phenomenon
-Dysmetria (heel-to-shin test) (also hypermetria/hypometria)
-Dysarthria, nystagmus, static tremor
-Lesion on left = deficits on left

Cortex lesion only
-Ataxia, tremor (static/kinetic), unsteady gait, dysmetria
-Lesion on left = deficits on left
-Deficits usually transient, full recovery commonly seen

Midline lesion
-Lesion usually bilateral
-Truncal ataxia, wide-based stance
-Unable to walk-in-tandem or on heels or on toes
-Titubation, nystagmus

Principal olivary nucleus

Dorsal accessory olivary nucleus

Medial accessory olivary nucleus

8-38B Representative lesions of the cerebellum and of cerebellothalamic fibers in the midbrain (and the adjacent red nucleus) and the deficits (in pink boxes) that correlate with each lesion. It is important to remember that the motor deficits seen in patients with cerebellar lesions are expressed through the corticospinal tract. Consequently, if a lesion is proximal to the decussation of the superior cerebellar peduncle, the deficits are ipsilateral to the lesion; if a lesion is distal to the decussation, the deficits are on the contralateral side. Note that the laterality (R/L) of the deficits is determined by whether the lesion is on the left or right side of the MRI; this reinforces important clinical concepts. For additional information on deficits related to cerebellar lesions, see Figure 8-36 on p. 246.

Blank Master Drawing for Efferent Cerebellar Connections

8-39 Blank master drawing for pathways projecting to the cerebellar cortex, and for efferent projections of cerebellar nuclei. This illustration is provided for self-evaluation of understanding of pathways to the cerebellar cortex and from the cerebellar nuclei, for the instructor to expand on cerebellar afferent/efferent pathways not covered in the atlas, or both.

NOTES

8-39 Blank Master Drawing for Efferent Cerebellar Connections

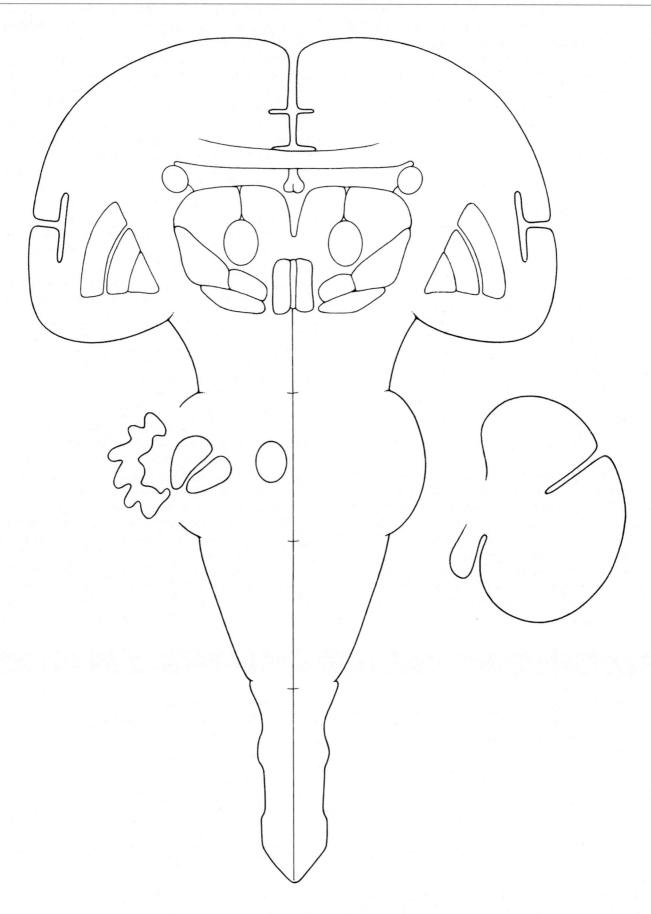

Striatal Connections in Anatomical Orientation

8-40 The origin, course, and distribution of **afferent fibers to,** and **efferent projections from,** the **neostriatum.** These projections are extensive, complex, and, in large part, topographically organized; only their general patterns are summarized here. Afferents to the caudate and putamen originate from the cerebral cortex (**corticostriate fibers**), from the intralaminar thalamic nuclei (**thalamostriate**), from the substantia nigra–pars compacta (**nigrostriate**), and from the raphe nuclei. Neostriatal cells send axons into the globus pallidus (paleostriatum) as **striopallidal fibers** and into the substantia nigra–pars reticulata as a **strionigral projection.**

Neurotransmitters

Glutamate (+) is found in corticostriate fibers, and serotonin is found in raphe striatal fibers from the nucleus raphe dorsalis. Four neuroactive substances are associated with striatal efferent fibers, these being γ-aminobutyric acid (GABA) (–), dynorphin, enkephalin (–), and substance P (+). Enkephalinergic and GABA-ergic striopallidal projections are numerous to the lateral pallidum (origin of pallidosubthalamic fibers), whereas GABA-ergic and dynorphin-containing terminals are more concentrated in its medial segment (source of pallidothalamic fibers). Enkephalin and GABA are also present in strionigral projections to the pars reticulata. Substance P and GABA are found in striopallidal *and* strionigral fibers. Dopamine is present in nigrostriatal projection neurons and in their terminals in the neostriatum.

Clinical Correlations

Degenerative changes, neuron loss, or loss of afferent fibers in the caudate nucleus, putamen, or substantia nigra result in movement disorders. Examples are seen in **Sydenham chorea (rheumatic chorea), Huntington disease** (a dominantly inherited disease), and **Wilson disease** (a genetic error in copper metabolism) and, **Parkinson disease** a loss of dopaminergic cells in the substantia nigra, pars compacta, and their neostriatial terminals.

Sydenham chorea is a disease seen in children between 5 and 15 years of age, resulting from infection with hemolytic streptococcus. The **choreiform movements** are brisk and flowing, irregular, and may involve muscles of the limbs, face, oral cavity, and trunk. **Dystonia** may be seen; muscle weakness is common. In most patients, the disease resolves after treatment of the infection.

Huntington disease is an inherited disorder; the symptoms appear at 35 to 45 years of age and are progressive. A feature of this disease is excessive CAG repeats on chromosome 4 (4p16.3); the greater the number of repeats, the earlier the onset, and more severe the disease. There is loss of GABA-ergic and enkephalinergic cells in the neostriatum (primarily the caudate) and cell loss in the cerebral cortex. Loss of neostriatal cell terminals in the lateral and medial segments of the globus pallidus correlates with the development of **choreiform movements** and later with **rigidity** and **dystonia.** Loss of cortical neurons correlates with personality changes and eventual **dementia. Huntington chorea** is rapid, unpredictable, and may affect muscles of the extremities, face, and trunk. Patients commonly attempt to mask the abnormal movement by trying to make it appear to be part of an intended movement (**parakinesia**).

Symptoms in **Wilson disease (hepatolenticular degeneration)** appear between 10 and 25 years of age. Copper accumulates in the basal nuclei and the frontal cortex, with resultant spongy degeneration in the putamen. These patients may show **athetoid movements, rigidity** and **spasticity, dysarthria, dysphagia, contractures,** and **tremor.** A unique movement of the hand and/or upper extremity in these patients is called a **flapping tremor** (**asterixis**) sometimes described as a **wing-beating tremor.** Copper also can be seen in the cornea (**Kayser-Fleischer ring**) in these patients.

In **Parkinson disease** (onset at 50 to 60 years of age), there is a progressive loss of dopaminergic cells in the substantia nigra–pars compacta, their terminals in the caudate and putamen, and their dendrites that extend into the substantia nigra–pars reticulata. Patients with Parkinson disease characteristically show a **resting tremor (pill-rolling), rigidity (cogwheel** or **lead-pipe),** and **bradykinesia** or **hypokinesia.** The slowness of movement also may be expressed in speech (**dysarthria, hypophonia, trachyphonia**) and writing (**micrographia**). These patients have a distinct stooped **flexed posture** and a **festinating gait.** Parkinson and Huntington diseases are neurodegenerative disorders.

Dystonia, as seen in some patients with basal nuclei disease, is characterized by increased/sustained muscle contractions, twisting of the trunk or extremities, and abnormal postures. These patients may have unusual and repetitive movements of the extremities or neck (**cervical dystonia** or **spasmodic torticollis**). Dystonia may be an inherited progressive disease or have other causes. The symptoms may initially appear during movements or when talking, but in later stages may be present at rest.

ABBREVIATIONS

CaNu	Caudate nucleus	**RaSt**	Raphestriatal fibers
CorSt	Corticostriate fibers	**SNpc**	Substantia nigra, pars compacta
GPL	Globus pallidus, lateral segment	**SNpr**	Substantia nigra, pars reticulata
GPM	Globus pallidus, medial segment	**StNig**	Striatonigral fibers
IC	Internal capsule	**StPal**	Striatopallidal fibers
NigSt	Nigrostriatal fibers	**SThNu**	Subthalamic nucleus
Put	Putamen	**ThSt**	Thalamostriatal fibers
RaNu	Raphe nuclei	**ZI**	Zona incerta

Review of Blood Supply to Caudate, Putamen, SN, CC, and IC	
Structures	**Arteries**
Caudate, Putamen, and **IC**	Medial striate artery for head of caudate and lateral striate branches of middle cerebral for Put and IC (see Figure 6-41)
SN and **CC**	Paramedian branches of basilar bifurcation, short circumferential branches of posterior cerebral and some from superior cerebellar (see Figure 6-30)

8-40 Striatal Connections in Anatomical Orientation

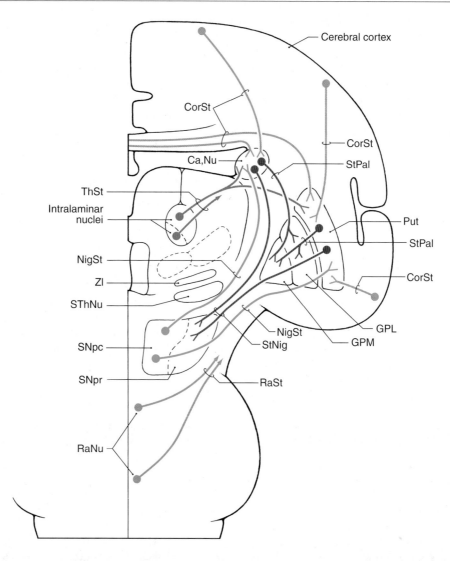

Cerebral cortex

CorSt

CorSt

Ca,Nu

StPal

ThSt

Intralaminar nuclei

Put

StPal

NigSt

CorSt

ZI

SThNu

NigSt

StNig

GPL

SNpc

GPM

SNpr

RaSt

RaNu

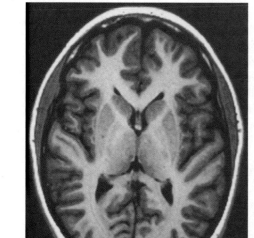

Normal axial T1 MRI

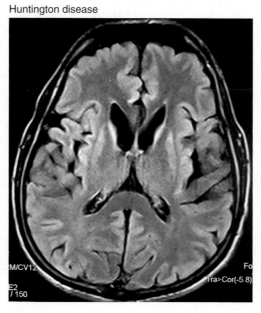

Huntington disease

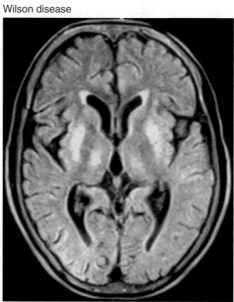

Wilson disease

Pallidal Efferents and Nigral Connections in Anatomical Orientation

8-41 The origin, course, and distribution of **efferent projections of the globus pallidus** (upper illustration), and **connections of the substantia nigra** (lower drawing) that were not shown in relation to the pallidum or in Figure 8-40 on p. 255 (see also Figure 8-42A on p. 258). The **ansa lenticularis** (dashed line) arches around the internal capsule and passes caudally to join in the formation of the thalamic fasciculus. **Pallidosubthalamic fibers** originate primarily from the lateral pallidal segment, but pallidothalamic projections, via the ansa lenticularis and **lenticular fasciculus**, arise mainly from its medial segment. The substantia nigra has extensive connections, the clinically most important being the **dopaminergic nigrostriatal fibers**. The globus pallidus influences motor activity by way of **pallidothalamic–thalamocortical–corticospinal** (and corticonuclear) pathways.

Neurotransmitters

γ-Aminobutyric acid (–)–containing cells in the globus pallidus give rise to pallidonigral projections, which end primarily in the substantia nigra–pars reticulata. Although GABA is also found in some subthalamopallidal axons, this latter projection contains many glutaminergic (+) fibers.

Dopamine-, GABA (–)-, and glycine (–)-containing cells are present in the substantia nigra. Of these, dopamine is found in pars compacta neurons, which give rise to nigrostriatal, nigroamygdaloid, and several other projections; GABA in pars reticulata cells, which give rise to nigrocollicular and nigrothalamic fibers; and glycine in some local circuit nigral neurons. Glutamate (+) is found in corticonigral fibers, and serotonin (–) is associated with raphenigral fibers; these latter fibers originate primarily from the nucleus raphe dorsalis.

The dopaminergic projections to the frontal cortex, shown here as arising only from SNpc, originate from this cell group as well as from the immediately adjacent ventral tegmental area. Excessive activity in neurons comprising this projection may play a partial role in **schizophrenia**.

Clinical Correlations

Movement disorders associated with lesions in the neostriatum and substantia nigra are reviewed in Figures 8-40 and 8-42B on pp. 254 and 259. **Hemorrhage** into, the occlusion of vessels serving, or a tumor within, the subthalamic nucleus will result in violent flailing movements of the extremities, a condition called **hemiballismus**. Through subthalamopallidal fibers to the medial segment of the globul pallidus and pallidothalamic fibers to the ipsilateral VL of the thalamus, the subthalamic nucleus influences the motor cortex on the same side, which, in turn, influences spinal motor neurons on the side opposite the primary lesion.

Hemiballistic movements are seen contralateral to the lesion because the motor expression of this lesion is through the corticospinal tract. Lesions confined to the globus pallidus, as in hemorrhage of lenticulostriate arteries, may result in **hypokinesia** and **rigidity** without tremor.

ABBREVIATIONS

AmyNig	Amygdalonigral fibers	**PedPonNu**	Pedunculopontine nucleus
AmyNu	Amygdaloid nucleus (complex)	**Put**	Putamen
AnLent	Ansa lenticularis	**RaNu**	Raphe nuclei
CaNu	Caudate nucleus	**SC**	Superior colliculus
CM	Centromedian nucleus of thalamus	**SNpc**	Substantia nigra, pars compacta
CorNig	Corticonigral fibers	**SNpr**	Substantia nigra, pars reticulata
CSp	Corticospinal fibers	**SThFas**	Subthalamic fasciculus
GPL	Globus pallidus, lateral segment	**SThNig**	Subthalamonigral fibers
GPM	Globus pallidus, medial segment	**SThNu**	Subthalamic nucleus
LenFas	Lenticular fasciculus (H$_2$)	**ThCor**	Thalamocortical fibers
NigAmy	Nigroamygdaloid fibers	**ThFas**	Thalamic fasciculus (H$_1$)
NigCol	Nigrocollicular fibers	**VA**	Ventral anterior nucleus of thalamus
NigTec	Nigrotectal fibers	**VL**	Ventral lateral nucleus of thalamus
NigSTh	Nigrosubthalamic fibers	**VM**	Ventromedial nucleus of thalamus
NigTh	Nigrothalamic fibers	**ZI**	Zona incerta
PalNig	Pallidonigral fibers		

Review of Blood Supply to Pallidum, Subthalamic Area, and SN

Structures	Arteries
GPM/GPL	Lateral striate branches of middle cerebral and branches of anterior choroidal (see Figure 6-41)
SThNu	Posteromedial branches of posterior cerebral and posterior communicating (see Figure 6-41)
SN	Branches of basilar bifurcation, medial branches of posterior cerebral and posterior communicating, short circumferential branches of posterior cerebral (see Figure 6-30)

8-41 Pallidal Efferents and Nigral Connections in Anatomical Orientation

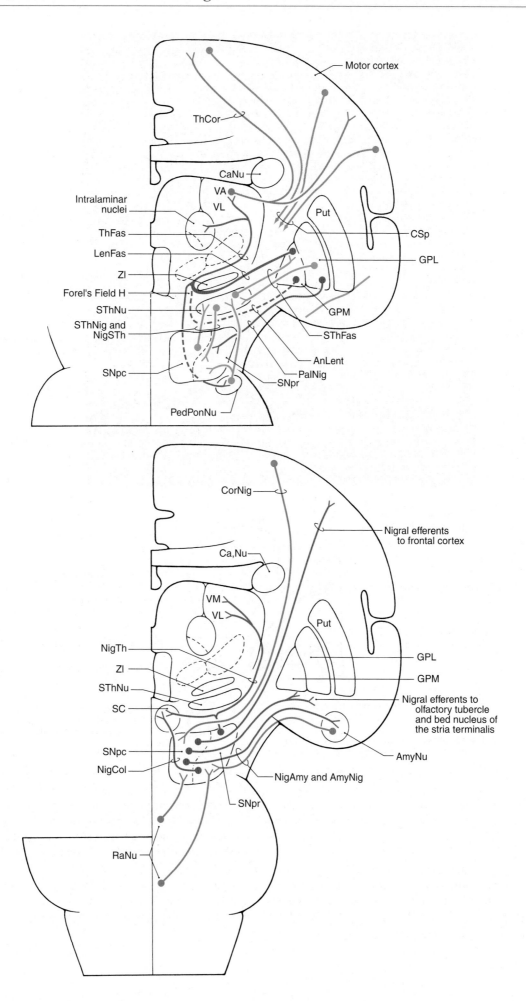

Pallidal Efferents, Subthalamic, and Nigral Connections in Clinical Orientation

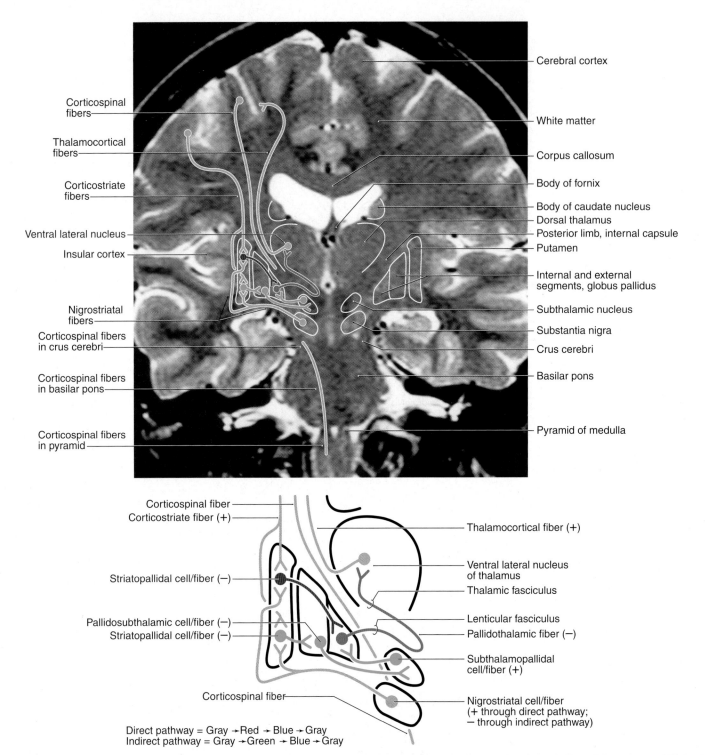

Direct pathway = Gray → Red → Blue → Gray
Indirect pathway = Gray → Green → Blue → Gray

8-42A The **direct and indirect pathways through the basal nuclei,** **subthalamic nucleus,** and **substantia nigra** superimposed on MRI (forebrain, T2-weighted MRI) shown in clinical orientation. The exploded view below the MRI illustrates the specific fiber types, by name, that comprise these two pathways and specifies whether the synaptic influences are excitatory (+) or inhibitory (−).

The direct pathway essentially functions as follows. The **corticostriatal (+) fiber** excites the **striatopallidal (−) fiber,** which inhibits the **pallidothalamic (−) fiber.** In this situation, the **thalamus is disinhibited** (removed from the inhibition of the pallidothalamic fiber), and the activity of the **thalamus and motor cortex is up-regulated.**

The indirect pathway functions in the following way. The **corticostriatal (+) fiber** excites the **striatopallidal (−) fiber,** which inhibits the **pallidosubthalamic (−) fiber.** In this situation, the **subthalamic nucleus is disinhibited** (removed from the inhibition of the pallidosubthalamic fiber), and the **subthalamopallidal (+) fiber** excites the **pallidothalamic (−) fiber,** which inhibits the thalamus; the activity of the **thalamus and the motor cortex is down-regulated.**

These two pathways work together. However, their influence takes into account the different number of synapses in each pathway; the respective messages are temporally separated.

Pallidal Efferents, Subthalamic, and Nigral Connections in Clinical Orientation: Representative Lesions and Deficits

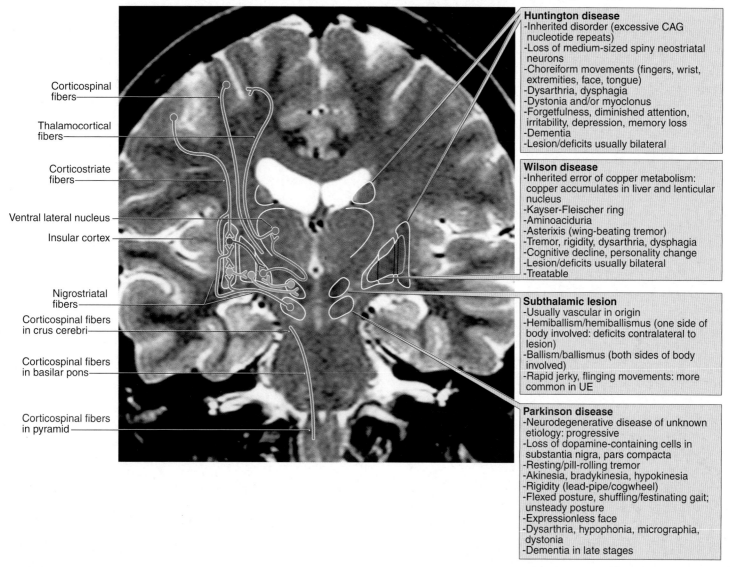

Corticospinal fibers

Thalamocortical fibers

Corticostriate fibers

Ventral lateral nucleus

Insular cortex

Nigrostriatal fibers

Corticospinal fibers in crus cerebri

Corticospinal fibers in basilar pons

Corticospinal fibers in pyramid

Huntington disease
-Inherited disorder (excessive CAG nucleotide repeats)
-Loss of medium-sized spiny neostriatal neurons
-Choreiform movements (fingers, wrist, extremities, face, tongue)
-Dysarthria, dysphagia
-Dystonia and/or myoclonus
-Forgetfulness, diminished attention, irritability, depression, memory loss
-Dementia
-Lesion/deficits usually bilateral

Wilson disease
-Inherited error of copper metabolism: copper accumulates in liver and lenticular nucleus
-Kayser-Fleischer ring
-Aminoaciduria
-Asterixis (wing-beating tremor)
-Tremor, rigidity, dysarthria, dysphagia
-Cognitive decline, personality change
-Lesion/deficits usually bilateral
-Treatable

Subthalamic lesion
-Usually vascular in origin
-Hemiballism/hemiballismus (one side of body involved: deficits contralateral to lesion)
-Ballism/ballismus (both sides of body involved)
-Rapid jerky, flinging movements: more common in UE

Parkinson disease
-Neurodegenerative disease of unknown etiology: progressive
-Loss of dopamine-containing cells in substantia nigra, pars compacta
-Resting/pill-rolling tremor
-Akinesia, bradykinesia, hypokinesia
-Rigidity (lead-pipe/cogwheel)
-Flexed posture, shuffling/festinating gait; unsteady posture
-Expressionless face
-Dysarthria, hypophonia, micrographia, dystonia
-Dementia in late stages

8-42B **Representative lesions of the basal nuclei, subthalamic nucleus, and substantia nigra** and the deficits (in pink boxes) that correlate with lesions at each of these locations. As was the case with the cerebellum, motor deficits resulting from lesions of the basal nuclei and related structures are expressed through the corticospinal tract. Note that the laterality (R/L) of the deficits is determined by whether the lesion is on the left or right side of the MRI; this reinforces important clinical concepts.

Blank Master Drawing for Connections of the Basal Nuclei

8-43 Blank master drawing for connections of the basal nuclei. This illustration is provided for self-evaluation of understanding of basal nuclei connections, for the instructor to expand on basal nuclei pathways not covered in this atlas, or both.

NOTES

8-43 Blank Master Drawing for Connections of the Basal Nuclei

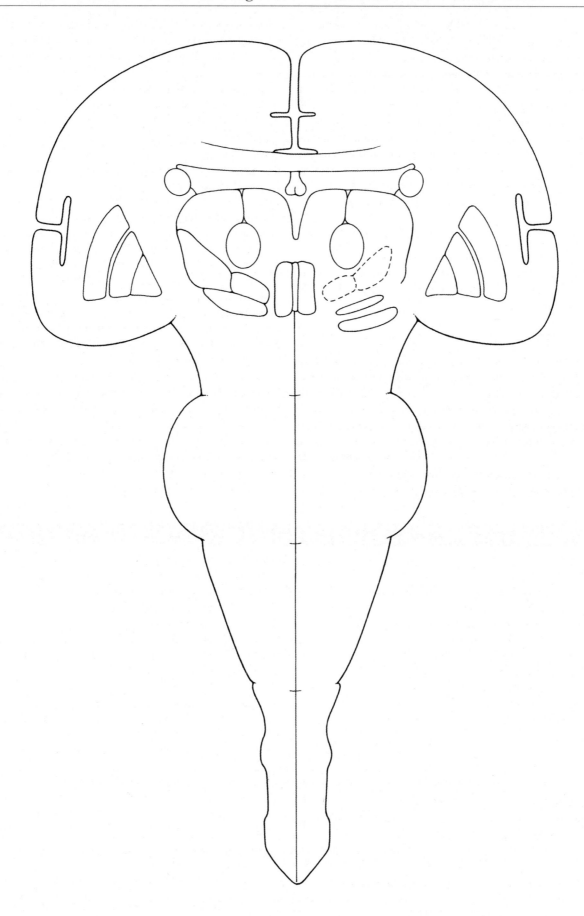

Pupillary Pathways

8-44 The origin, course, and distribution of fibers involved in the pathway for the **pupillary light reflex**. In addition, the pathway for **sympathetic innervation of the dilator muscle of the iris** is also depicted. The **intermediolateral cell column** of the spinal cord receives input predominately from the paraventricular nucleus and also from cells in the lateral hypothalamic zone and posterior hypothalamus. This projection may be supplemented, in a minor way, by descending fibers through the reticular formation of the brainstem. **Postganglionic sympathetic fibers** to the head originate from the **superior cervical ganglion**. Although not shown, descending projections to the intermediolateral cell column also originate from various hypothalamic areas and nuclei (hypothalamospinal fibers), some of which receive retinal input.

Neurotransmitters

Acetylcholine is the transmitter found in the preganglionic and post-ganglionic autonomic fibers shown in this illustration. In addition, N-acetyl-aspartyl-glutamate is present in some retinal ganglion cells (**retinogeniculate projections**).

Clinical Correlations

Total or partial **blindness** in one or both eyes may result from a variety of causes (e.g., **gliomas, meningiomas, strokes, aneurysms, infections,** and **demyelinating diseases**); lesions may occur at any locus along the visual pathway. A complete lesion (i.e., a transection) of the optic nerve will result in **blindness** and loss of the **pupillary light reflex** (**direct response**) in the eye on the injured side and a loss of the **pupillary light reflex** (**consensual response**) in the opposite eye **when shining a light in the blind eye**. On the other hand, **shining a light in the normal eye** will result in a **pupillary light reflex** (**direct response**) in that eye *and* a consensual response in the blind eye. See also Figure 8-32 on p. 239. A **pituitary adenoma** may damage the crossing fibers in the optic chiasm (producing a **bitemporal hemianopia**) or damage the uncrossed fibers in the right (or left) side of the optic chiasm. These lateral lesions produce a **right** (**or left**) **nasal hemianopia**.

Optic (geniculocalcarine) radiations (see Figs. 8-45 and 8-47 on pp. 264 and 266) may pass directly caudal to the upper lip (cuneus) of the calcarine sulcus or follow an arching route (the **Meyer**, or **Meyer-Archambault loop**) through the temporal lobe to the lower bank (lingual gyrus) of the calcarine sulcus. Temporal lobe lesions involving the Meyer-Archambault loop, or involving fibers entering the lingual gyrus, can produce a **homonymous superior quadrantanopia**. A **homonymous inferior quadrantanopia** is seen in patients with damage to upper (parietal) parts of the geniculocalcarine radiations or to these fibers as they enter the cuneus. See Figure 8-47B on p. 267 for additional lesions of the visual pathways and the corresponding visual field deficits.

Damage to the visual cortex adjacent to the calcarine sulcus (distal posterior cerebral artery occlusion) results in a **right** (or **left**) **homonymous hemianopia**. With the exception of macular sparing, this deficit is the same as that seen in optic tract lesions. See Figure 8-47B on p. 267 for additional lesions of the optic radiations and visual cortex and the corresponding visual field deficits.

Vascular lesions (e.g., the **lateral medullary syndrome**), tumors (e.g., **brainstem gliomas**), or **syringobulbia** may interrupt the descending projections from hypothalamus (hypothalamospinal fibers) and midbrain to the intermediolateral cell column at upper thoracic levels. This may result in a **Horner syndrome** (**ptosis, miosis,** and **anhidrosis**) on the ipsilateral side. The **enophthalmos** (a slight sinking of the eyeball into the orbit) frequently mentioned in relation to Horner syndrome is not really very apparent in afflicted patients.

ABBREVIATIONS

CC	Crus cerebri	PoCom	Posterior commissure
CilGang	Ciliary ganglion	PrTecNu	Pretectal nucleus
EWpgNu	Edinger-Westphal preganglionic nucleus	PulNu	Pulvinar nuclear complex
ILCC	Intermediolateral cell column	RetF	Reticular formation
LGNu	Lateral geniculate nucleus	RNu	Red nucleus
MGNu	Medial geniculate nucleus	SC	Superior colliculus
ML	Medial lemniscus	SC, Br	Superior colliculus, brachium
OcNr	Oculomotor nerve	SCerGang	Superior cervical ganglion
OpCh	Optic chiasm	SN	Substantia nigra
OpNr	Optic nerve	WRCom	White ramus communicans
OpTr	Optic tract		

Review of Blood Supply to OpTr, MGNu, LGNu, SC, and Midbrain Tegmentum, Including PrTecNu	
Structures	**Arteries**
OpTr	Anterior choroidal (see Figure 6-41)
MGNu, LGNu	Thalamogeniculate branches of posterior cerebral (see Figure 6-41)
SC and PrTecNu	Long circumferential branches (quadrigeminal) of posterior cerebral, posterior choroidal, and some from superior cerebellar (to SC) (see Figures 6-30 and 6-41)
Midbrain Tegmentum	Paramedian branches of basilar bifurcation, medial branches of posterior cerebral and posterior communicating, short circumferential branches of posterior cerebral (see Figure 6-30)

8-44 Pupillary Pathways

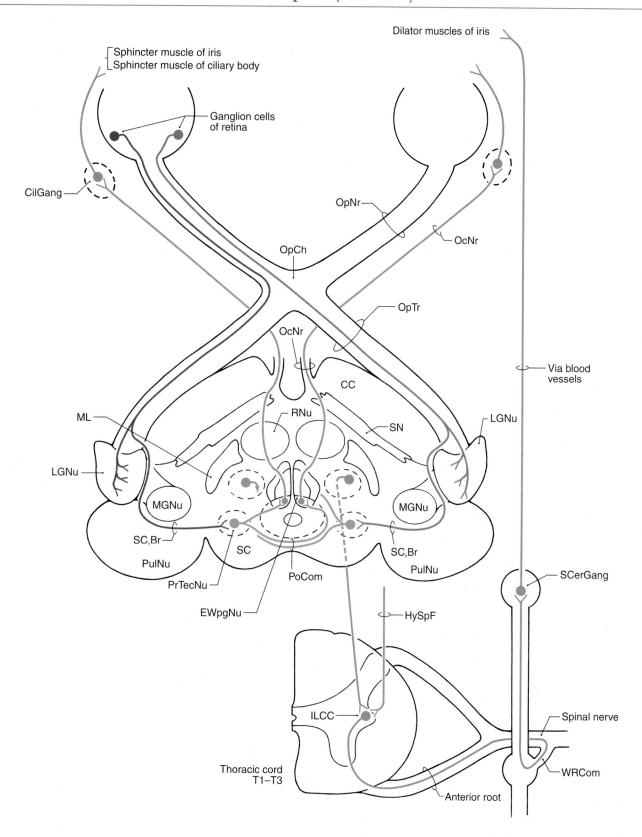

Sphincter muscle of iris
Sphincter muscle of ciliary body

Dilator muscles of iris

Ganglion cells of retina

CilGang

OpNr

OcNr

OpCh

OcNr

OpTr

CC

Via blood vessels

ML

RNu

SN

LGNu

LGNu

MGNu

MGNu

SC,Br

SC,Br

PulNu

SC

PulNu

PrTecNu

PoCom

EWpgNu

SCerGang

HySpF

Spinal nerve

ILCC

WRCom

Thoracic cord
T1–T3

Anterior root

Visual Pathways

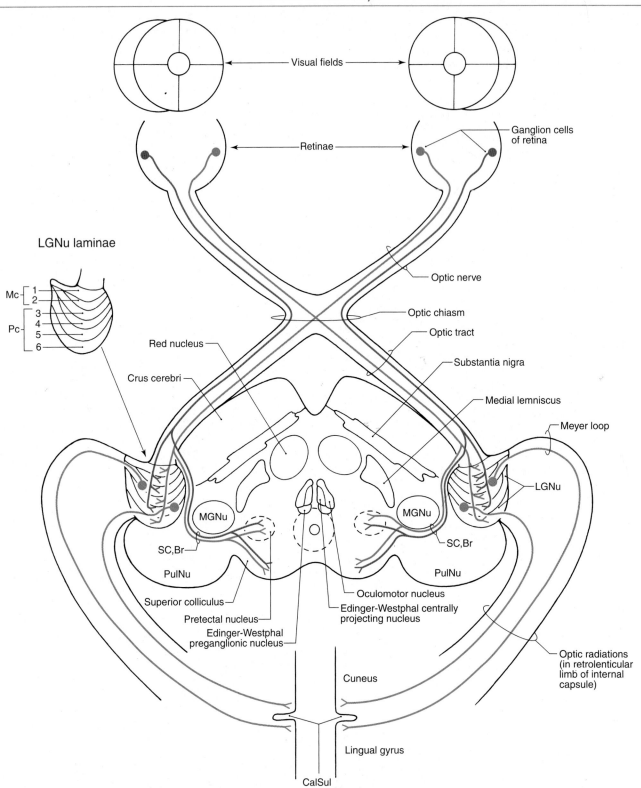

Visual fields

Retinae

Ganglion cells of retina

LGNu laminae

Mc — 1, 2
Pc — 3, 4, 5, 6

Optic nerve

Optic chiasm

Optic tract

Red nucleus

Substantia nigra

Crus cerebri

Medial lemniscus

Meyer loop

MGNu

LGNu

SC,Br

SC,Br

PulNu

PulNu

Superior colliculus

Oculomotor nucleus

Pretectal nucleus

Edinger-Westphal centrally projecting nucleus

Edinger-Westphal preganglionic nucleus

Optic radiations (in retrolenticular limb of internal capsule)

Cuneus

Lingual gyrus

CalSul

8-45 The **origin, course, and distribution of the visual pathway** are shown. Uncrossed **retinogeniculate fibers** terminate in laminae 2, 3, and 5, whereas crossed fibers end in laminae 1, 4, and 6. **Geniculocalcarine fibers** arise from laminae 3 through 6. Retinogeniculate and geniculocalcarine pathways are **retinotopically organized** (see facing page).

Neurotransmitters

Cholecystokinin (+) is present in some geniculocalcarine fibers. N-acetyl-aspartyl-glutamate is found in some retinogeniculate fibers, and in some lateral geniculate and visual cortex neurons.

Clinical Correlations

Deficits seen following lesions of various parts of visual pathways are described in Figures 8-44 and 8-47B on pp. 262 and 267.

ABBREVIATIONS	
CalSul	Calcarine sulcus
LGNu	Lateral geniculate nucleus
Mc	Magnocellular
Pc	Parvocellular
MGNu	Medial geniculate nucleus
PulNu	Pulvinar nuclear complex
SC, Br	Superior colliculus, brachium

Visual Pathways

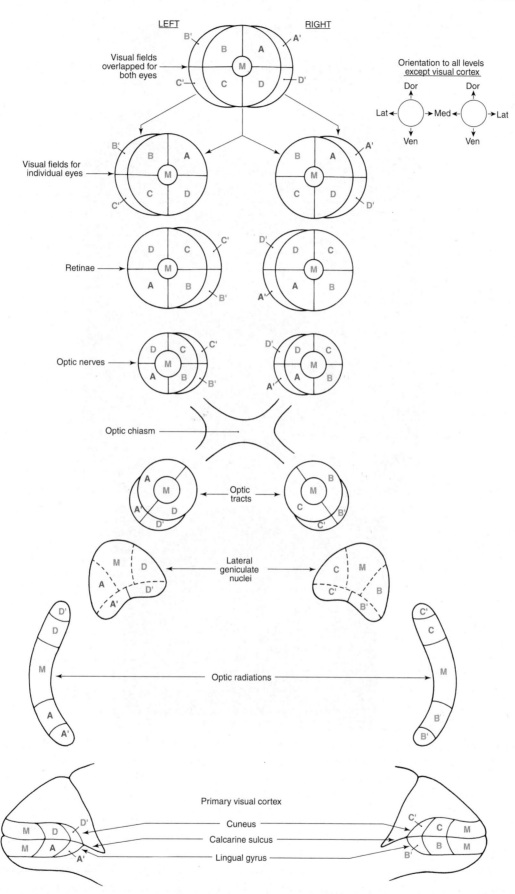

8-46 Semi-diagrammatic representation of the **retinographic arrangement of visual and retinal fields,** and the subsequent topography of these projections throughout the visual system. Upper case letters identify the binocular visual fields (A, B, C, D), the macula (M), and the monocular visual fields (A', B', C', D').

Clinical Correlations

Deficits seen following lesions of various parts of the visual pathway are described in Figures 8-44 and 8-47B on pp. 262 and 267.

Visual Pathways in Clinical Orientation

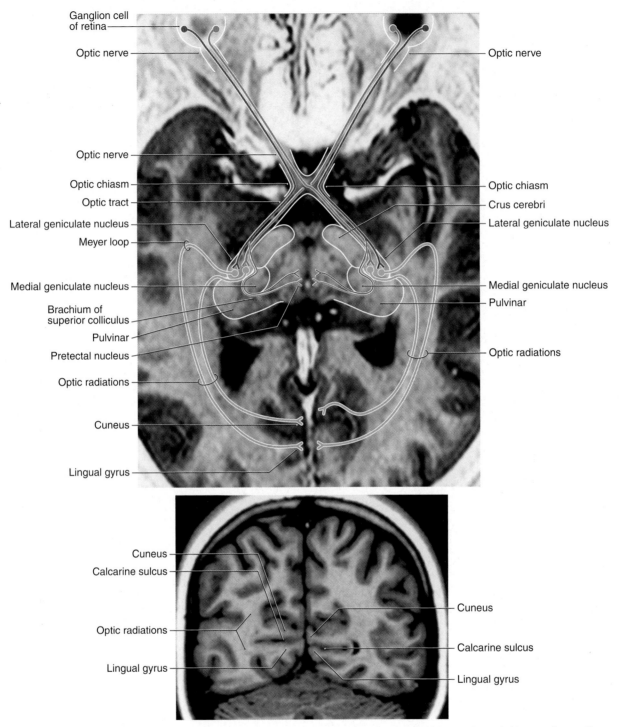

Ganglion cell of retina		Optic nerve
Optic nerve		Optic chiasm
Optic nerve		Crus cerebri
Optic chiasm		Lateral geniculate nucleus
Optic tract		
Lateral geniculate nucleus		Medial geniculate nucleus
Meyer loop		Pulvinar
Medial geniculate nucleus		Optic radiations
Brachium of superior colliculus		
Pulvinar		
Pretectal nucleus		
Optic radiations		
Cuneus		
Lingual gyrus		

Cuneus
Calcarine sulcus
Optic radiations
Lingual gyrus

Cuneus
Calcarine sulcus
Lingual gyrus

8-47A The **visual pathway from retina to primary visual cortex** superimposed on MRI in clinical orientation. The upper T1-weighted image is in the axial plane and the lower T1-weighted image is in the coronal plane. The red, blue, and gray fibers in the upper image correlate with those of the same color in Figure 8-45.

8-47B **Representative lesions** at 13 different locations in the **visual pathway** and the patterns of visual field deficits (in pink boxes) that correlate with each lesion. As indicated by the letters (A–I), some lesions, especially those caudal to the optic chiasm, may result in comparable visual field deficits even though the lesions may be at different locations within the pathway.

International clinical convention dictates that **Visual Field Deficits** are illustrated as the patient sees the environment. In this respect, the patient's right eye and visual field are on the right and the patient's left eye and visual field are on the left. Axial and coronal MRI and CT images are viewed as if the observer is standing at the patient's feet looking toward the head (axial) or looking at the patient's face

Visual Pathways in Clinical Orientation: Representative Lesions and Deficits

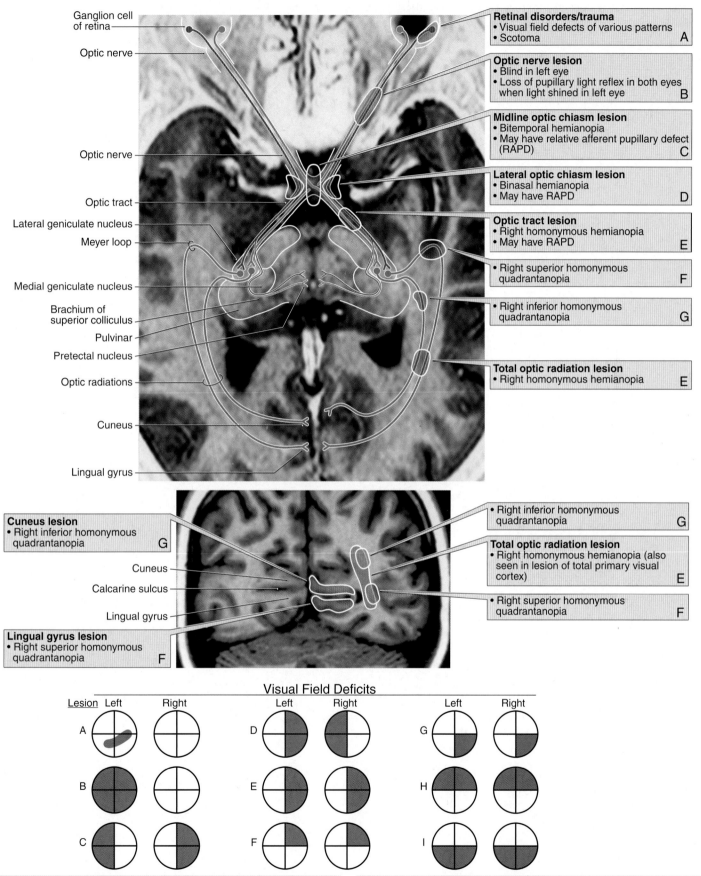

Ganglion cell of retina

Optic nerve

Optic nerve

Optic tract

Lateral geniculate nucleus

Meyer loop

Medial geniculate nucleus

Brachium of superior colliculus

Pulvinar

Pretectal nucleus

Optic radiations

Cuneus

Lingual gyrus

Retinal disorders/trauma
• Visual field defects of various patterns
• Scotoma   A

Optic nerve lesion
• Blind in left eye
• Loss of pupillary light reflex in both eyes when light shined in left eye   B

Midline optic chiasm lesion
• Bitemporal hemianopia
• May have relative afferent pupillary defect (RAPD)   C

Lateral optic chiasm lesion
• Binasal hemianopia
• May have RAPD   D

Optic tract lesion
• Right homonymous hemianopia
• May have RAPD   E

• Right superior homonymous quadrantanopia   F

• Right inferior homonymous quadrantanopia   G

Total optic radiation lesion
• Right homonymous hemianopia   E

Cuneus lesion
• Right inferior homonymous quadrantanopia   G

Cuneus

Calcarine sulcus

Lingual gyrus

Lingual gyrus lesion
• Right superior homonymous quadrantanopia   F

• Right inferior homonymous quadrantanopia   G

Total optic radiation lesion
• Right homonymous hemianopia (also seen in lesion of total primary visual cortex)   E

• Right superior homonymous quadrantanopia   F

Visual Field Deficits

Lesion   Left   Right   Left   Right   Left   Right
A   D   G
B   E   H
C   F   I

(coronal). In this case, when looking at MRI/CT, the observer's right is the patient's left and the observer's left is the patient's right. Understanding the reality of how these images are used and viewed in the clinical environment is absolutely essential to the diagnosis of the patient with visual system lesions and the corresponding visual field deficits.

Blank Master Drawing for Visual Pathways

8-48 Blank master drawing for visual pathways. This illustration is provided for self-evaluation of visual pathway understanding, for the instructor to expand on aspects of the visual pathways not covered in the atlas, or both.

NOTES

8-48 Blank Master Drawing for Visual Pathways

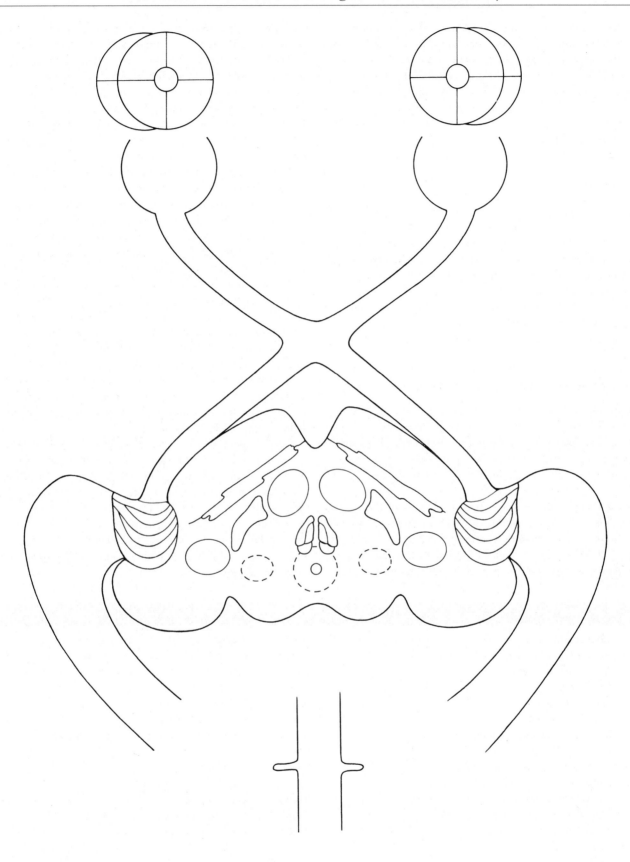

Auditory Pathways in Anatomical Orientation

8-49 The origin, course, and distribution of the fibers collectively composing the **auditory pathway**. Central to the **cochlear nerve** and **dorsal and ventral cochlear nuclei**, this system is, largely, bilateral and multisynaptic, as input is relayed to the auditory cortex. Synapse and crossing (or re-crossing) of information can occur at several levels in the neuraxis. Consequently, central lesions rarely result in a total unilateral hearing loss. The **medial geniculate body** is the thalamic station for the relay of auditory information to the temporal cortex.

Neurotransmitters

Glutamate (+) and aspartate (+) are found in some spiral ganglion cells and in their central terminations in the cochlear nuclei. Dynorphin-containing and histamine-containing fibers are also present in the cochlear nuclei; the latter arises from the hypothalamus. A noradrenergic projection to the cochlear nuclei and the inferior colliculus originates from the nucleus locus ceruleus. Cells in the superior olive that contain cholecystokinin and cells in the nuclei of the lateral lemniscus that contain dynorphin project to the inferior colliculus. Although the olivocochlear bundle is not shown, it is noteworthy that enkephalin is found in some of the cells that contribute to this projection.

Clinical Correlations—Categories of Deafness

Conductive deafness is caused by problems of the external ear (obstruction of the canal, wax build-up) or disorders of the middle ear (otitis media, **otosclerosis**). **Nerve deafness (sensorineural hearing loss)** results from diseases involving the cochlea or the cochlear portion of the vestibulocochlear nerve. **Central deafness** results from damage to the cochlear nuclei or their central connections.

Hearing loss may result from trauma (e.g., **fracture of the petrous bone**), demyelinating diseases, **tumors**, certain medications (**streptomycin**), or **occlusion of the labyrinthine artery**. Damage to the cochlear part of the eighth nerve (e.g., **vestibular schwannoma**) results in **tinnitus** and/or **deafness** (partial or total) in the ipsilateral ear. High-frequency hearing losses (**presbyacusis**), such as a woman's voice or discrimination between sounds, are more commonly seen in older patients.

The **Weber test** and **Rinne test** are used to differentiate between neural hearing loss and conduction hearing loss, and to lateralize the deficit. In the **Weber test**, a tuning fork (512 Hz) is applied to the midline of the forehead or apex of the skull. In the normal patient, the sound (conducted through the skull bones) is heard the same in each ear. In the case of **nerve deafness** (cochlea or cochlear nerve lesions), the sound is best heard in the normal ear, whereas in **conductive deafness**, the sound is best heard in the abnormal ear. In the **Rinne test**, a tuning fork (512 Hz) is placed against the mastoid process. When the sound is no longer perceived, the prongs are moved close to the external acoustic meatus, where the sound is again heard; this is the situation in a normal individual (positive Rinne test). In middle ear disease, the sound is not heard at the external meatus after it has disappeared from touching the mastoid bone (abnormal or negative Rinne test). Therefore, a negative Rinne test signifies conductive hearing loss in the ear tested. In mild nerve deafness (cochlea or cochlear nerve lesions), the sound is heard by application of the tuning fork to the mastoid and movement to the ear (the Rinne test is positive). In severe nerve deafness, the sound may not be heard at either position.

In addition to hearing loss and tinnitus, large vestibular schwannomas may result in nausea, vomiting, ataxia/unsteady gait (vestibular root involvement), facial muscle weakness (facial root), altered facial sensations, and a diminished corneal reflex (trigeminal root). There also may be general signs associated with increased intracranial pressure (lethargy, headache, and vomiting).

Central lesions (e.g., gliomas or vascular occlusions) rarely produce unilateral or bilateral hearing losses that can be detected, the possible exception being pontine lesions, which damage the trapezoid body and nuclei. Injury to central auditory pathways and/or primary auditory cortex may diminish auditory acuity, decrease the ability to hear certain tones, or make it difficult to precisely localize sounds in space. Patients with damage to the secondary auditory cortex in the temporal lobe experience difficulty in understanding and/or interpreting sounds (**auditory agnosia**).

ABBREVIATIONS

AbdNu	Abducens nucleus	**MLF**	Medial longitudinal fasciculus
ACNu	Anterior (ventral) cochlear nucleus	**PCNu**	Posterior (dorsal) cochlear nucleus
ALS	Anterolateral system	**PulNu**	Pulvinar nuclear complex
CC	Crus cerebri	**RB**	Restiform body
FacNu	Facial nucleus	**RetF**	Reticular formation
IC	Inferior colliculus	**SC**	Superior colliculus
IC, Br	Inferior colliculus, brachium	**SCP, Dec**	Superior cerebellar peduncle, decussation
IC, Com	Inferior colliculus, commissure	**SO**	Superior olive
IC, SL	Internal capsule, sublenticular limb	**SpGang**	Spiral ganglion
LGNu	Lateral geniculate nucleus	**SpTTr**	Spinal trigeminal tract
LL	Lateral lemniscus	**TrapB**	Trapezoid body
LL, Nu	Lateral lemniscus, nucleus	**TrapNu**	Trapezoid nucleus
MGNu	Medial geniculate nucleus	**TTGy**	Transverse temporal gyrus
ML	Medial lemniscus		

Review of Blood Supply to Cochlear Nuclei, LL (and Associated Structures), Pontine Tegmentum, IC, and MGNu

Structures	Arteries
Cochlear Nuclei	Anterior inferior cerebellar (see Figure 6-16)
LL, SO in Pons	Long circumferential branches of basilar (see Figure 6-23)
IC	Long circumferential branches (quadrigeminal branches) of basilar, superior cerebellar (see Figure 6-30)
MGNu	Thalamogeniculate branches of posterior cerebral (see Figure 6-41)

8-49 Auditory Pathways in Anatomical Orientation

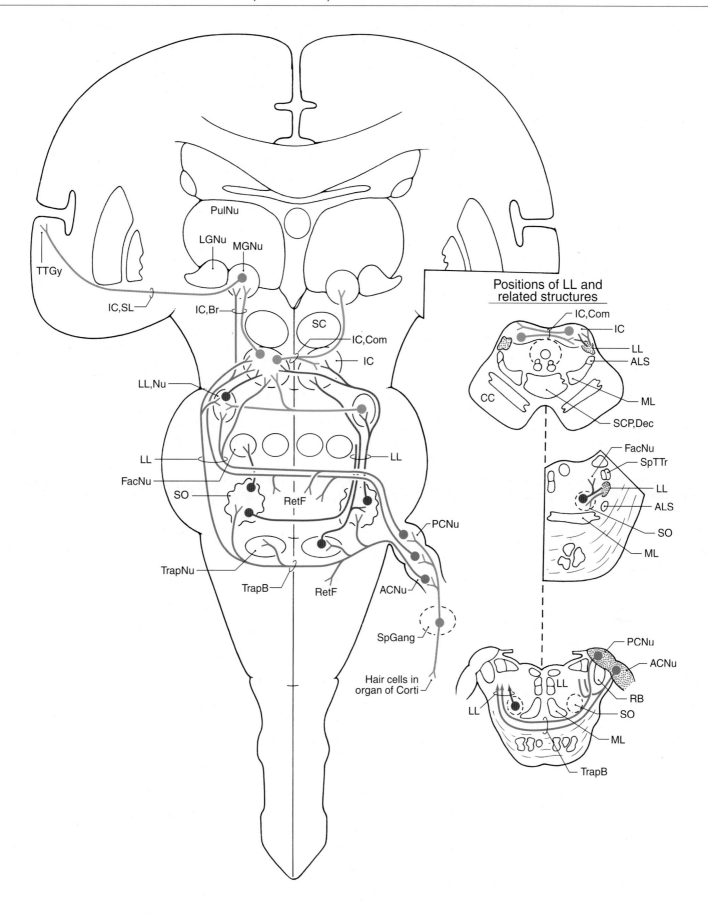

PulNu

LGNu MGNu

TTGy

IC,SL   IC,Br

SC

IC,Com

IC

LL,Nu

LL   LL

FacNu

SO   RetF

TrapNu

TrapB   RetF   ACNu

PCNu

SpGang

Hair cells in
organ of Corti

Positions of LL and
related structures

IC,Com

IC

LL
ALS

CC

ML

SCP,Dec

FacNu

SpTTr

LL

ALS

SO

ML

LL

PCNu

ACNu

LL

RB

SO

ML

TrapB

Vestibular Pathways in Anatomical Orientation

8-50 The origin, course, and distribution of the main **afferent and efferent connections of the vestibular nuclei** (see also Figs. 8-16, 8-36, and 8-37 on pp. 220, 246 and 248). **Primary vestibular afferent fibers** may end in the **vestibular nuclei** or pass to cerebellar structures via the **juxtarestiform body**. **Secondary vestibulocerebellar axons** originate from the vestibular nuclei and follow a similar path to the cerebellum. Efferent projections from the vestibular nuclei also course to the spinal cord through **vestibulospinal tracts** (see Figs. 8-16, 8-36, and 8-37), as well as to the **motor nuclei** of the **oculomotor, trochlear,** and **abducens nerves** via the MLF. Cerebellar structures most extensively interconnected with the vestibular nuclei include the lateral regions of the vermal cortex of anterior and posterior lobes, the **flocculonodular lobe,** and the fastigial (medial) cerebellar nucleus.

Neurotransmitters

γ-Aminobutyric acid (–) is the transmitter associated with many cerebellar corticovestibular fibers and their terminals in the vestibular complex; this substance is also seen in cerebellar corticonuclear axons. The medial vestibular nucleus also has fibers that are dynorphin-positive and histamine-positive; the latter arise from cells in the hypothalamus.

Clinical Correlations

The vestibular part of the eighth nerve can be damaged by many of the same insults that affect the cochlear nerve. Damage to vestibular receptors of the **vestibular nerve** commonly results in **vertigo**. The patient may feel that his or her body is moving (**subjective vertigo**) or that objects in the environment are moving (**objective vertigo**). They have equilibrium problems, an **unsteady (ataxic) gait,** and a tendency to fall to the lesioned side but do not have cerebellar signs such as an **intention tremor.** Deficits seen in nerve lesions, or in brainstem lesions involving the vestibular nuclei, include **nystagmus, nausea,** and **vomiting,** along with **vertigo** and gait problems.

Vestibular schwannoma represents about 8%–10% of CNS tumors, commonly results in hearing loss (95+%), is frequently characterized by disequilibrium and tinnitus (65%–70%), and is sometimes related to headache and facial numbness (about 30%); the latter indicates that the lesion is large (generally > 2 cm in size), and has encroached on the trigeminal nerve root. Facial weakness (**facial palsy**) occurs in about 10% of cases. These vestibular deficits, along with partial or complete deafness, are seen in **Ménière disease.** A patient that presents with **bilateral vestibular schwannomas** should be evaluated for **neurofibromatosis type 2.** These lesions are genetic in origin (autosomal dominant), may be accompanied by lesions elsewhere in the body (but less than NFT-Type 1), and are sometimes called **bilateral acoustic neurofibromatosis.**

Lesions of those parts of the cerebellum with which the vestibular nerve and nuclei are most intimately connected (**flocculonodular lobe** and **fastigial nucleus**) result in **nystagmus, truncal ataxia, ataxic gait,** and a propensity to fall to the injured side. The nystagmus seen in patients with vestibular lesions and the **internuclear ophthalmoplegia** seen in some patients with **multiple sclerosis** are signs that correlate with the interruption of vestibular projections to the motor nuclei of III, IV, and VI via the MLF.

ABBREVIATIONS

AbdNu	Abducens nucleus	**OcNu**	Oculomotor nucleus
ALS	Anterolateral system	**PAG**	Periaqueductal gray
Cbl	Cerebellar	**Py**	Pyramid
Cbl-CoVes	Cerebellar corticovestibular fibers	**RB**	Restiform body
CblNu	Cerebellar nuclei	**RNu**	Red nucleus
HyNu	Hypoglossal nucleus	**SC**	Superior colliculus
IC	Inferior colliculus	**SCP, Dec**	Superior cerebellar peduncle, decussation
InfVNu	Inferior (spinal) vestibular nucleus	**SN**	Substantia nigra
JRB	Juxtarestiform body	**SolNu**	Solitary nucleus
LVesSp	Lateral vestibulospinal tract	**SolTr**	Solitary tract
LVNu	Lateral vestibular nucleus	**SpTTr**	Spinal trigeminal tract
MesNu	Mesencephalic nucleus	**SVNu**	Superior vestibular nucleus
ML	Medial lemniscus	**TroNu**	Trochlear nucleus
MLF	Medial longitudinal fasciculus	**VesGang**	Vestibular ganglion
MVesSp	Medial vestibulospinal tract	**VesCbl, Prim**	Vestibulocerebellar fibers, primary
MVNu	Medial vestibular nucleus	**VesCbl, Sec**	Vestibulocerebellar fibers, secondary

Review of Blood Supply to Vestibular Nuclei, TroNu, and OcNu	
Structures	**Arteries**
Vestibular Nuclei	Posterior inferior cerebellar in medulla (see Figure 6-16), long circumferential branches of basilar in pons (see Figure 6-23)
TroNu and **OcNu**	Paramedian branches of basilar bifurcation, medial branches of posterior cerebral and posterior communicating, short circumferential branches of posterior cerebral (see Figure 6-30)

8-50 Vestibular Pathways in Anatomical Orientation

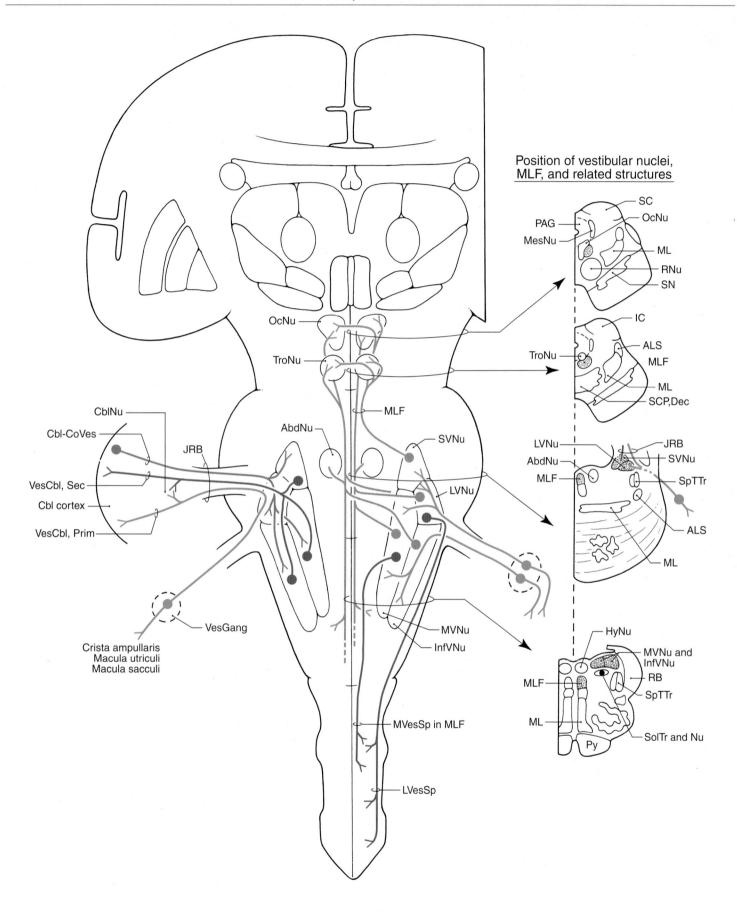

Position of vestibular nuclei, MLF, and related structures

Blank Master Drawing for Auditory or Vestibular Pathways

8-51 Blank master drawing for auditory or vestibular pathway. This illustration is provided for self-evaluation of auditory or vestibular pathway understanding, for the instructor to expand on aspects of these pathways not covered in the atlas, or both.

NOTES

8-51 Blank Master Drawing for Auditory or Vestibular Pathways

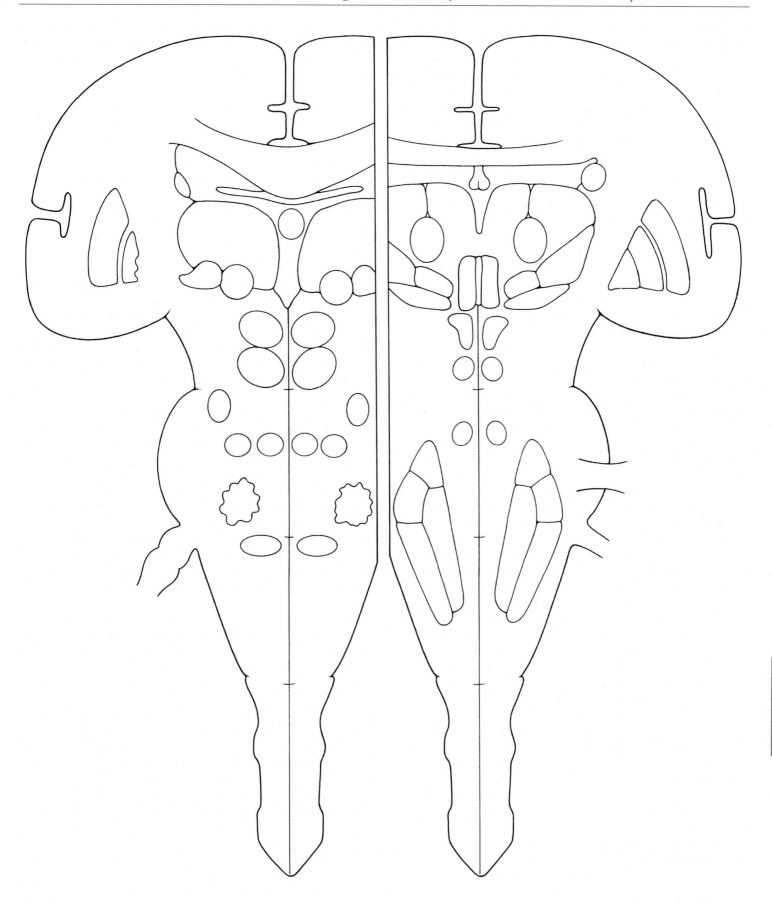

The Internal Capsule: Relationships and Contents

8-52 The **internal capsule**, its relationship to the basal nuclei and thalamus, and its major constituent fiber bundles in the axial plane. Pathways conveying sensory information (with the exception of olfaction) from the entire body and pathways influencing motor activity of cranial nerves and the extremities all traverse some part of the internal capsule.

The **internal capsule** is divided into five parts, called **limbs**, which are most easily recognized in the axial plane (see facing page). Each limb has a characteristic relationship to adjacent structures and largely contains particular fiber groups.

Anterior limb: The **anterior limb** is located between the head of the caudate nucleus and the lenticular nucleus. The major fiber populations found in the anterior limb are **frontopontine fibers**, the **anterior thalamic radiations** (medial and anterior thalamic projections to the frontal and cingulate cortex), and, adjacent to the genu, small fascicles of descending fibers from the frontal eye fields.

Genu: The positions of the **column of the fornix**, the **interventricular foramen**, the **venous angle**, and the **anterior tubercle of the thalamus** indicate the location of the **genu of the internal capsule**. The most clinically significant fiber bundles in the genu are **corticonuclear fibers** projecting to the motor nuclei of cranial nerves (see also Figures 8-13 and 8-14 on pp. 214–217).

Posterior limb: The **posterior limb** is the largest part of the internal capsule, is located **between the thalamus and the lenticular nucleus**, and contains a number of important fiber populations. These larger bundles include **corticospinal fibers, superior thalamic radiations** (ventral anterior, ventral lateral, ventral posteromedial, and posterolateral projections to motor and sensory cortices), and, in its more caudal region, **parietopontine fibers**. Smaller bundles of fibers including **corticorubral, corticoreticular, corticonigral, corticosubthalamic**, the general category of corticotegmental fibers, and **pallidothalamic fibers** that arise in the medial segment of the globus pallidus, traverse the posterior limb.

Sublenticular limb: The **sublenticular limb** is difficult to identify, although its trajectory and contents are well known. It extends between the medial geniculate nucleus and the temporal lobe, particularly the auditory cortex, and contains **auditory radiations (geniculotemporal radiations), temporopontine fibers**, and **corticotectal fibers**.

Retrolenticular limb: The **retrolenticular limb** is that large mass of fibers located immediately caudal the lenticular nucleus; hence its name, retrolenticular. The larger fiber bundles within this limb are **visual radiations (geniculocalcarine or optic radiations)** and occipitopontine fibers; the smaller bundles comprise **corticotectal, corticotegmental**, and some **corticorubral fibers**.

Recall that the **optic radiations** are composed of fibers that arise in the **lateral geniculate nucleus** and pass caudally directly to the **primary visual cortex**, and of fibers that arise in the lateral geniculate nucleus, arch forward into the temporal lobe, turn sharply caudal (as the **Meyer loop**), and then proceed to the primary visual cortex. These two portions of the optic radiations are conveying information from different parts of the visual fields; lesions of these parts result in specific visual deficits (see Figs. 8-44 through 8-47 on pp. 262–267).

General note: Most of the limbs of the internal capsule also contain **thalamocortical projections** (other than those mentioned above), **corticothalamic fibers** (from all cortical areas to their respective thalamic nuclei), and **corticostriate fibers**.

Neurotransmitters

There are no nuclei within the internal capsule, only fibers of passage conveying a variety of motor and sensory information, and fibers that are integrative in nature. The major transmitters associated with fibers within the internal capsule are **glutamate** (most cortical efferent fibers, thalamocortical fibers) and **GABA** (pallidothalamic fibers), and smaller populations of **cholinergic, dopaminergic, serotoninergic, histaminergic**, and **GABA-ergic fibers**.

Clinical Correlations

Lesions of the internal capsule are usually expressed as **movement disorders** related to involvement of **corticospinal or corticonuclear fibers** (depending on the general location of the lesion) and **somatosensory losses** related to damage to **thalamocortical projections**. A general characteristic of forebrain lesions is motor and sensory deficits that are all on the same side (the side of the body opposite the location of the lesion). Cranial nerve deficits are usually lacking unless the damage involves the genu of the internal capsule.

A lesion in the **genu of the internal capsule** results in deficits that generally reflect damage to corticonuclear fibers to the **facial** and **hypoglossal nuclei**, and to the **nucleus ambiguus**. The facial muscles are weak on the lower half of the face opposite the lesion (a **central seven** as opposed to a **Bell palsy**), the **tongue deviates** to the opposite side on attempted protrusion, and the **uvula deviates** toward the lesioned side when the patient makes an "ah" sound. In addition, the patient may not be able to elevate the ipsilateral shoulder against resistance (**trapezius weakness**) or to rotate the head to the contralateral side against resistance (**sternocleidomastoid weakness**) assuming injury to fibers of the accessory nucleus. This combination of deficits is unique to genu lesions and is clearly different from cranial nerve deficits resulting from brainstem lesions.

Damage to the posterior limb of the internal capsule may result in a frank **contralateral hemiplegia** or **hemiparesis** (-plegia refers to paralysis and -paresis refers to weakness or incomplete paralysis) affecting upper and lower extremities and a **hemianesthesia** on the same side as the weakness. This sensory loss may affect the body only or the body plus the head.

The **anterior choroidal artery syndrome** (also called **von Monakow syndrome**) is characterized by a **hemiplegia** and a **homonymous hemianopia**, both contralateral to the side of the lesion. If this lesion (which is in the lower portion of the posterior limb) extends upward, it may also involve thalamocortical fibers from sensory relay nuclei, producing a **hemianesthesia** on the same side as the other deficits. This vessel serves portions of the genu, and corticonuclear deficits may sometimes be seen.

ABBREVIATIONS	
f.	Fibers
rad.	Radiations

Review of Blood Supply to the Internal Capsule	
Structures	**Arteries**
Anterior Limb	Lateral striate branches of middle cerebral; medial striate branches of anterior cerebral (see Figure 6-41)
Genu	Lateral striate branches of middle cerebral; anterior choroidal artery (see Figure 6-41)
Posterior Limb	Lateral striate branches of middle cerebral; anterior choroidal artery (see Figure 6-41)
Sublenticular Limb	Penetrating branches of middle cerebral (temporal, angular branches)
Retrolenticular Limb	Posterior cerebral; small branches from anterior choroidal

8-52 The Internal Capsule: Relationships and Contents

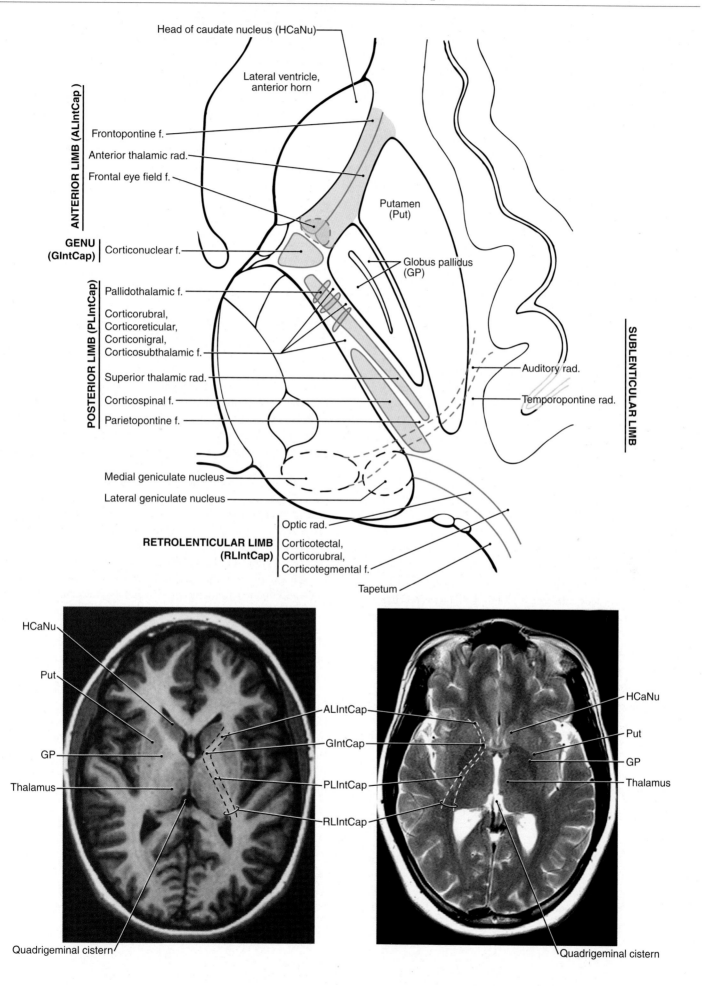

The Topography of Thalamocortical Connections

8-53 The major nuclei of the **dorsal thalamus,** commonly called the **thalamus,** and their major cortical targets. The thalamic nuclei may generally be divided into **association nuclei, relay nuclei,** and **intralaminar nuclei. Association nuclei** project to multiple cortical regions and receive input from similarly diverse regions (e.g., pulvinar, centromedian). **Relay nuclei** are those which receive a specific type of information (discriminative touch, vision) and send this information on to a precise cortical target (primary somatosensory cortex, primary visual cortex); examples are: the ventral posterolateral nucleus and the lateral geniculate nucleus. **Intralaminar nuclei** are located within the internal medullary lamina; the most obvious is the centromedian nucleus; smaller intralaminar nuclei include the central lateral, central medial, and the parafascicular nuclei. The **thalamic reticular nucleus** is a group of neurons forming a shell around the thalamus, separated from it by the internal medullary lamina, and located medial to the internal capsule.

The thalamic nuclei receive information from many sources and project to the cerebral cortex. The more important thalamic nuclei, their afferents, and the cortical areas/gyri to which they project are summarized below and illustrated in Figure 8-53 on the facing page. Some generalizations are made for clarity.

Association nuclei:

Dorsomedial nucleus: **afferents**—amygdala, pallidum, temporal and orbitofrontal cortex, olfactory system, basal forebrain; **efferents**—orbital cortex, medial and lateral frontal lobe (excluding the motor cortex)

Pulvinar: **afferents**—superior colliculus, visual cortex (areas 17, 18, 19), temporal and occipital cortex; **efferents**—superior colliculus, visual cortex (areas 17, 18, 19), temporal and occipital cortex

Relay nuclei:

Anterior thalamic nuclei: **afferents**—medial mammillary nucleus, hippocampal formation; **efferents**—cingulate gyrus, small amount to limbic and orbitofrontal cortex

Ventral anterior nucleus: **afferents**—globus pallidus, substantia nigra, cortical areas 6 and 8; **efferents**—frontal cortex (excluding area 4), orbital cortex

Ventral lateral nucleus: **afferents**—globus pallidus, cerebellar nuclei, motor cortex (area 4); **efferents**—motor cortex (area 4), supplemental motor cortex

Ventral posterolateral nucleus: **afferents**—posterior column–medial lemniscus system, anterolateral system; **efferents**—primary somatosensory cortex (areas 3, 1, 2)

Ventral posteromedial nucleus: **afferents**—spinal and principal sensory nuclei, solitary nucleus (taste); **efferents**—face area of primary somatosensory cortex (areas 3, 1, 2), frontal operculum and adjacent insular cortex (taste areas)

Medial geniculate nucleus: **afferent**—inferior colliculus; **efferents**—transverse temporal gyrus (of Heschl, area 41)

Lateral geniculate nucleus: **afferents**—portions of both retina, visual area 17; **efferents**—primary visual cortex (area 17, some to 18 and 19)

Intralaminar nuclei:

Centromedian nucleus: **afferents**—frontal, limbic and motor cortex, pallidum, cerebellar nuclei, reticular formation, spinal cord, sensory cortex; **efferents**—corpus striatum (putamen, globus pallidus, caudate), subthalamic nucleus, substantia nigra, frontal lobe

Other intralaminar nuclei: **afferents**—cerebral cortex, brainstem reticular formation, nucleus accumbens, olfactory tubercle; **efferents**—similar to centromedian, cingulate gyrus

Other:

Thalamic reticular nucleus: **afferents**—collaterals of thalamocortical, corticothalamic, thalamostriate, and pallidothalamic fibers; **efferents**—thalamic nuclei

Clinical Correlations

The thalamus receives extensive sensory and motor messages, has an equally extensive projection to all parts of the cerebral cortex, and receives reciprocal connections from the cerebral cortex. Consequently, a variety of deficits is seen resultant to lesions of the thalamus. While thalamic lesions may present as **tumors** (such as **astrocytoma**), **neural degenerative,** or encephalopathic, they are most commonly vascular in origin.

Hemorrhage into the thalamogeniculate territory damages the sensory relay nuclei (VPM and VPL) and may result in the **thalamic syndrome** (syndrome of **Déjèrine-Roussy**). The characteristics of this syndrome are: (1) loss of all somatic sensation on the contralateral side of the body, or a **dissociated sensory loss** (position/vibratory loss greater than pain/thermal loss, or vice versa); (2) with recovery, the occurrence of a perception of pain (**paresthesia, hyperpathia**) sometimes intense and/or long-lasting; and, (3) may present with a **homonymous hemianopia** and/or **hemiplegia** of the UE and LE, all on the contralateral side; these may resolve with time. The hemiplegia may relate to hemorrhage impinging on the laterally adjacent internal capsule or pressure from the primary lesion.

In addition to variations of the thalamic syndrome, hemorrhagic thalamic lesions may extend into the midbrain and produce various **oculomotor deficits** (third nerve or nucleus damage), **pupil dilation,** and an absent or diminished **pupillary light reflex.** These hemorrhagic lesions may also invade the subthalamic nucleus and contribute abnormal movements to the overall clinical picture.

Lesions in more anterior and medial portions of the dorsal thalamus may produce deficits that are generally more global. The patient may experience **ataxia** (thalamic ataxia) of a transient nature and possibly **aphasia** .In the case of a lesion in the thalamic territory of an azygous thalamoperforating territory (see Figure 2-44, p. 39), the pathway of the ascending reticular activating system is interrupted, and the patient may be difficult to arouse, stuporous, or in a coma.

Review of Blood Supply to the Dorsal Thalamus	
Structures	**Arteries**
Anterior Thalamic Areas	Thalamoperforating branches of P_1 (see Figure 6-41)
Posterior Thalamic Areas	Thalamogeniculate branches of P_2 (see Figure 6-41)
Caudomedial Thalamic Area	Medial posterior choroidal artery, P_2 branch (see Figure 6-41)

8-53 The Topography of Thalamocortical Connections

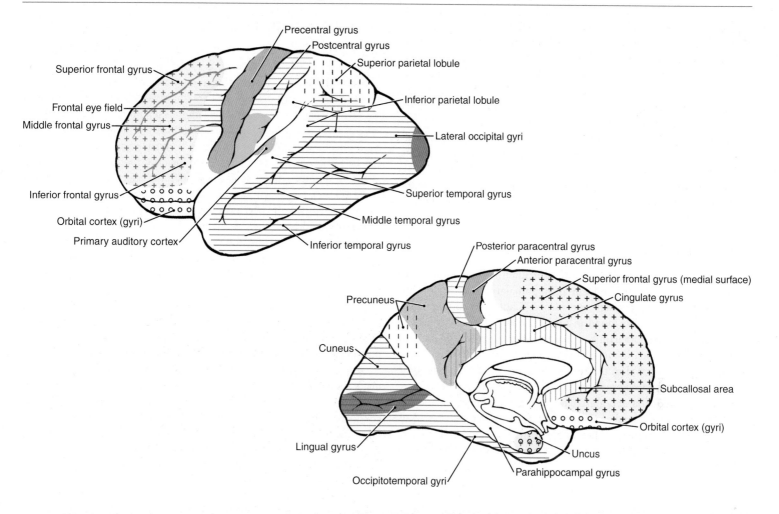

Precentral gyrus
Postcentral gyrus
Superior parietal lobule
Superior frontal gyrus
Inferior parietal lobule
Frontal eye field
Middle frontal gyrus
Lateral occipital gyri
Inferior frontal gyrus
Superior temporal gyrus
Orbital cortex (gyri)
Middle temporal gyrus
Primary auditory cortex
Inferior temporal gyrus

Posterior paracentral gyrus
Anterior paracentral gyrus
Superior frontal gyrus (medial surface)
Precuneus
Cingulate gyrus
Cuneus
Subcallosal area
Orbital cortex (gyri)
Lingual gyrus
Uncus
Parahippocampal gyrus
Occipitotemporal gyri

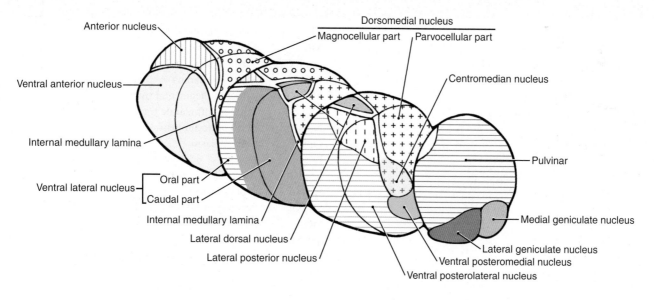

Dorsomedial nucleus
Anterior nucleus
Magnocellular part   Parvocellular part
Ventral anterior nucleus
Centromedian nucleus
Internal medullary lamina
Ventral lateral nucleus — Oral part
                         Caudal part
Pulvinar
Internal medullary lamina
Lateral dorsal nucleus
Medial geniculate nucleus
Lateral posterior nucleus
Lateral geniculate nucleus
Ventral posteromedial nucleus
Ventral posterolateral nucleus

Hippocampal Connections in Anatomical Orientation

8-54 Selected **afferent and efferent connections of the hippocampus** (upper) and the **mammillary body** (lower) with emphasis on the **circuit of Papez.** The hippocampus receives input from, and projects to, diencephalic nuclei (especially the mammillary body via the **postcommissural fornix**), the septal region, and amygdala. The hippocampus receives cortical input from the superior and middle frontal gyri, superior temporal and cingulate gyri, precuneus, lateral occipital cortex, occipitotemporal gyri, and subcallosal cortical areas. The mammillary body is connected with the dorsal and ventral tegmental nuclei, anterior thalamic nucleus (via the **mammillothalamic tract**), septal nuclei, and through the **mammillotegmental tract,** to the tegmental pontine and reticulotegmental nuclei.

Neurotransmitters

Glutamate (+)-containing cells in the subiculum and Ammon's horn project to the mammillary body, other hypothalamic centers, and the lateral septal nucleus through the fornix. Cholecystokinin (+) and somatostatin (−) are also found in hippocampal cells that project to septal nuclei and hypothalamic structures. The septal nuclei and the nucleus of the diagonal band give rise to cholinergic afferents to the hippocampus that travel in the fornix. In addition, a γ-aminobutyric acid (−) septohippocampal projection originates from the medial septal nucleus. Enkephalin and glutamate containing hippocampal afferent fibers arise from the adjacent entorhinal cortex; the locus ceruleus gives origin to noradrenergic fibers to the dentate gyrus, Ammon horn, and subiculum; and serotoninergic fibers arise from the rostral raphe nuclei.

Clinical Correlations

Dysfunction associated with damage to the hippocampus is seen in patients with **trauma** to the temporal lobe, as a sequel to **alcoholism,** and as a result of **neurodegenerative changes** seen in the dementing diseases (e.g., **Alzheimer disease** and **Pick disease**). Bilateral injury to the hippocampus results in loss of recent memory (remote memory is unaffected), impaired ability to remember recent (new) events, and difficulty in turning a new experience (something just done or experienced) into a longer-term memory that can be retrieved at a later time. Also, memory that depends on visual, tactile, or auditory discrimination is noticeably affected. These represent **visual agnosia, tactile agnosia,** and **auditory agnosia,** respectively.

In the **Korsakoff psychosis (amnestic confabulatory syndrome, Korsakoff syndrome)** there is memory loss, dementia, amnesia, and a tendency to give confabulated responses. This type of response is fluent (the patient's response is immediate, smooth, and in appropriate cadence), but consists of a string of unrelated, or even made up, "memories" that never actually occurred or make no sense (hence, the **confabulation**). This may lead to an incorrect conclusion that the patient is suffering from **dementia.** In addition to lesions in the hippocampus in these patients, the mammillary bodies and dorsomedial nucleus of the thalamus are noticeably affected. Korsakoff psychosis is irreversible.

Wernicke encephalopathy (Wernicke-Korsakoff syndrome, or Wernicke syndrome) is seen in patients who are long-term alcoholics, and presents with a variety of **eye movement deficits, pupil changes, ataxia, confusion,** and **tremor.** Degenerative changes, or cell loss, are seen in many areas but especially in the hippocampus, mammillary nuclei, and dorsomedial nucleus of the thalamus. This condition is treatable with therapeutic doses of thiamin and dietary improvements.

ABBREVIATIONS

AC	Anterior commissure	**LT**	Lamina terminalis
AmHrn	Ammon horn	**MB**	Mammillary body
Amy	Amygdaloid nucleus (complex)	**MedFCtx**	Medial frontal cortex
AntNu	Anterior nucleus of thalamus	**MedTh**	Medial thalamus
CC, G	Corpus callosum, genu	**MTegTr**	Mammillotegmental tract
CC, Spl	Corpus callosum, splenium	**MtTr**	Mammillothalamic tract
Cing	Cingulum	**NuAcc**	Nucleus accumbens
CingGy	Cingulate gyrus	**OpCh**	Optic chiasm
CorHip	Corticohippocampal fibers	**Pi**	Pineal
DenGy	Dentate gyrus	**RSplCtx**	Retrosplenial cortex
EnCtx	Entorhinal cortex	**SepNu**	Septal nuclei
For	Fornix	**SMNu**	Supramammillary nucleus
GyRec	Gyrus rectus	**Sub**	Subiculum
Hip	Hippocampus	**TegNu**	Tegmental nuclei
Hyth	Hypothalamus	**VmNu**	Ventromedial hypothalamic nucleus
IC, G	Internal capsule, genu		

Review of Blood Supply to Hip, MB, Hyth, and CingGy	
Structures	**Arteries**
Hip	Anterior choroidal (see Figure 6-41)
MB, Hyth	Branches of circle of Willis (see Figure 2-21)
AntNu	Thalamoperforating (see Figure 6-41)
CingGy	Branches of anterior cerebral

8-54 Hippocampal Connections in Anatomical Orientation

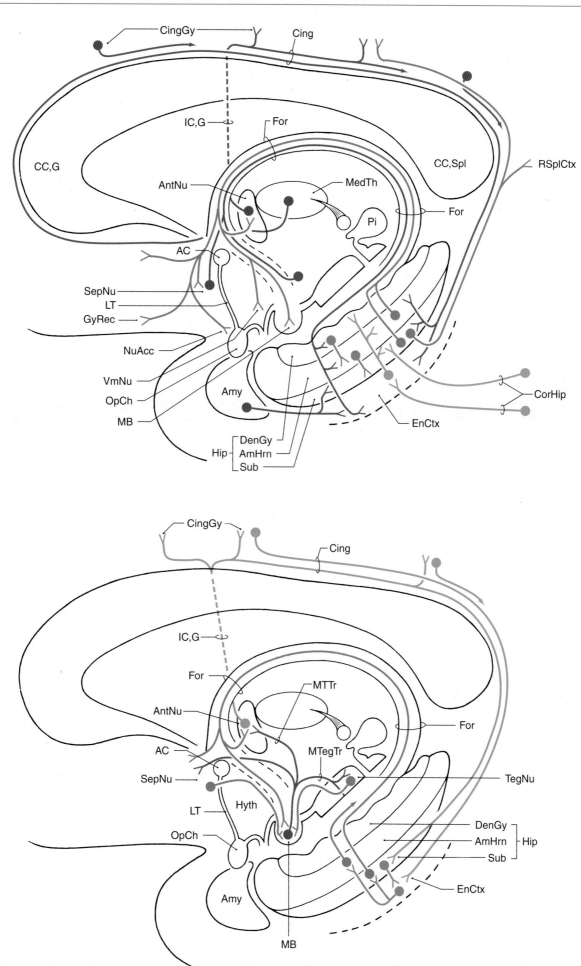

Amygdaloid Connections in Anatomical Orientation

8-55 The origin, course, and distribution of selected **afferent and efferent connections of the amygdaloid nuclear complex** in sagittal (upper) and coronal (lower) planes. The amygdala receives input from, and projects to, brainstem and forebrain centers via the **stria terminalis** and the **ventral amygdalofugal pathway**. Corticoamygdaloid and amygdalocortical fibers interconnect the basal and lateral amygdaloid nuclei with select cortical areas.

Neurotransmitters

Cells in the amygdaloid complex contain vasoactive intestinal polypeptide (VIP, +), neurotensin (NT), somatostatin (SOM, −), enkephalin (ENK, −), and substance P (SP, +). These neurons project, via the stria terminalis or the ventral amygdalofugal path, to the septal nuclei (VIP, NT), the bed nucleus of the stria terminalis (NT, ENK, SP), the hypothalamus (VIP, SOM, SP), the nucleus accumbens septi, and the caudate and putamen (NT). Serotonergic amygdaloid fibers originate from the nucleus raphe dorsalis and the superior central nucleus, dopaminergic axons from the ventral tegmental area and the substantia nigra–pars compacta, and noradrenalin-containing fibers from the locus ceruleus. Glutamate (+) is found in olfactory projections to the prepiriform cortex and the amygdaloid complex. Acetylcholine is present in afferents to the amygdala from the substantia innominata, as well as from the septal area. In patients with Alzheimer disease and the associated dementia, there is a marked loss of acetylcholine-containing neurons in the basal nucleus of the substantia innominata, the cortex, and the hippocampus.

Clinical Correlations

Dysfunctions related to damage to the **amygdaloid complex** are seen in patients with trauma to the temporal lobes, **herpes simplex encephalitis**, bilateral temporal lobe surgery to treat intractable epileptic activity, and in some CNS degenerative disorders (e.g., **Alzheimer disease** and **Pick disease**). The behavioral changes seen in individuals with what are usually bilateral amygdala lesions collectively form the **Klüver-Bucy syndrome**. In humans these changes/deficits are: 1) **hyperorality**; 2) **visual, tactile**, and **auditory agnosia**; 3) **placidity**; 4) **hyperphagia** or other dietary manifestations; 5) an intense desire to explore the immediate environment (**hypermetamorphosis**); and 6) what is commonly called **hypersexuality**. These changes in sexual attitudes are usually in the form of comments, suggestions, and and inept attempts at actual contact rather than attempts at inappropriate behavior. These patients also may show **aphasia, dementia**, and **amnesia**.

ABBREVIATIONS

AC	Anterior commissure	NuRa, d	Nucleus raphe, dorsalis
Amy	Amygdaloid nuclear complex	NuRa, m	Nucleus raphe, magnus
AmyCor	Amygdalocortical fibers	NuRa, o	Nucleus raphe, obscurus
AmyFugPath	Amygdalofugal pathway	NuRa, p	Nucleus raphe, pallidus
AntHyth	Anterior hypothalamus	NuStTer	Nucleus of the stria terminalis
Ba-LatNu	Basal and lateral nuclei	OlfB	Olfactory bulb
CaNu	Caudate nucleus	OpCh	Optic chiasm
Cen-MedNu	Central, cortical and medial nuclei	PAG	Periaqueductal (central) gray
CorAmy	Corticoamygdaloid fibers	PbrNu	Parabrachial nuclei
DVagNu	Dorsal motor vagal nucleus	PfNu	Parafascicular nucleus
EnCtx	Entorhinal cortex	Pi	Pineal
For	Fornix	POpNu	Preoptic nucleus
GP	Globus pallidus	PPriCtx	Prepiriform cortex
Hyth	Hypothalamus	Put	Putamen
LT	Lamina terminalis	SepNu	Septal nuclei
LHAr	Lateral hypothalamic area	SNpc	Substantia nigra, pars compacta
MedThNu	Medial thalamic nuclei	SolNu	Solitary nucleus
MGNu	Medial geniculate nucleus	StTer	Stria terminalis
MidTh	Midline thalamic nuclei	Sub	Subiculum
NuAcc	Nucleus accumbens	SubLn	Substantia innominata
NuCen, s	Nucleus centralis, superior	VenTegAr	Ventral tegmental area
NuCer	Nucleus ceruleus	VmNu	Ventromedial hypothalamic nucleus

Review of Blood Supply to Amy and Related Centers	
Structures	**Arteries**
Amy	Anterior choroidal (see Figure 6-41)
Hyth	Branches of circle of Willis (see Figure 6-41)
Brainstem	(see Figures 6-16, 6-23, and 6-30)
Thalamus	Thalamoperforating, thalamogeniculate (see Figure 6-41)

8-55 Amygdaloid Connections in Anatomical Orientation

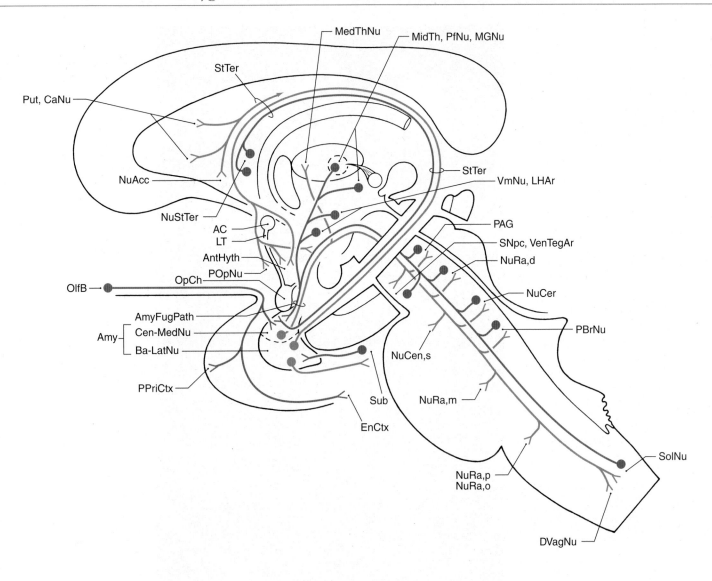

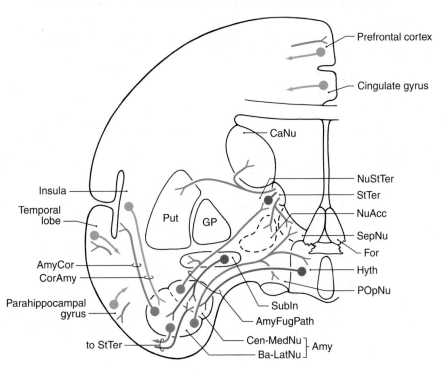

Hippocampal and Amygdaloid Efferents in Clinical Orientation

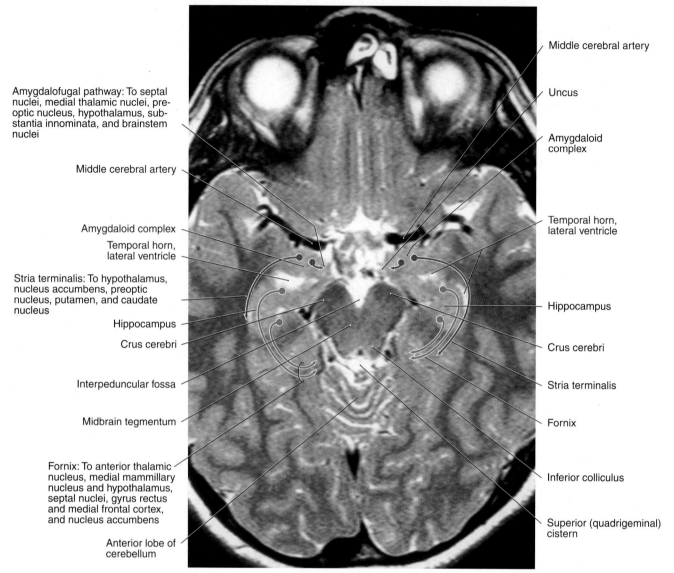

Amygdalofugal pathway: To septal nuclei, medial thalamic nuclei, pre-optic nucleus, hypothalamus, sub-stantia innominata, and brainstem nuclei

Middle cerebral artery

Amygdaloid complex

Temporal horn, lateral ventricle

Stria terminalis: To hypothalamus, nucleus accumbens, preoptic nucleus, putamen, and caudate nucleus

Hippocampus

Crus cerebri

Interpeduncular fossa

Midbrain tegmentum

Fornix: To anterior thalamic nucleus, medial mammillary nucleus and hypothalamus, septal nuclei, gyrus rectus and medial frontal cortex, and nucleus accumbens

Anterior lobe of cerebellum

Middle cerebral artery

Uncus

Amygdaloid complex

Temporal horn, lateral ventricle

Hippocampus

Crus cerebri

Stria terminalis

Fornix

Inferior colliculus

Superior (quadrigeminal) cistern

8-56A The **principal efferent projections of the amygdaloid nucleus and the hippocampal formation** superimposed on MRI in clinical orientation. This axial image is a T2-weighted MRI. The arrowheads on the efferent fibers, and the targets indicated for these fibers, indicate that these pathways have extensive and wide-spread connections.

Hippocampal and Amygdaloid Efferents in Clinical Orientation: Representative Lesions and Deficits

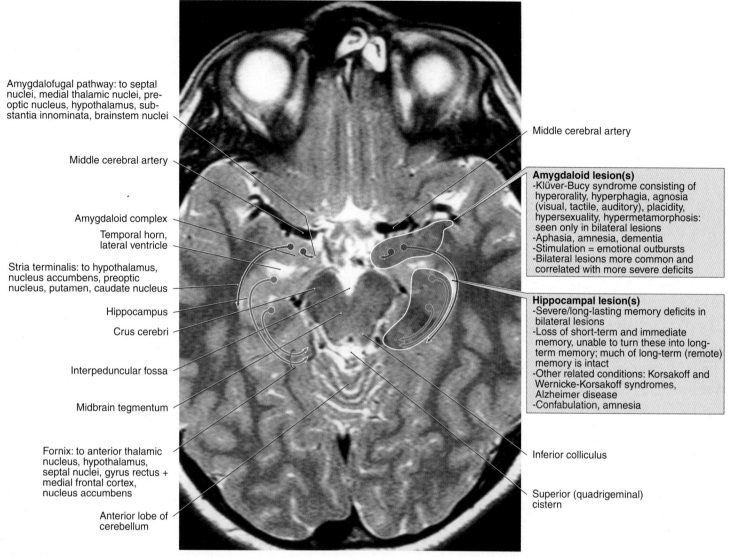

Amygdalofugal pathway: to septal nuclei, medial thalamic nuclei, pre-optic nucleus, hypothalamus, substantia innominata, brainstem nuclei

Middle cerebral artery

Amygdaloid complex

Temporal horn, lateral ventricle

Stria terminalis: to hypothalamus, nucleus accumbens, preoptic nucleus, putamen, caudate nucleus

Hippocampus

Crus cerebri

Interpeduncular fossa

Midbrain tegmentum

Fornix: to anterior thalamic nucleus, hypothalamus, septal nuclei, gyrus rectus + medial frontal cortex, nucleus accumbens

Anterior lobe of cerebellum

Middle cerebral artery

Amygdaloid lesion(s)
-Klüver-Bucy syndrome consisting of hyperorality, hyperphagia, agnosia (visual, tactile, auditory), placidity, hypersexuality, hypermetamorphosis: seen only in bilateral lesions
-Aphasia, amnesia, dementia
-Stimulation = emotional outbursts
-Bilateral lesions more common and correlated with more severe deficits

Hippocampal lesion(s)
-Severe/long-lasting memory deficits in bilateral lesions
-Loss of short-term and immediate memory, unable to turn these into long-term memory; much of long-term (remote) memory is intact
-Other related conditions: Korsakoff and Wernicke-Korsakoff syndromes, Alzheimer disease
-Confabulation, amnesia

Inferior colliculus

Superior (quadrigeminal) cistern

8-56B Representative lesions of the amygdaloid nucleus and hippocampal formation and the deficits (in pink boxes) that correlate with each lesion. Damage to these regions of the rostral and medial temporal lobes is most frequently bilateral; motor vehicle collisions are common causes. Although there may be damage to only one side, as in stroke, deficits are most severe in situations of bilateral damage.

Blank Master Drawing for Limbic Pathways

8-57 Blank master drawing for limbic pathways. This illustration is provided for self-evaluation of limbic pathways or connections, for the instructor to expand on aspects of these pathways not covered in the atlas, or both.

NOTES

8-58 Hypothalamic Structures and Connections: Stained Sections

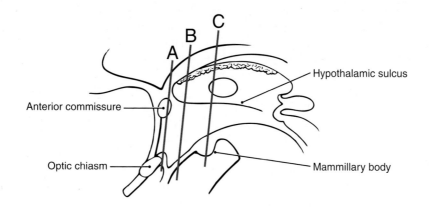

Anterior commissure

Hypothalamic sulcus

Optic chiasm

Mammillary body

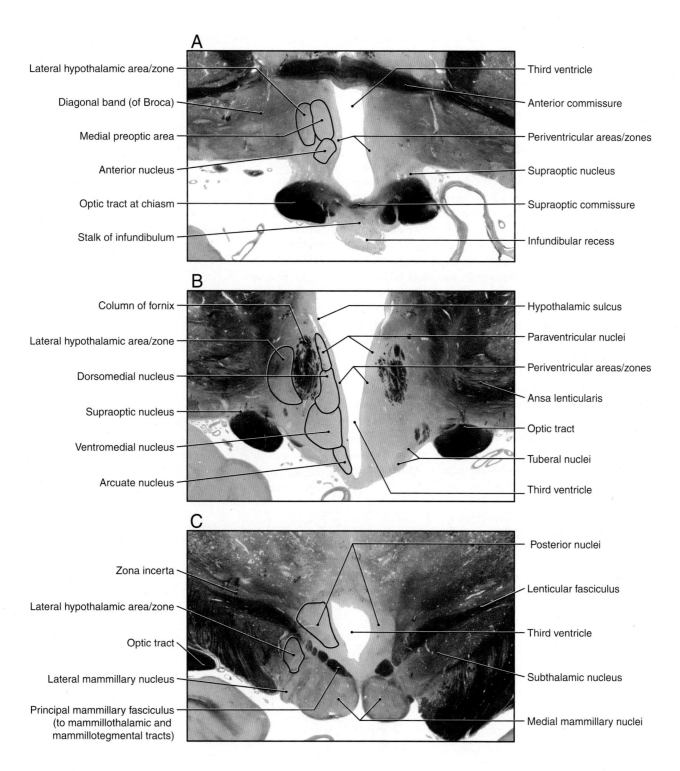

A

Lateral hypothalamic area/zone — Third ventricle

Diagonal band (of Broca) — Anterior commissure

Medial preoptic area — Periventricular areas/zones

Anterior nucleus — Supraoptic nucleus

Optic tract at chiasm — Supraoptic commissure

Stalk of infundibulum — Infundibular recess

B

Column of fornix — Hypothalamic sulcus

Lateral hypothalamic area/zone — Paraventricular nuclei

Dorsomedial nucleus — Periventricular areas/zones

Supraoptic nucleus — Ansa lenticularis

Ventromedial nucleus — Optic tract

Arcuate nucleus — Tuberal nuclei

Third ventricle

C

Posterior nuclei

Zona incerta — Lenticular fasciculus

Lateral hypothalamic area/zone — Third ventricle

Optic tract — Subthalamic nucleus

Lateral mammillary nucleus — Medial mammillary nuclei

Principal mammillary fasciculus
(to mammillothalamic and
mammillotegmental tracts)

Hypothalamic Structures and Connections: Projections

8-59 The structure of the **hypothalamus** represented in the axial plane showing the **three zones,** the **regions of each zone,** and their major afferent and efferent connections. The connections of the hypothalamus are complex and widespread within the brain. In addition, many of these connections are reciprocal: structures that project to the hypothalamus frequently receive input from the hypothalamus. An effort is made here to illustrate the hypothalamus in axial plane, its principal nuclei, and its major afferent and efferent pathways, all in a diagrammatic format. Hypothalamic afferents are shown in red (on right), efferents in blue (on left).

Zones: The **lateral zone** (shaded blue) contains diffuse cell groups, the tuberal nuclei, and the fibers of the medial forebrain bundle. The **medial zone** is organized into the **supraoptic region** (shaded green), the **tuberal region** (shaded red), and the **mammillary region** (shaded gray); each region is composed of several named nuclei. The **periventricular zone** (unshaded/white) is a thin sheet of cells in the wall of the hypothalamic portion of the third ventricle. See also Figure 8-58.

Retinohypothalamic fibers: Axons arising from ganglion cells of the retina project bilaterally to the **suprachiasmatic nucleus** via the optic nerve and tract. These projections are essential to the **maintenance of circadian rhythms.**

Amygdalohypothalamic fibers: The amygdala projects to the hypothalamus via the **ventral amygdalofugal pathway (VAF)** and the **stria terminalis (ST).** VAF fibers arise in the **basolateral amygdala,** course medially and inferior to the lenticular nucleus, to end in the septal area, lateral zone, and preoptic areas. Fibers forming the ST arise in the **corticomedial amygdala,** form a small bundle medial to the caudate and accompanied by the thalamostriate vein, and distribute to the septal area and nuclei of the supraoptic and tuberal regions.

Hippocampohypothalamic fibers: Cells of the hippocampal formation coalesce to form the **fornix.** The **precommissural fornix** is diffusely arranged and distributes to septal, preoptic, and anterior hypothalamic nuclei, whereas the primary target of the **postcommissural fornix,** which is compactly arranged is the medial mammillary nucleus with lesser projections to the dorsomedial nucleus and lateral hypothalamic zone.

Brainstem-hypothalamic fibers: Afferents to the hypothalamus that arise within the brainstem and ascend mainly in the **mammillary peduncle** and **posterior (dorsal) longitudinal fasciculus,** with fewer fibers traversing the **medial forebrain bundle.** These projections arise in the tegmental and raphe nuclei of the midbrain, the locus coeruleus, and the lateral parabrachial nucleus and terminate in the lateral zone and in many of the nuclei of the medial and paraventricular zones. Serotinergic fibers arise from the raphe nuclei, and monoaminergic projections originate from the locus coeruleus.

Other afferent fibers: The hypothalamus also receives **spinohypothalamic fibers** via the anterolateral system and **corticohypothalamic fibers** from widespread areas of the cerebral cortex including occipital, frontal, and parietal, and from the cortices of the limbic lobe.

Efferent hypothalamic connections: The double-headed arrows on the left signify the fact that the amygdaloid nuclear complex and the hippocampal formation receive input from the hypothalamic nuclei to which they project. This also applies to the fact that many of the cortical areas that give rise to a corticohypothalamic projection also receive hypothalamocortical fibers.

The **posterior (dorsal) longitudinal fasciculus** contains fibers arising in various nuclei of the periventricular and medial zones and projects to the midbrain tegmentum, tectum, and the central gray of the brainstem; some of these fibers target visceral motor nuclei.

The **principal mammillary fasciculus** is the bundle that passes out of the mammillary nuclei, then immediately divides into the **mammillothalamic tract** and the **mammillotegmental tract.** The former projects to the anterior thalamic nucleus, and the latter projects mainly to the midbrain tegmental nuclei.

Descending fibers that arise in the paraventricular and posterior hypothalamic nuclei (emphasis on the paraventricular) and in the lateral hypothalamic zone, influence brainstem visceral motor and sensory nuclei, parts of the nucleus ambiguus, the ventrolateral medullary regions, and the spinal cord (specifically the **interomediolateral cell column).** Through these descending fibers to visceral nuclei of the brainstem, the hypothalamus influences a wide range of essential activities controlled by these brainstem regions. Damage to these hypothalamospinal fibers results in a **Horner syndrome (ptosis, myosis, anhydrosis** on the ipsilateral side) along with other deficits characteristic of the lesion be it in the midbrain, lateral pontine tegmentum, lateral medulla, or cervical spinal cord.

The **medial forebrain bundle** is diffusely arranged and contains fibers arising in the lateral zone and ascending to hypothalamic, olfactory, and other basal forebrain areas and of some descending fibers to the brainstem.

Clinical Correlations

In addition to the clinical comments made above, a number of further clinical examples of hypothalamic lesions are described in Figure 8-58 on p. 288. It is important to recall that hypothalamic lesions may initially present with the patient complaining of various **visual deficits;** a thorough examination and evaluation will reveal the hypothalamic source of the primary lesion.

ABBREVIATIONS	
n.	nucleus
tr.	tract

Review of Blood Supply to the Hypothalamus	
Structures	**Arteries**
Anterior Hypothalamus	Anteromedial group from A_1 and ACom (see Figure 2-21)
Mid/Caudal Hypothalamus	Posteromedial group from PCom and P_1 (see Figure 2-21)

8-59 Hypothalamic Structures and Connections: Projections

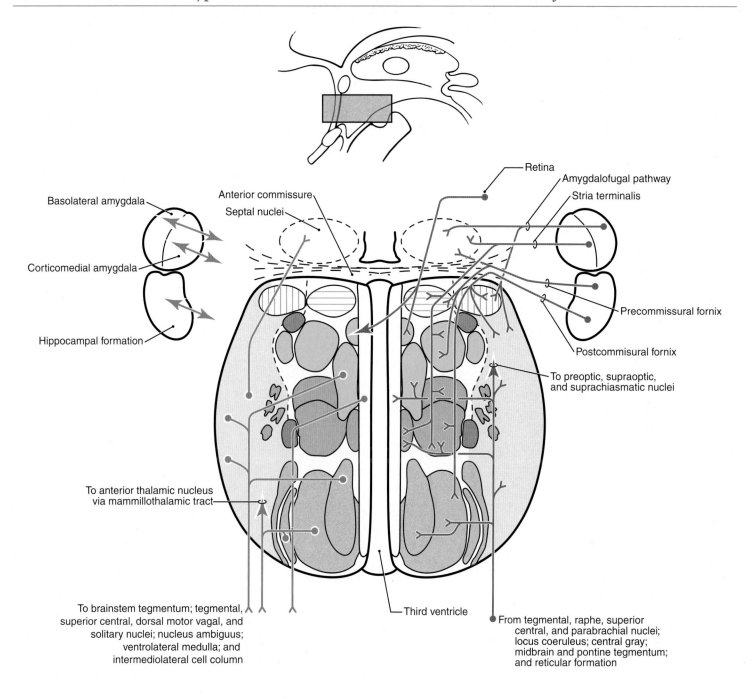

Retina
Amygdalofugal pathway
Stria terminalis
Anterior commissure
Septal nuclei
Basolateral amygdala
Corticomedial amygdala
Hippocampal formation
Precommissural fornix
Postcommisural fornix
To preoptic, supraoptic, and suprachiasmatic nuclei
To anterior thalamic nucleus via mammillothalamic tract
Third ventricle
To brainstem tegmentum; tegmental, superior central, dorsal motor vagal, and solitary nuclei; nucleus ambiguus; ventrolateral medulla; and intermediolateral cell column
From tegmental, raphe, superior central, and parabrachial nuclei; locus coeruleus; central gray; midbrain and pontine tegmentum; and reticular formation

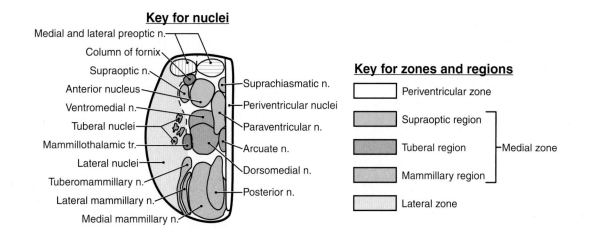

Key for nuclei

Medial and lateral preoptic n.
Column of fornix
Supraoptic n.
Anterior nucleus
Ventromedial n.
Tuberal nuclei
Mammillothalamic tr.
Lateral nuclei
Tuberomammillary n.
Lateral mammillary n.
Medial mammillary n.

Suprachiasmatic n.
Periventricular nuclei
Paraventricular n.
Arcuate n.
Dorsomedial n.
Posterior n.

Key for zones and regions

☐	Periventricular zone
☐	Supraoptic region
☐	Tuberal region
☐	Mammillary region
☐	Lateral zone

Medial zone

Blank Master Drawing for Hypothalamic Structures and Connections

8-60 Hypothalamic structures and connections are complex. This illustration is provided in the recognition that the instructor may wish to provide a less detailed, or a more detailed, treatment of the structure and connections of the hypothalamus than is covered in this atlas.

NOTES

8-60 Blank Master Drawing for Hypothalamic Structures and Connections

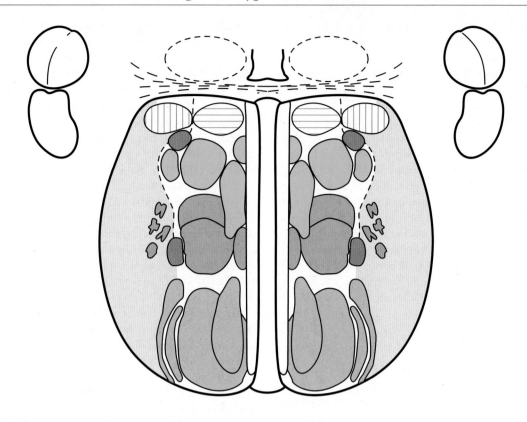

The Pituitary Gland

8-61 The structure, relationships, and **major pathways of the pituitary gland** in the sagittal plane. The **pituitary gland**, also called the **hypophysis**, consists of two parts: one that arises from the developing oral cavity (**adenohypophysis, anterior lobe**) and the other that arises from the developing neural tube (**neurohypophysis, posterior lobe**).

The **adenohypophysis**, commonly called the anterior lobe of the pituitary, consists of a larger portion called the **pars distalis** (or **pars anterior**), a small portion, the **pars intermedia**, and the **pars tuberalis**, which is a small extension of the anterior lobe that wraps around the infundibular stalk. The **neurohypophysis**, also called the posterior lobe of the pituitary, consists of a **neural lobe**, the **pars nervosa**, and the **infundibulum**, or **infundibular stalk**, which joins the neural lobe with the hypothalamus.

The pituitary gland sits in the **sella turcica** of the sphenoid bone; the **diaphragma sellae**, a small extension of the dura, forms a donut-shaped structure through which the infundibular stalk passes. The anterior and posterior intercavernous sinuses pass across the midline (and between the cavernous sinuses) at the attachment of the diaphragma sellae to the sphenoid bone.

Hormones

There are numerous hormones and neuroactive substances associated with the hypothalamus and pituitary. Of particular importance to the pituitary gland are those substances found in the **supraopticohypophyseal** and the **tuberoinfundibular** (or **tuberohypophyseal**) **tracts**.

The peptides **oxytocin** and **vasopressin** (**antidiuretic hormone**) are synthesized in the paraventricular and supraoptic nuclei and transported to the posterior lobe via the supraopticohypophyseal tract. Oxytocin is released during coitus, parturition, suckling, and regression of the uterus after birth. Vasopressin (ADH) is involved in the regulation of fluid homeostasis within the body and may either increase or reduce the production of urine.

A variety of **releasing hormones** are synthesized in the periventricular zone and in the arcuate nucleus, with further contributions coming from the paraventricular, medial preoptic, tuberal, and suprachiasmatic nuclei. These hormones are transported to the hypophyseal portal system and to the anterior lobe where they enter the vascular system.

Clinical Correlations

Due to its location, lesions of the pituitary may present as **endocrine disorders, visual deficits** (**bitemporal hemianopia** is most common), features of **increased intracranial pressure, diplopia**, and **headache** related to activation of nerves of the diaphragma sellae. In addition, lesions of the pituitary may be classified according to size: **microadenomas** (less than or equal to 1.0 cm in size) or **macroadenomas** (greater than 1.0 cm), or as **secreting** (excess hormone production) or **nonsecreting** (no hormone secretion). Hypersecreting tumors are those commonly seen in the clinical setting.

Excessive production of **growth hormone** may produce either **gigantism** or **acromegaly**. In the former, excessive hormone is produced before the growth plates have closed; the patient is abnormally tall and has large, but weak, muscles. In the latter, excessive hormone is produced after the growth plates have closed; the patient has large facial features, a large nose and thick lips, large hands and feet, and cardiac problems (hypertension, heart failure).

A female patient that presents with headache (common), **visual deficits, amenorrhea**, and **vertigo** ("dizziness") may have an **empty sella syndrome**. This may result from increased intracranial pressure, an untreated pituitary tumor, or arachnoid herniation into the sella. The pituitary may be compressed or displaced.

Excessive production of **corticotropin** results in **Cushing disease**. The patient has **truncal obesity**, a rounded ("moonlike") face, **hypertension, acne, osteoporosis**, violet stretch marks, and **diabetes mellitus**. Excessive production of **luteinizing hormone** may result in **hypogonadism** in males (testes may be present, but may not function normally) or disruption of the ovarian cycle in females.

Excessive production of **prolactin** in females results in **gallactorrhea** (milk production when not pregnant) and **amenorrhea** (absent menstrual cycles). **Hyperprolactinemia** in men may be signaled by infertility, decreased libido, or a combination of these signs and symptoms.

A patient presents with frequent urination (**polyuria**) and the need for large amounts of water (**polydipsia**), particularly cold water, following an automobile collision. CT reveals a **traumatic brain injury** (**TBI**) and consequent brain swelling within the skull. Shearing of the infundibular stalk and resultant **diabetes insipidus** (**DI**), in this case, may relate to: 1) sudden violent movement of the brain within the skull; 2) brain swelling in a supratentotrial compartment with a shift from one side to the other; or 3) **transtentorial** (**central**) **herniation**, in which the brain is extruded downward through the tentorial notch (see Chapter 9). **Basal skull fracture** involving the sella turcica or the clivus may cause DI due to vascular compromise; clivus fractures may also damage the larger vertebrobasilar arteries. In addition, DI may be a consequence of hemorrhage into the pituitary, or into a tumor located within the pituitary.

Excessive production of **vasopressin** (**antidiuretic hormone**) produces **hyponatremia** (low blood sodium levels and decreased urine excretion) and **natriuresis** (enhanced excretion of sodium in the urine). These patients may have hypotension, dehydration, headache, or may have more serious problems, such as **coma** and **seizures**.

Review of Blood Supply to the Pituitary Gland

The arterial blood supply to the pituitary comes from the **inferior hypophyseal arteries** (branches of the cavernous part of the internal carotid) and from the **superior hypophyseal arteries** (branches of the cerebral part of the internal carotid, A_1, and P_1). The venous drainage is via the **hypophyseal portal system** and **inferior hypophyseal veins** into locally adjacent dural sinuses.

8-61 The Pituitary Gland

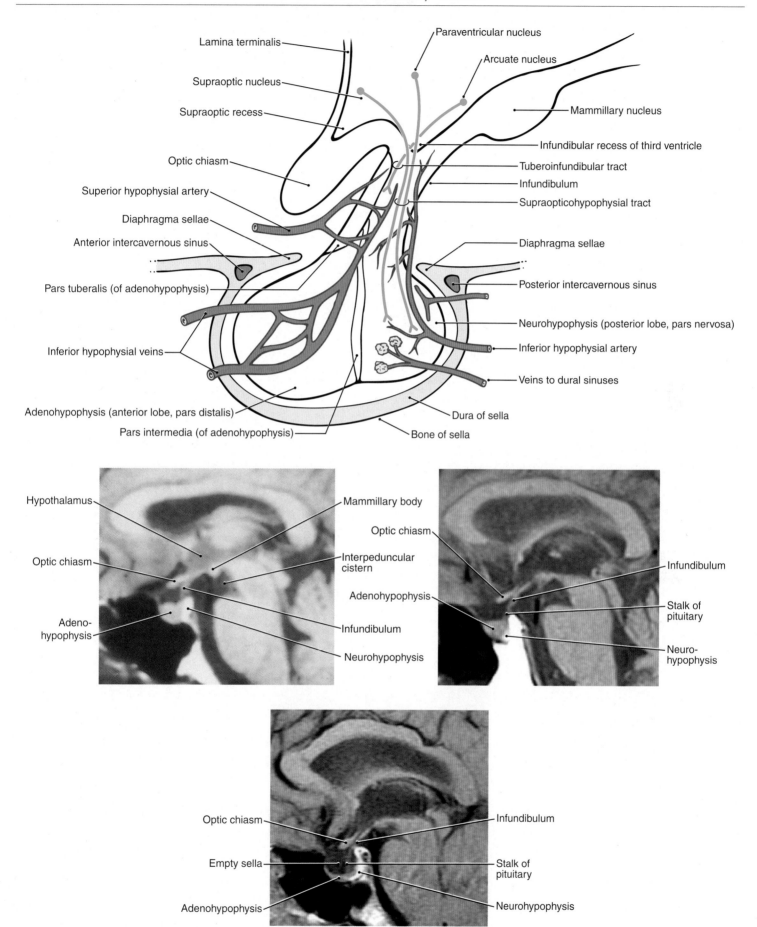

Lamina terminalis

Paraventricular nucleus

Arcuate nucleus

Supraoptic nucleus

Supraoptic recess

Mammillary nucleus

Optic chiasm

Infundibular recess of third ventricle

Tuberoinfundibular tract

Superior hypophysial artery

Infundibulum

Supraopticohypophysial tract

Diaphragma sellae

Anterior intercavernous sinus

Diaphragma sellae

Posterior intercavernous sinus

Pars tuberalis (of adenohypophysis)

Neurohypophysis (posterior lobe, pars nervosa)

Inferior hypophysial artery

Inferior hypophysial veins

Veins to dural sinuses

Adenohypophysis (anterior lobe, pars distalis)

Dura of sella

Pars intermedia (of adenohypophysis)

Bone of sella

Hypothalamus

Mammillary body

Optic chiasm

Interpeduncular cistern

Optic chiasm

Adenohypophysis

Infundibulum

Adeno-hypophysis

Infundibulum

Neurohypophysis

Optic chiasm

Infundibulum

Adenohypophysis

Stalk of pituitary

Neuro-hypophysis

Optic chiasm

Infundibulum

Empty sella

Stalk of pituitary

Adenohypophysis

Neurohypophysis

NOTES

Herniation Syndromes: Brain and Spinal Discs

Introduction and Compartments

The cranial cavity contains brain, cerebrospinal fluid (CSF), and blood (within vessels) all within a vault of unforgiving bone. This is good in that it offers essential protection to the soft, almost gelatinous, brain when there is a minor bump to the head. At the same time, this is bad when there is trauma to the skull that may result in brain damage (resultant edema, bleeding) or an intracranial event (hemorrhage, rapidly growing mass); all of which may increase intracranial pressure that attempts to displace the brain.

As a mass increases in size within a particular intracranial compartment, it displaces CSF and, to a lesser extent, blood within vessels, and raises the pressure within that compartment when compared to the adjacent compartments. When a mass increases to the point where the CSF space is exhausted, the pressure differential between the compartment containing the mass (higher) and the adjacent compartments (lower) may result in a herniation of brain from the region of higher pressure into one of lower pressure. These events, and resultant deficits, are called **herniation syndromes**.

A wide variety of clinical events may precede the development of a **herniation syndrome**, such as **hemorrhage** (epidural, subdural, parenchymatous), **mass lesion/tumor** (primary or secondary), **trauma, brain infarcts** or **abscess, infections**, and a variety of **metabolic conditions**. One thing that is common, to varying degrees, to all of these, is the **brain edema** that usually accompanies these events; it can be a major element in the resulting herniation or its propagation.

The **supratentorial space**, the space above the tentorium, is divided into **right** (Figure 9-1, pink) and **left** (Figure 9-1, blue) **compartments** by the midline position of the **falx cerebri**. The space below the **tentorium cerebelli** is not subdivided but presents as a single **infratentorial compartment** (Figure 9-1, green). The continuation of the supratentorial compartments with the infratentorial compartment is through the **tentorial notch**, which contains the midbrain and large vessels. Although not specifically described as a compartment, the cranial subarachnoid space, and its CSF, is continuous with the spinal subarachnoid space and represents the anatomical basis for herniation through the foramen magnum (Figure 9-2).

While brain herniation syndromes may be characterized on the basis of their own specific features, one herniation may morph, with clinical deterioration, into another. For example, a **subfalcine herniation** may, as the mass enlarges, become a **central herniation**, or a central herniation contributes to a **tonsillar herniation**. In a real sense, brain herniation is a dynamic process that may change as the clinical picture changes.

Spinal cord injuries, particularly those resulting from **extruded intervertebral discs**, or trauma, share similarities with brain herniations: mechanical impingement on neural structures with predictable deficits. Recognizing these features in common, selected samples of intervertebral disc extrusions and other spinal cord syndromes or lesions are included here to offer a more complete picture of this important clinical problem.

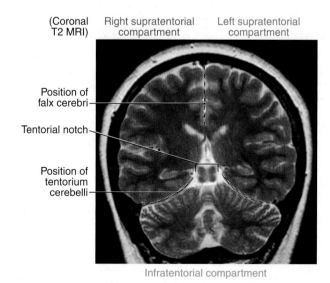

(Coronal T2 MRI) Right supratentorial compartment — Left supratentorial compartment — Position of falx cerebri — Tentorial notch — Position of tentorium cerebelli — Infratentorial compartment

9-1

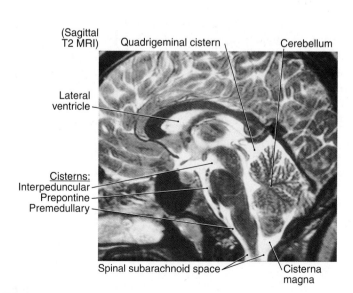

(Sagittal T2 MRI) Quadrigeminal cistern — Cerebellum — Lateral ventricle — Cisterns: Interpeduncular, Prepontine, Premedullary — Spinal subarachnoid space — Cisterna magna

9-2

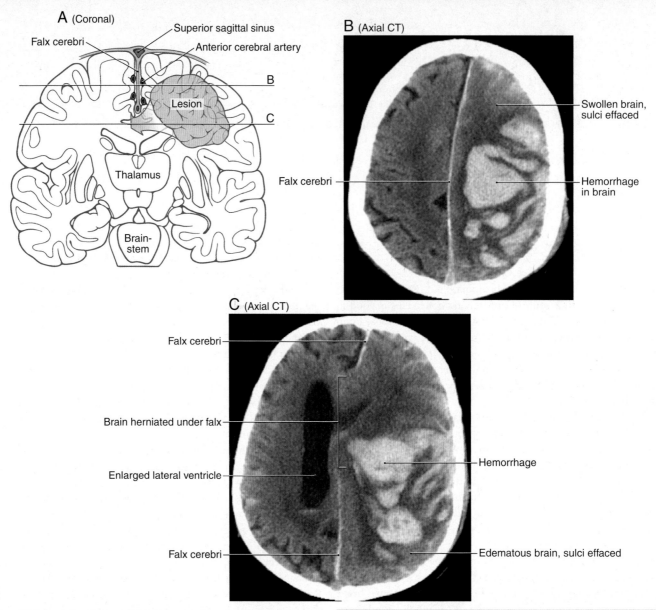

A (Coronal)

Falx cerebri
Superior sagittal sinus
Anterior cerebral artery
B
Lesion
C
Thalamus
Brain-stem

B (Axial CT)

Falx cerebri
Swollen brain, sulci effaced
Hemorrhage in brain

C (Axial CT)

Falx cerebri
Brain herniated under falx
Enlarged lateral ventricle
Falx cerebri
Hemorrhage
Edematous brain, sulci effaced

9-3 **Subfalcine (cingulate or falcine) herniation.** An expanding mass in the supratentorial compartment on one side may force the cingulate gyrus against, and/or under, the edge of the falx cerebri (**A**). These lesions are frequently located in the more superior area of the hemisphere, such as the **parietal lobe**, but may also occur in **parietofrontal areas**.

Several features generally characterize a subfalcine herniation. *First,* with the exception of the general symptoms of increased intracranial pressure (**headache, nausea, vomiting**), the event may be initially "silent" in that the patient has no long tract or focal signs. *Second,* this herniation may compromise the **anterior cerebral artery** (**ACA**) against the falx cerebri on the side of the mass, on the opposite side, or on both sides (**A, B**). The resulting deficits reflect damage to the lower extremity regions of the primary motor and somatosensory cortices (weakness, loss of proprioception and exteroceptive sense in a lower extremity). Depending on which ACA is occluded, the deficits may be on the side of the mass, the opposite side, or bilateral. *Third,* as the herniation progresses, the brain is pushed underneath the edge of the falx cerebri (**A, C**). When this takes place, the superior areas of the diencephalon may be involved and the internal cerebral veins may be compressed resulting in **venous stasis, edema,** or **venous infarcts** in the areas served by these veins. *Fourth,* with enlargement of the mass, a subfalcine herniation may evolve into a **central,** or **transtentorial, herniation** with the consequent clinical deficits. *Fifth,* damage to the cingulate gyrus may also result in alterations in behavior, but these are masked by other more obvious deficits.

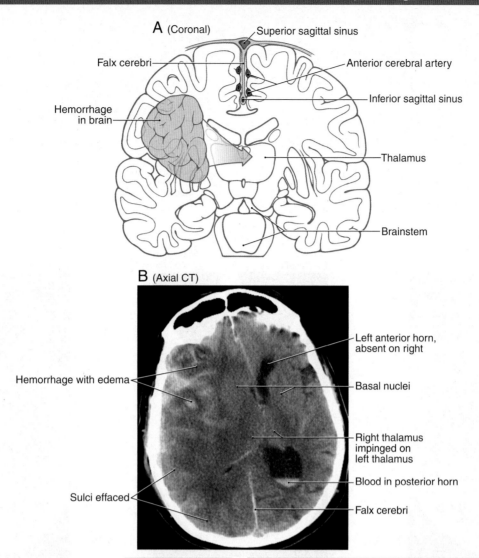

A (Coronal)

Superior sagittal sinus

Falx cerebri

Anterior cerebral artery

Inferior sagittal sinus

Hemorrhage in brain

Thalamus

Brainstem

B (Axial CT)

Hemorrhage with edema

Left anterior horn, absent on right

Basal nuclei

Right thalamus impinged on left thalamus

Blood in posterior horn

Sulci effaced

Falx cerebri

9-4 **Diencephalic stage** of **central herniation.** Expanding masses in frontal, parietal, and, to a lesser degree, occipital lobes, or in the central region of the hemisphere (basal nuclei, internal capsule, lateral thalamus) may result in brain displacement toward the opposite side: this is the **diencephalic (thalamic) stage** of **central herniation (A, B).**

A supratentorial mass within the hemisphere that enlarges and impinges on the contralateral side of the brain will result in a cascade of deficits characteristic of the structures damaged. The affected hemisphere is significantly swollen, sulci usually obliterated, and the midline clearly effaced (**A, B**). These signs and symptoms include a **decrease in the level consciousness** (reflecting compromise of the ascending reticular activating system), **potential onset of diabetes insipidus** (if the pituitary stalk is damaged as the brain shifts), a general **increase in muscle tone,** and respiratory changes accompany these motor symptoms. Breathing may initially be normal with occasional yawns or sighs but followed by the potential onset of ascending and descending rhythmic patterns characteristic of **Cheyne-Stokes respiration** (breathing that increases in depth then decreases followed by a period of **apnea**). In this stage, the pupils are small but minimally reactive, both eyes rotate to

the side opposite a head rotation (**doll's eyes maneuver**), and both eyes look toward the ear irrigated by cold water (**cold caloric test**). A noxious stimulus results in a movement of the upper extremity to deflect the offending source. Based on the extent of the damage the patient may have unilateral, contralateral, or bilateral **Babinski reflexes** (extension, fanning of the toes), and a **hemiparesis** of upper and lower extremities (compromise of corticospinal fibers; the Babinski is on the same side as the weakness).

A likely outcome of an enlarging supratentorial mass is **decorticate rigidity** (also called **decorticate posturing**). The level of consciousness, alertness, and arousability is decreased. The **lower extremities, trunk and neck musculature are extended** (**opisthotonos,** representing increased activity in reticulospinal and vestibulospinal fibers to extensor motor neurons in the spinal cord), and the **upper extremities are flexed** (increased activity in rubrospinal fibers to flexor motor neurons in the cervical spinal cord). With the removal of cortical modulation (**decortication**), brainstem nuclei are driven to higher levels of activity by infratentorial centers such as the cerebellum, vestibular nuclei, and spinal cord.

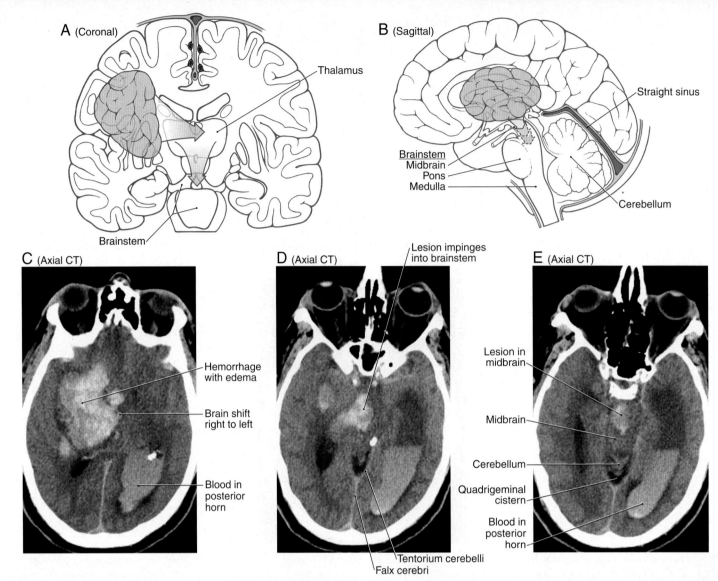

9-5 **Transtentorial** or **central herniation.** As a supratentorial mass enlarges, and in the absence of an opportunity to control or reverse the pressure, the brain will be displaced downward through the tentorial notch; this is **transtentorial** or **central herniation (A, B).** The brain is displaced from a region of greater pressure (above the tentorium) into a region of lower pressure (below the tentorium).

When the capacity of the supratentorial compartments is exceeded, the brain will herniate downward and compromises the midbrain and even lower levels. In this example, a large supratentorial mass **(C)** extends through the tentorial notch and into the brainstem **(D, E).** This may happen suddenly or unexpectedly, or be predictable based on the clinical deterioration during the diencephalic/thalamic stage.

The **decorticate rigidity,** that may appear during the diencephalic stage, may convert to **decerebrate rigidity** (also called **decerebrate posturing**). In this situation, there is total body rigidity; the lower extremities, trunk and neck, and the upper extremities are extended. This reflects increased influence of vestibulospinal and reticulospinal tracts, especially the latter, on extensor spinal motor neurons, and loss of the red nucleus (midbrain damage) and its influence on cervical flexor spinal motor neurons. Consequently, spinal extensor motor neuron activity prevails.

Respiratory patterns are irregular and may range from **tachypnea** (rapid breathing) to **Cheyne-Stokes** (breathing that increases in depth then decreases followed by a period of **apnea**). The pupils are fixed, dilated to midposition, or irregular in shape, and there may be visual losses resultant to compression of the posterior cerebral artery within the tentorial notch. Head rotation or cold caloric irrigation of an ear generally results in **dysconjugate eye movements.** After central herniation has occurred, the chance of a meaningful recovery is low (less than 5%) even if a treatment can be instituted and is successful.

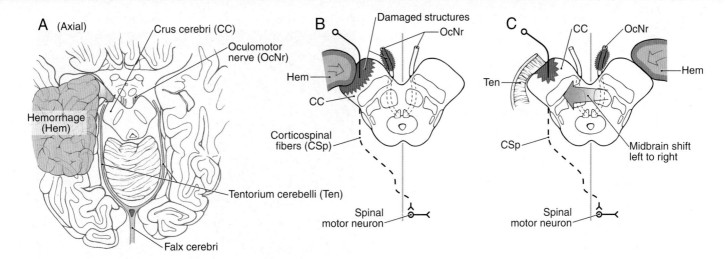

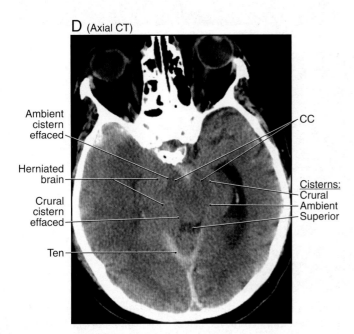

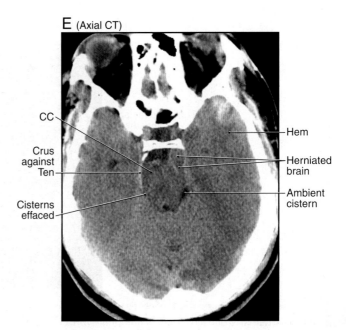

9-6 **Uncal herniation.** A rapidly expanding mass, such as a hematoma, neoplasm, or infarction with resultant edema, located in the temporal lobe may result in uncal herniation. The uncus, and frequently portions of the parahippocampal gyrus, are extruded over the edge of tentorium cerebelli, through the tentorial notch, and impinge on the midbrain (**A**). An early sign is a dilated pupil that responds slowly; if unilateral, the side of the dilated pupil predicts the side of the herniation in about 90% of cases. The dilated pupil may also be fixed, unresponsive to stimuli. Respiration is usually normal (**eupneic**) in early stages, and there is an appropriate response to a noxious stimuli; the patent may **hyperventilate** as herniation progresses. Consequent to pupillary dilation, most eye movement is absent (third nerve palsy), and eye movements in head rotation or cold caloric irrigation may be **dysconjugate**. In the same interval, the patient may become **hemiparetic** (damage to corticospinal fibers in the crus cerebri) with a Babinski reflex on the hemiparetic side, experience visual deficits (compression of the posterior cerebral artery serving the visual cortex), and

have a decreased level of consciousness or arousability (somnolence or stupor).

There are two variations on this theme. The *first* is a herniation that damages the midbrain (third root, crus cerebri) on the side of the herniation resulting in oculomotor deficits on the side of the herniation and hemiparesis on the contralateral side (with additional symptoms) (**B, D**). This is essentially a **Weber syndrome**; a **superior crossed** (or **alternate**) **hemiplegia**. The *second* is a herniation that shifts the midbrain from one side toward the other, damaging the oculomotor root on the side of the herniation and causing damage to the crus cerebri (and corticospinal fibers) on the opposite side (**C, E**) sometimes by impinging on the edge of the tentorium (**E**). *This results in oculomotor deficits on the side of the herniation and a hemiparesis of the upper and lower extremities on the same side.* The damage to the crus opposite the herniation is the cause of the corticospinal deficits on the same side as the oculomotor deficits (**C**). This is a **Kernohan syndrome**, also called the **Kernohan phenomenon**. In this case, the corticospinal deficits are a **false localizing sign**.

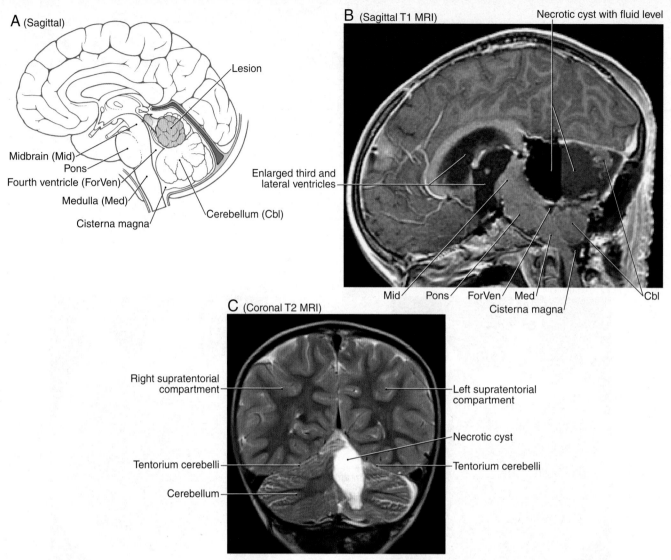

A (Sagittal)

Lesion

Midbrain (Mid)
Pons
Fourth ventricle (ForVen)
Medulla (Med)
Cisterna magna
Cerebellum (Cbl)

B (Sagittal T1 MRI)

Necrotic cyst with fluid level

Enlarged third and
lateral ventricles

Mid   Pons   ForVen   Med   Cbl
Cisterna magna

C (Coronal T2 MRI)

Right supratentorial
compartment

Left supratentorial
compartment

Necrotic cyst

Tentorium cerebelli

Tentorium cerebelli

Cerebellum

9-7 **Upward cerebellar herniation.** A posterior fossa (infratentorial) mass, particularly one in the cerebellum, may force brain structures upward through the tentorial incisure (notch) (**A**). A lesion in the posterior fossa may present with cardinal signs/symptoms of **increased intracranial pressure: headache, nausea,** and/or **vomiting.** In addition, an **abducens palsy** and **papilledema** (the latter seen after 4–6 days) may be present; both are exacerbated by increased intracranial pressure. In this example, the lesion involves primarily medial cerebellar structures with a consequent presentation of a **wide-based gait, titubation,** and **vertigo** (**B, C**).

Additional potential consequences of this type of lesion include the following: entrapment of the PCA (potential visual deficits, **homonymous** **hemianopia**), compression of the SCA between the tentorium and the cerebellum (infarct of cerebellar cortex and nuclei, cerebellar motor signs/symptoms), occlusion of the cerebral aqueduct (increased intracranial pressure, **hydrocephalus**), and compression of the caudal midbrain (impaired voluntary upward gaze, horizontal gaze intact; the **Parinaud syndrome**). Recognizing that about 450 cc of cerebrospinal fluid is produced every 24 hours in a normal healthy individual, and much of this in the lateral and third ventricles, a sudden occlusion of the cerebral aqueduct may quickly become a medical emergency. The medical urgency is created because only about 150 cc (of the 450 cc) of cerebrospinal fluid is needed at any given time; the remainder must circulate and be reabsorbed, or significant complications may occur.

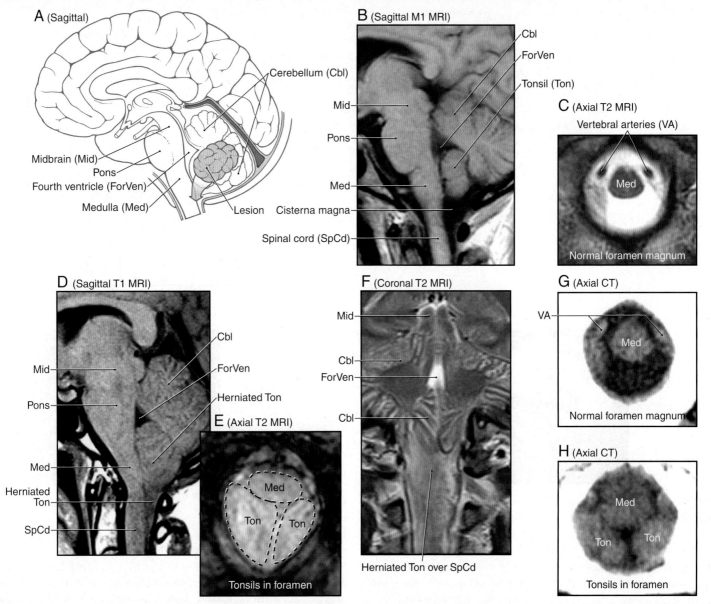

A (Sagittal)

Cerebellum (Cbl)

Midbrain (Mid)
Pons
Fourth ventricle (ForVen)
Medulla (Med)
Lesion

B (Sagittal M1 MRI)

Cbl
ForVen
Tonsil (Ton)
Mid
Pons
Med
Cisterna magna
Spinal cord (SpCd)

C (Axial T2 MRI)

Vertebral arteries (VA)
Med
Normal foramen magnum

D (Sagittal T1 MRI)

Mid
Pons
Med
Herniated Ton
SpCd
Cbl
ForVen
Herniated Ton

E (Axial T2 MRI)

Med
Ton　Ton
Tonsils in foramen

F (Coronal T2 MRI)

Mid
Cbl
ForVen
Cbl
Herniated Ton over SpCd

G (Axial CT)

VA
Med
Normal foramen magnum

H (Axial CT)

Med
Ton　Ton
Tonsils in foramen

9-8　Tonsillar herniation. Herniation of the cerebellar tonsils through the foramen magnum may be a sequel to an enlarging cerebellar mass (**A**) or to a supratentorial lesion descending through the tentorial notch and resulting in a pressure cone directed toward the foramen magnum. There are, however, situations where the tonsils may be found in the foramen, and below, without neurologic signs or symptoms. This may be the case where the tonsils descended during development or over long periods of time.

Normally the posterior fossa cisterns are open and the foramen magnum contains the medulla, vertebral and posterior inferior cerebellar arteries, and CSF (**B, C, G**). With herniation, the tonsils descend through the cistern magna and into the foramen and eventually the spinal subarachnoid space (**D–F, H**).

Sudden herniation may compress the medulla, compromise cardiac and respiratory centers therein, and result in rapid clinical deterioration. Initially, there is an immediate increase in blood pressure, followed by equally rapid increases in heart rate (**tachycardia**) and respiratory rate (**tachypnea**), followed by an equally rapid decline. Tonsillar herniation may occur suddenly and may be rapidly fatal if not treated as a medical emergency. Lumbar puncture (**LP**) should generally be avoided if elevated intracranial pressure is suspected.

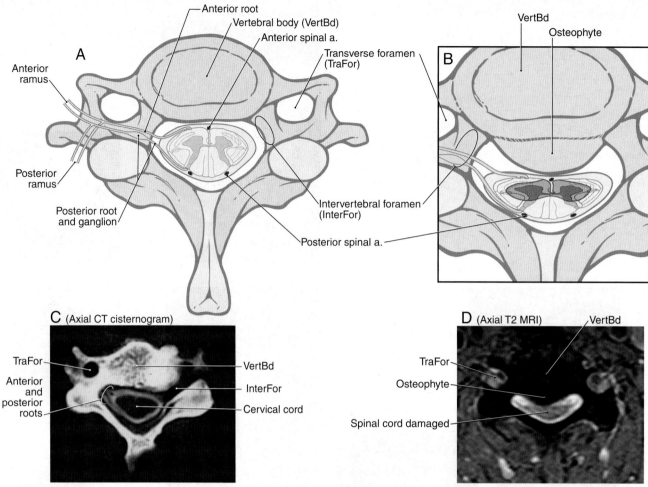

A

Anterior ramus

Posterior ramus

Posterior root and ganglion

Anterior root

Vertebral body (VertBd)

Anterior spinal a.

Transverse foramen (TraFor)

Intervertebral foramen (InterFor)

Posterior spinal a.

B

VertBd

Osteophyte

C (Axial CT cisternogram)

TraFor

Anterior and posterior roots

VertBd

InterFor

Cervical cord

D (Axial T2 MRI)

VertBd

TraFor

Osteophyte

Spinal cord damaged

9-9 **Central cord syndrome.** The normal cervical spinal cord is oval shaped, located within the dura, and separated from the bony vertebral canal by an epidural space (**A, C**). The **central cord syndrome** is an **incomplete spinal cord injury** (some motor/sensory function survives three or more segments below the level of the injury) and is the most commonly seen incomplete spinal cord injury. Contributing factors to this syndrome are hyperextension of the vertebral column (common in cervical levels) in older patients with **stenosis** of the vertebral canal complicated by **osteophytes** or hypertrophy of the ligamentum flavum (**B, D**). In younger patients, the hyperextension may occur during sport injuries or blows to the face/forehead with or without fractures.

A central cord syndrome presents as **weakness of the extremities** (greater in the upper extremity [UE], less in the lower extremity [LE]), **irregular sensory deficits** (pain and thermal sense), and **urinary retention**. These deficits correlate primarily with damage to the anterior horn at cervical levels and to the medial fibers of the lateral corticospinal tract (**bilateral weakness of the UEs**), damage to the anterolateral system taking into account its somatotopy (**irregular loss of pain and thermal sense**), and descending visceromotor fibers in the central areas of the cord (**sphincter dysfunction/urine retention**). Compromise of the anterior spinal artery may be a contributing factor in some cases. As these patients recover (about 90% may ambulate with assistance in 4–6 days) the LEs come back first, the bladder next, followed by the UEs, with sensation returning intermittently. Younger patients fare much better than elderly patients (about 95%+ versus 40%+ recovery).

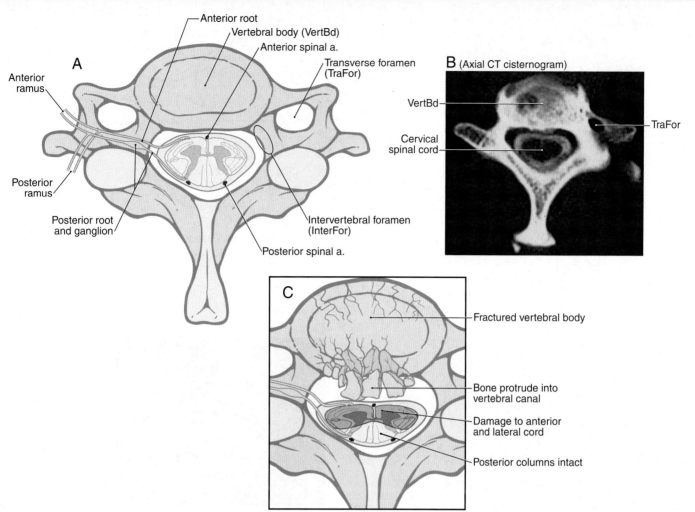

A

Anterior root
Vertebral body (VertBd)
Anterior spinal a.
Transverse foramen (TraFor)

Anterior ramus

Posterior ramus

Posterior root and ganglion

Intervertebral foramen (InterFor)

Posterior spinal a.

B (Axial CT cisternogram)

VertBd

Cervical spinal cord

TraFor

C

Fractured vertebral body

Bone protrude into vertebral canal

Damage to anterior and lateral cord

Posterior columns intact

9-10 **Anterior cord syndrome.** The morphological features of the cervical spinal cord and its relationships are described in Figure 9-9 and further shown here (**A, B**). The **anterior cord syndrome** (**ACS**) not only involves the territory of the anterior spinal artery, but is more inclusive in that it involves all cord regions except the posterior columns; this is also an **incomplete spinal cord injury** since there is surviving sensory function (discriminative touch, vibratory sense, proprioception in the posterior columns) below the level of the lesion. A common cause of ACS is vascular surgery, particularly that which may compromise branches of the aorta that ultimately serve the spinal cord. Precipitating events may also include anterior spinal cord compression pursuant to trauma resulting in intervertebral disc or bone fragments

(from a fracture of a vertebral body) that impinge on the cord (**C**). This pattern of compression may compromise the anterior spinal artery, the arterial vasocorona on the anterolateral surface of the cord, and/or the cord itself.

The deficits present as **paralysis** below the level of the lesion (bilateral corticospinal fiber damage): **paraplegia** if at thoracic cord levels and below, **quadriplegia** if at cervical cord levels. Additional deficits include a **bilateral loss of pain and thermal sensation** (bilateral ALS damage), and **bowel and bladder dysfunction** (descending visceromotor fibers). Posterior column function (proprioception, discriminative touch, vibratory sense) remains intact. The prognosis is grave; only about 15% recover to a functional level.

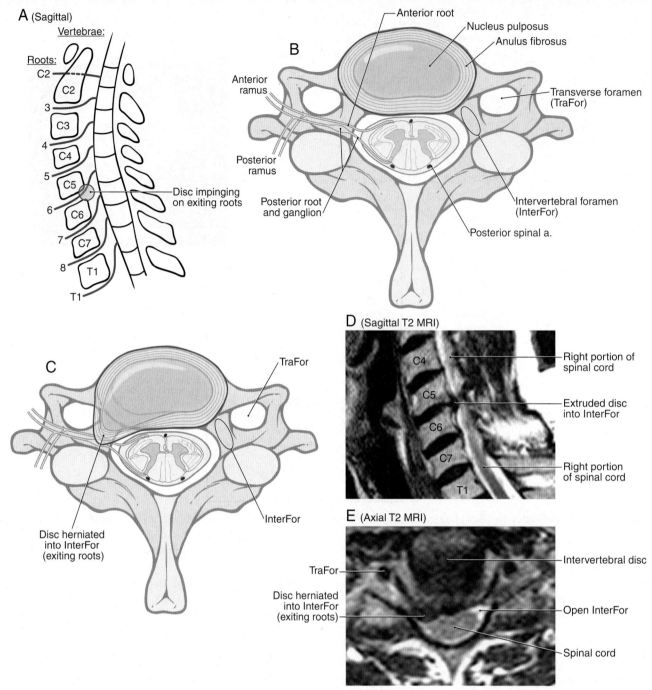

A (Sagittal)

Vertebrae:

Roots:
C2
C2
3   C3
4   C4
5   C5
6   C6
7   C7
8   T1
T1

Disc impinging on exiting roots

B

Anterior root
Nucleus pulposus
Anulus fibrosus

Anterior ramus

Transverse foramen (TraFor)

Posterior ramus

Posterior root and ganglion

Intervertebral foramen (InterFor)

Posterior spinal a.

C

TraFor

Disc herniated into InterFor (exiting roots)

InterFor

D (Sagittal T2 MRI)

C4
C5
C6
C7
T1

Right portion of spinal cord

Extruded disc into InterFor

Right portion of spinal cord

E (Axial T2 MRI)

TraFor

Disc herniated into InterFor (exiting roots)

Intervertebral disc

Open InterFor

Spinal cord

9-11 **Exiting roots** at **cervical levels.** The cervical spinal nerves exit the spinal cord and course laterally, and just slightly caudad, to their respective intervertebral spaces (see Figures 2-1 and 2-2). This relationship means that the vast majority of disc herniations in cervical levels involve the **exiting root.** The cervical spinal nerves exit the cord superior to their respectively numbered vertebrae; C1 between the C1 vertebrae and skull base, the C4 root above the C4 vertebrae at the C3–C4 interspace, the C6 root above the C6 vertebrae at the C5–C6 interspace, and so on (**A**). The C8 root exits between the C7 and the T1 vertebrae; consequently, below T1 all spinal nerves exit caudal to their respectively numbered vertebrae (e.g., the T1 root below the T1 vertebrae at the T1–T2 interspace).

An example of a lesion involving an **exiting root** is a disc protrusion at the C5–C6 interspace that impinges on the C6 root (**B–D**). The extruded disc clearly invades the intervertebral space on the right side, especially when compared to the left (**D, E**). In this case, the deficits reflect damage to the C6 root and include **weakness of forearm and wrist extensors, inability to flex (dorsiflex) the wrist,** and **sensory loss in the C6 dermatome** (back of the shoulder, lateral aspect of UE, thumb). The losses reflect the damage to the root at that level; not above or below; the root exiting at that level.

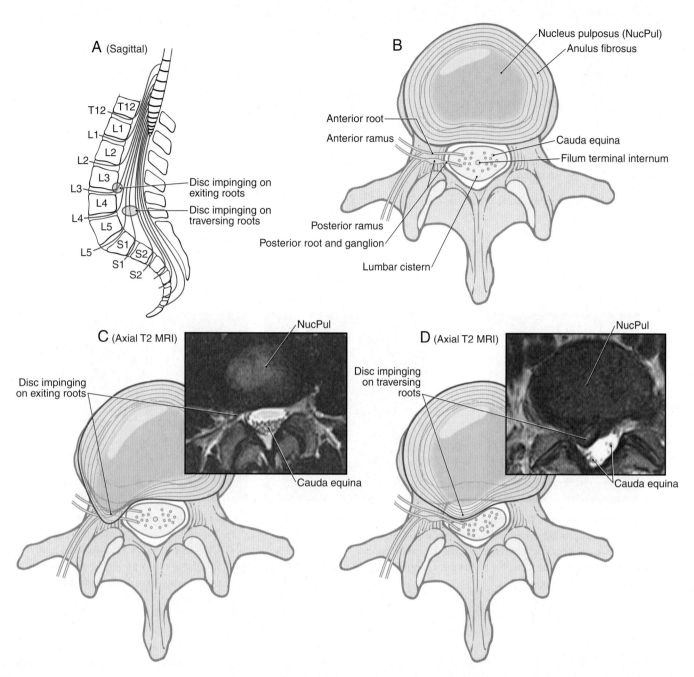

Exiting and **traversing roots** at **lumbosacral levels.** Depending on the direction of the disc extrusion, herniations at the lumbosacral levels may damage either an **exiting** root or **traversing** roots (**A, B**).

A herniated lumbar disc that protrudes superiorly or laterally and into the subarticular space of one intervertebral level damages the **exiting root** at that level; this root has a limited distribution. For example, a herniation superiorly or far laterally at the L3–L4 interspace damages the L3 root resulting in **weakness of knee extension**, pain over the anterior thigh and **decreased sensation** on the medial distal thigh, and a **diminished knee jerk** (patellar tendon) reflex (**A, C**).

Lesions that may damage **traversing roots** are commonly seen at lumbosacral levels; most disc extrusions occur at L4–L5 or L5–S1,

those extending posterolaterally may compress traversing roots. This reflects the descending nature of roots at these levels to form the cauda equina (see Figure 2-4). For example, a disc extruded medial to the subarticular zone/space at the L4–L5 interspace may avoid the L4 root (the root at that level) and compress roots that are descending to exit at lower levels such as L5 and S1–S5 (**A, D**). In this example, the deficits reflect damage to these traversing roots resulting in **weakness of knee flexion; plantarflexion of the ankle and extension of the great toe; loss of the Achilles, bulbocavernosus, and anal-cutaneous (anal wink) reflexes; and a loss of sensation in these respective dermatomes (buttock, posterior thigh and leg, lateral leg, and most of foot).** These losses reflect damage to roots descending and exiting at lower levels, not to roots at the level of the extruded disc.

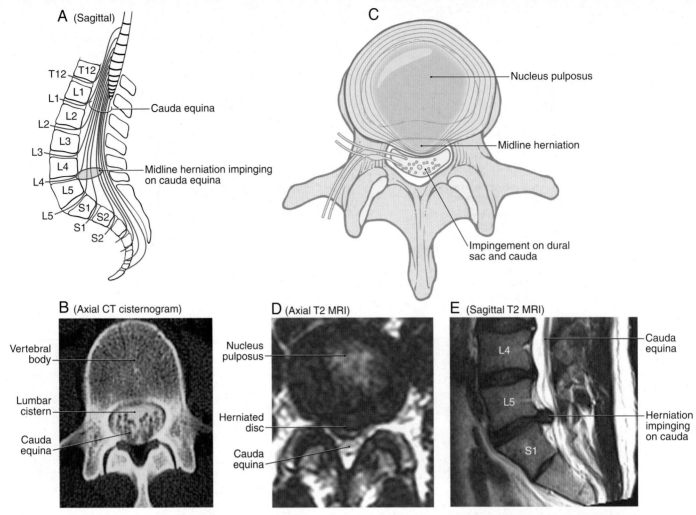

A (Sagittal)

T12 — T12
L1 — L1
— Cauda equina
L2 — L2
L3 — L3
L4 — L4
— Midline herniation impinging on cauda equina
L5 — L5
S1 — S1, S2
S1
S2

C

— Nucleus pulposus

— Midline herniation

— Impingement on dural sac and cauda

B (Axial CT cisternogram)

Vertebral body

Lumbar cistern

Cauda equina

D (Axial T2 MRI)

Nucleus pulposus

Herniated disc

Cauda equina

E (Sagittal T2 MRI)

Cauda equina

L4

L5

Herniation impinging on cauda

S1

9-13 **Cauda equina syndrome.** The **lumbar cistern** is located between about the L1/L2 and S2 vertebral levels and contains descending anterior and posterior roots that collectively form the cauda equina (**A, B**). This cistern is the primary avenue for retrieving a sample of cerebrospinal fluid for diagnostic purposes.

Intervertebral disc extrusions take place at the L4–L5 and at the L5–S1 levels in about the same numbers (about 45% each level). Large disc ruptures at the midline at L4–L5 are a major cause of cauda equina syndrome, followed by other events such as metastatic tumors, bone fragments from spinal trauma, spinal epidural hematoma, or the complication of infections (vascular compromise, compression). The protruded disc, or other mass/fragments within the vertebral column, may compress the dural sac and the roots located therein (**C–E**).

Bladder and bowel problems (**urinary retention, overflow incontinence; decreased anal sphincter tone**) are early and usually consistent findings. Other characteristic features include **saddle anesthesia** (sensory loss over perineum, genitals, anus, buttocks, and inner thighs, reflecting the Coc root and S2–S5 roots), **lower extremity weakness** (damage to multiple motor roots), potential loss of the Achilles reflex (S1 level), pain in the lower back or **sciatica** (pain radiating down the posterior thigh and leg) and, **sexual dysfunction** (a later finding).

Q&A for this chapter is available online on thePoint

Anatomical–Clinical Correlations: Cerebral Angiogram, MRA, and MRV

10

A

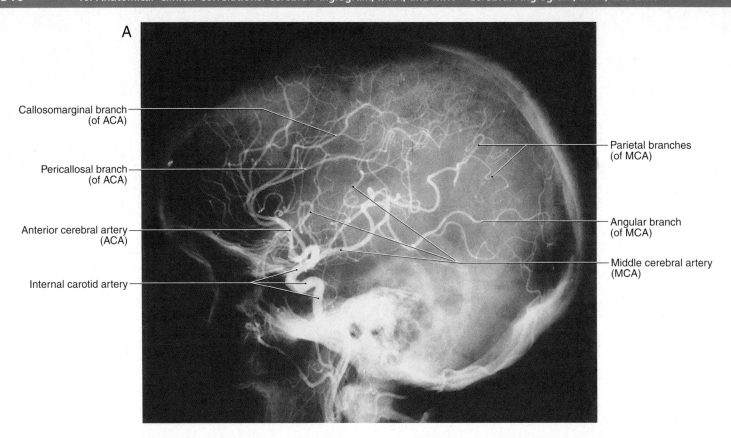

Callosomarginal branch (of ACA)

Pericallosal branch (of ACA)

Anterior cerebral artery (ACA)

Internal carotid artery

Parietal branches (of MCA)

Angular branch (of MCA)

Middle cerebral artery (MCA)

B

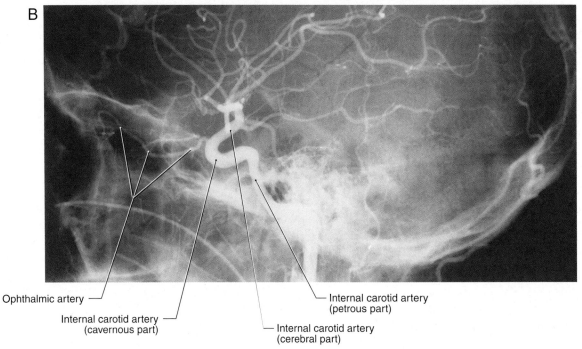

Ophthalmic artery

Internal carotid artery (cavernous part)

Internal carotid artery (cerebral part)

Internal carotid artery (petrous part)

10-1 Internal carotid angiogram (left lateral projection, arterial phase) showing the general patterns of the internal carotid, middle, and anterior cerebral arteries (**A, B**) and an image with especially good filling of the ophthalmic artery (**B**). The **ophthalmic artery** leaves the cerebral part of the internal carotid and enters the orbit via the optic canal. This vessel gives rise to the **central artery of the retina**, which is an important source of blood supply to the retina. Occlusion of the ophthalmic artery may result in blindness in the eye on that side.

The terminal branches of the ophthalmic artery anastomose with superficial vessels around the orbit. The venous drainage of the orbit generally mirrors that of the arteries serving the orbit. Orbital veins receive tributaries from the face and coalesce to form the **ophthalmic vein**, which ends in the cavernous sinus. This is a potential route through which infections of the face around the orbit, or within the orbit, may access the central nervous system. Compare with Figures 2-12 (p. 17), 2-21 (p. 23), 2-25 (p. 25), and 3-2 (p. 47).

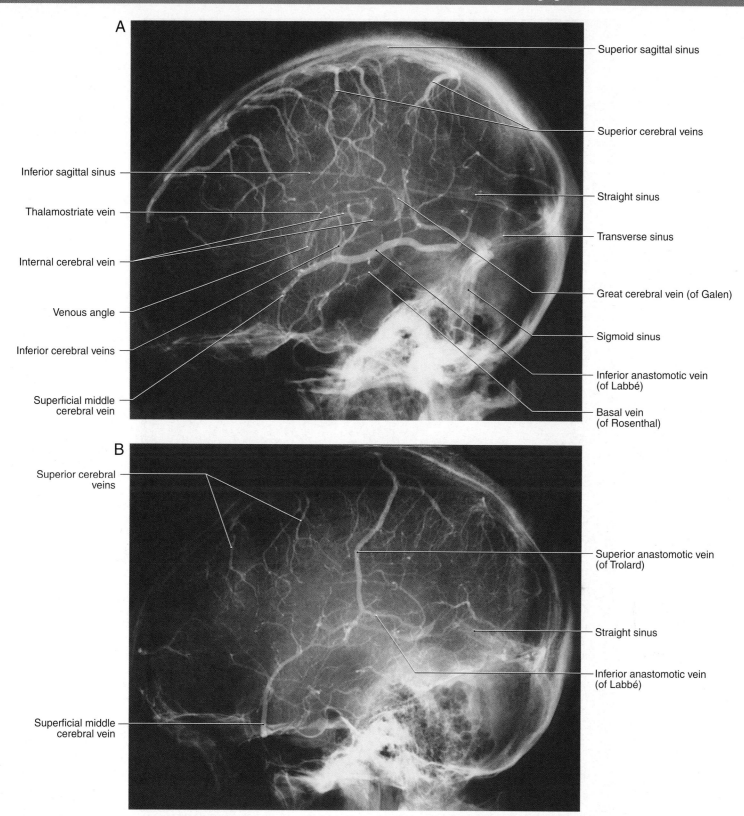

A

Superior sagittal sinus

Superior cerebral veins

Inferior sagittal sinus

Thalamostriate vein

Internal cerebral vein

Venous angle

Inferior cerebral veins

Superficial middle
cerebral vein

Straight sinus

Transverse sinus

Great cerebral vein (of Galen)

Sigmoid sinus

Inferior anastomotic vein
(of Labbé)

Basal vein
(of Rosenthal)

B

Superior cerebral
veins

Superficial middle
cerebral vein

Superior anastomotic vein
(of Trolard)

Straight sinus

Inferior anastomotic vein
(of Labbé)

10-2 Two internal carotid angiograms (left lateral projection, venous phase). Superficial and deep venous structures are clear in (**A**), but (**B**) shows a particularly obvious vein of Trolard. The thalamostriate vein (**A**) at this location is also called the superior thalamostriate vein. The junction of the superior thalamostriate vein with the internal cerebral vein is called the **venous angle** (**A**). The interventricular foramen is located immediately rostral to this point; small tumors at this location (such as a **colloid cyst,** or a small **choroid plexus papilloma**) may block the flow of cerebrospinal fluid from one or both lateral ventricles and result in **hydrocephalus** (see Figure 2-26 on p. 26 for a colloid cyst and enlarged ventricles). Compare these images with the drawings of veins and sinuses in Figures 2-13 (p. 17), 2-19 (p. 21), and 2-28 (p. 27).

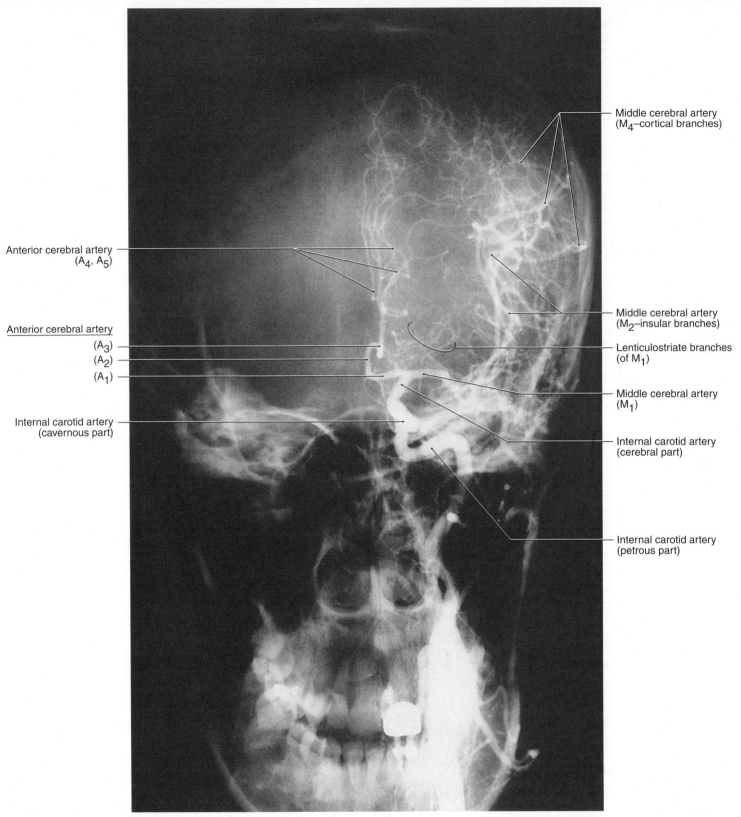

Anterior cerebral artery
(A₄, A₅)

Anterior cerebral artery
(A₃)
(A₂)
(A₁)

Internal carotid artery
(cavernous part)

Middle cerebral artery
(M₄–cortical branches)

Middle cerebral artery
(M₂–insular branches)

Lenticulostriate branches
(of M₁)

Middle cerebral artery
(M₁)

Internal carotid artery
(cerebral part)

Internal carotid artery
(petrous part)

10-3 Internal carotid angiogram (anterior–posterior projection, arterial phase). Note general distribution patterns of anterior and middle cerebral arteries and the location of lenticulostriate branches. The A_1 segment of the anterior cerebral artery is located between the internal carotid bifurcation and the anterior communicating artery. The distal portion of the anterior cerebral artery (ACA) immediately rostral to the anterior communicating artery and inferior to the rostrum of the corpus callosum is the A_2 segment (infracallosal). The portion of the ACA arching around the genu of the corpus callosum is the A_3 segment (precallosal) and the A_4 (supracallosal) and A_5

(postcallosal) **segments** are located superior (above), and caudal, to the corpus callosum.

The M_1 **segment** of the middle cerebral artery is located between the internal carotid bifurcation and the point at which this vessel branches into superior and inferior trunks on the insular cortex. As branches of the middle cerebral artery pass over the insular cortex, they are designated as M_2, as M_3 when these branches are located on the inner surface of the frontal, parietal, and temporal opercula, and as M_4 where they exit the lateral sulcus and fan out over the lateral aspect of the cerebral hemisphere. Compare with vascular figures in Chapter 2.

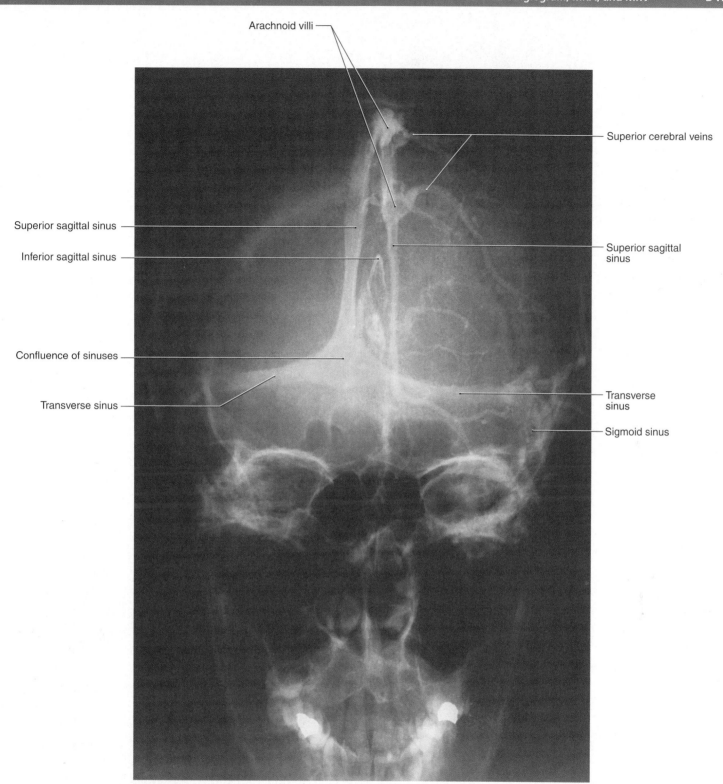

Arachnoid villi

Superior cerebral veins

Superior sagittal sinus

Superior sagittal sinus

Inferior sagittal sinus

Confluence of sinuses

Transverse sinus

Transverse sinus

Sigmoid sinus

10-4 Internal carotid angiogram (anterior–posterior projection, venous phase). The patient's head is tilted slightly; this shows the arching shapes of the superior and inferior sagittal sinuses to full advantage. In many individuals, the superior sagittal sinus turns predominately to the right at the confluence to form the right transverse sinus (Figure 10-6 on p. 315), and the straight sinus turns mainly to the left to form the left transverse sinus. In some individuals, there is a true confluence of sinuses where both transverse sinuses and the superior sagittal and the straight sinuses meet. Note the other venous structures in this image and compare with the arterial phase shown in Figure 10-3 (facing page) and the images in Figures 10-5 and 10-6 on pp. 314–315. Also compare with Figure 2-28 on p. 27.

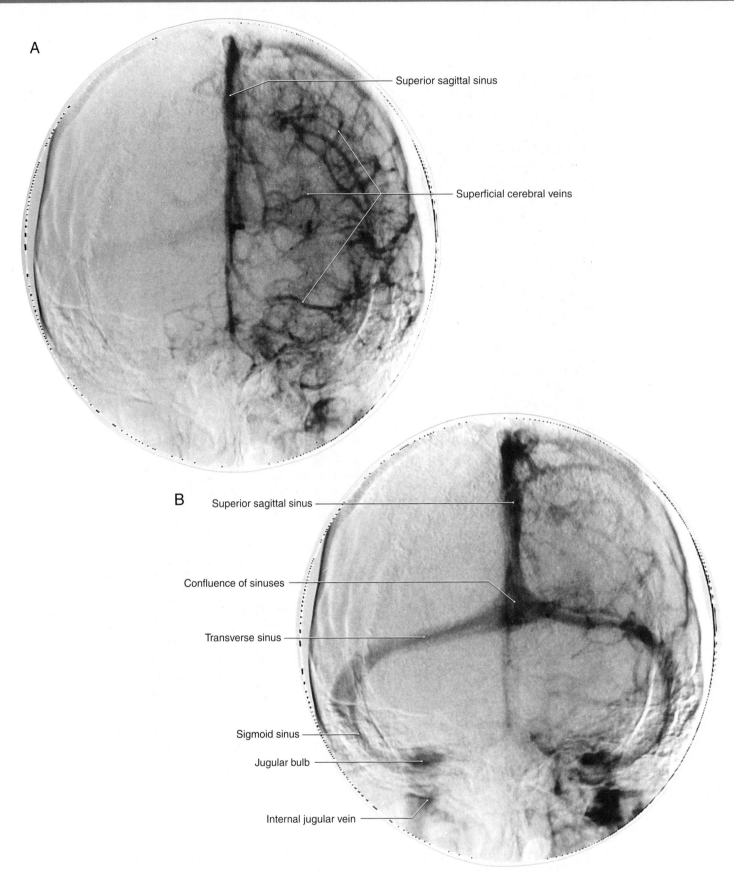

A

— Superior sagittal sinus

— Superficial cerebral veins

B   Superior sagittal sinus ———

Confluence of sinuses ———

Transverse sinus ———

Sigmoid sinus ———

Jugular bulb ———

Internal jugular vein ———

10-5 Digital subtraction image of an internal carotid angiogram (anterior–posterior projection, venous phase). Image (**A**) is early in the venous phase (greater filling of cortical veins), whereas image (**B**) is later in the venous phase (greater filling of the sinuses and jugular vein). Both images are of the same patient.

The **jugular bulb** is a dilated portion of internal jugular vein (IJV) in the jugular fossa at the point where the sigmoid sinus is continuous with the IJV; this continuity is through the jugular foramen. The jugular foramen also contains the roots of cranial nerves IX, X, and XI, the continuation of inferior petrosal sinus with the IJV and several small arteries. There are several syndromes that signify damage to the contents of the jugular foramen (such as the **Vernet syndrome**), or damage to these structures plus the hypoglossal root (**Collet-Sicard syndrome**). Recall that the jugular foramen and the hypoglossal canal are immediately adjacent, one to the other, in the posterior fossa. Compare with Figures 2-16 (p. 19) and 2-19 (p. 21).

A

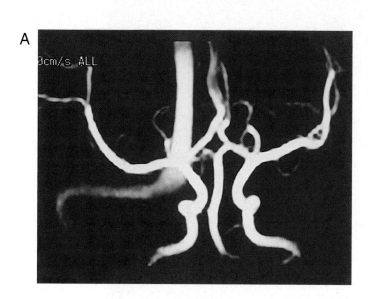

0cm/s ALL

B

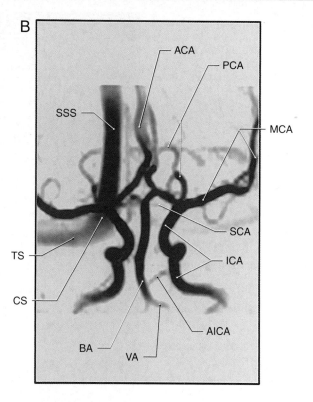

C

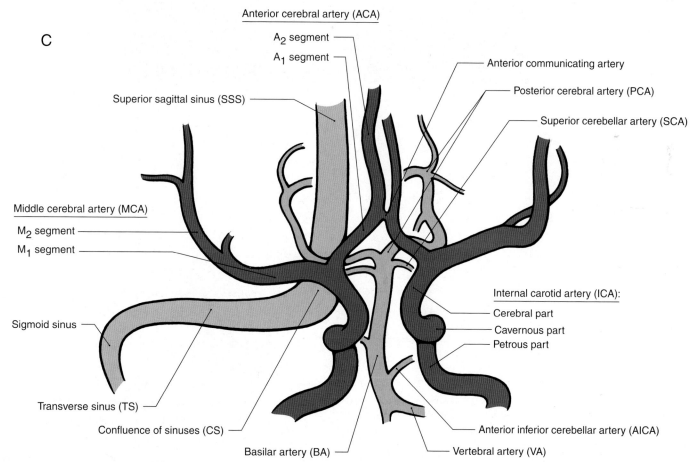

Anterior cerebral artery (ACA)

A₂ segment

A₁ segment

Superior sagittal sinus (SSS)

Anterior communicating artery

Posterior cerebral artery (PCA)

Superior cerebellar artery (SCA)

Middle cerebral artery (MCA)

M₂ segment

M₁ segment

Internal carotid artery (ICA):

Cerebral part

Cavernous part

Petrous part

Sigmoid sinus

Transverse sinus (TS)

Confluence of sinuses (CS)

Basilar artery (BA)

Anterior inferior cerebellar artery (AICA)

Vertebral artery (VA)

10-6 Magnetic resonance angiography (MRA) is a noninvasive method for imaging cerebral arteries, veins, and sinuses simultaneously. A three-dimensional phase contrast MRA (**A**) and an inverted video image window (**B**) of the same view show major vessels and sinuses from anterior to posterior. C shows the relative position of the major vessels and dural sinuses as imaged in (**A**) and (**B**). The superior sagittal sinus, as seen in (**A**) and (**B**), is usually continuous with the right transverse sinus at the confluence of sinuses.

A

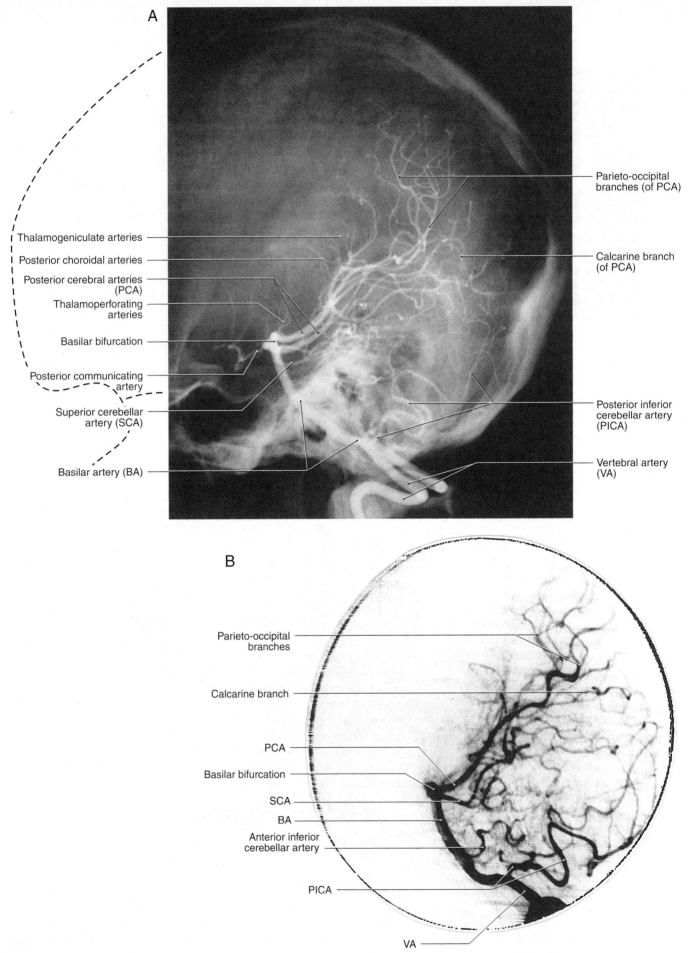

Thalamogeniculate arteries

Posterior choroidal arteries

Posterior cerebral arteries (PCA)

Thalamoperforating arteries

Basilar bifurcation

Posterior communicating artery

Superior cerebellar artery (SCA)

Basilar artery (BA)

Parieto-occipital branches (of PCA)

Calcarine branch (of PCA)

Posterior inferior cerebellar artery (PICA)

Vertebral artery (VA)

B

Parieto-occipital branches

Calcarine branch

PCA

Basilar bifurcation

SCA

BA

Anterior inferior cerebellar artery

PICA

VA

10-7 A vertebral artery angiogram (left lateral projection, arterial phase) is shown in (**A**), and the same view, but in a different patient, is shown in (**B**), using digital subtraction methods. Note the characteristic orientation of the major vessels, particularly the loop of PICA around the medulla and through the cisterna magna. Compare with Figures 2-21 (p. 23) and 2-24 (p. 25).

A

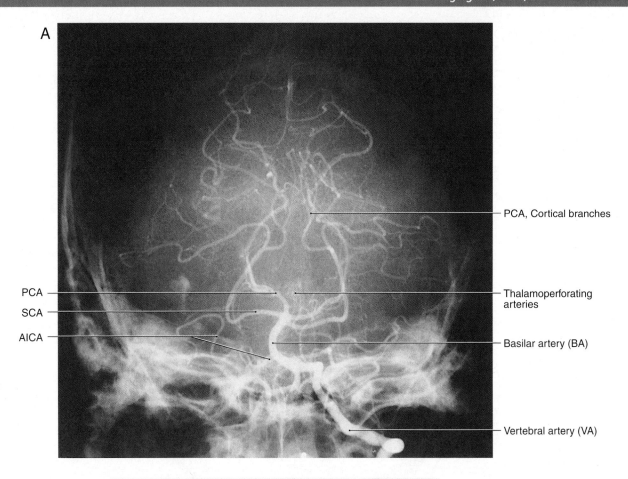

PCA, Cortical branches

PCA

SCA

AICA

Thalamoperforating
arteries

Basilar artery (BA)

Vertebral artery (VA)

B

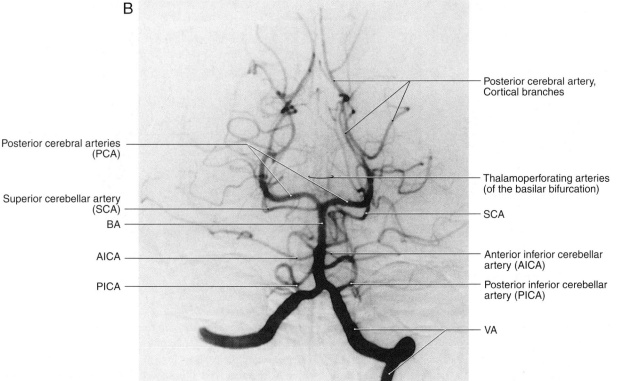

Posterior cerebral artery,
Cortical branches

Posterior cerebral arteries
(PCA)

Thalamoperforating arteries
(of the basilar bifurcation)

Superior cerebellar artery
(SCA)

SCA

BA

AICA

Anterior inferior cerebellar
artery (AICA)

PICA

Posterior inferior cerebellar
artery (PICA)

VA

10-8   A vertebral artery angiogram (anterior–posterior projection, arterial phase) is shown in (**A**); the same view, but in a different patient, is shown in (**B**), using digital subtraction methods. Even though the injection is into the left vertebral, there is bilateral filling of the vertebral arteries and branches of the basilar artery. The thalamoperforating arteries are important branches of P_1 that generally serve rostral portions of the diencephalon.

The root of the oculomotor (third) nerve, after exiting the inferior aspect of the midbrain, characteristically passes through the interpeduncular cistern and between the superior cerebellar and posterior cerebral arteries en route to its exit from the skull through the superior orbital fissure. In this position the third nerve may be damaged by large aneurysms of the rostral end of the basilar artery (called the **basilar tip**, or **basilar head**) that impinge on the nerve root. Compare with Figures 2-21 (p. 23), 3-2B (p. 47), and 3-3C (p. 48).

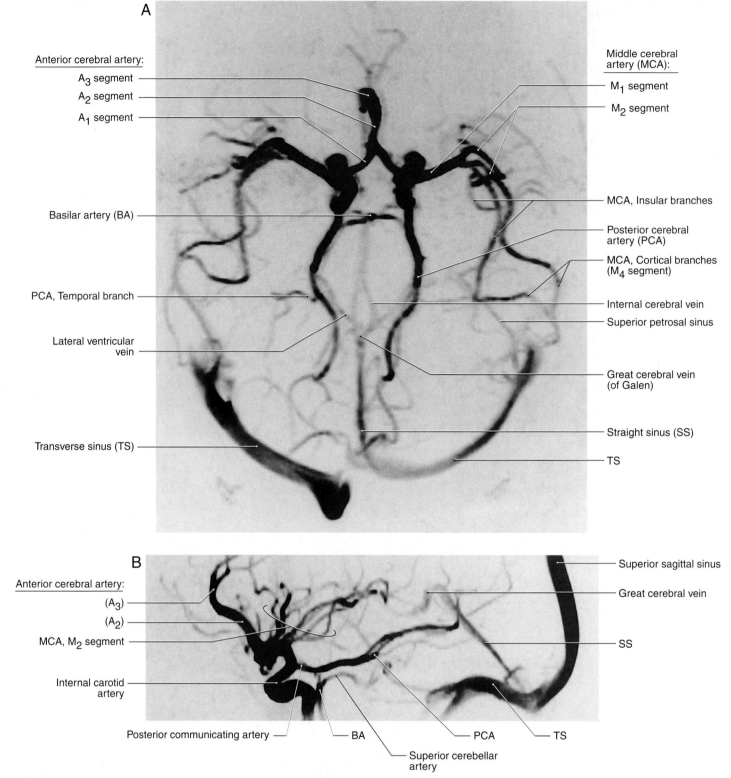

A

Anterior cerebral artery:
A₃ segment
A₂ segment
A₁ segment

Basilar artery (BA)

PCA, Temporal branch

Lateral ventricular vein

Transverse sinus (TS)

Middle cerebral artery (MCA):
M₁ segment
M₂ segment

MCA, Insular branches
Posterior cerebral artery (PCA)
MCA, Cortical branches (M₄ segment)
Internal cerebral vein
Superior petrosal sinus

Great cerebral vein (of Galen)

Straight sinus (SS)
TS

B

Anterior cerebral artery:
(A₃)
(A₂)
MCA, M₂ segment

Internal carotid artery

Posterior communicating artery — BA

Superior cerebellar artery

Superior sagittal sinus
Great cerebral vein
SS

PCA   TS

10-9 MRA images arteries, veins, and sinuses simultaneously, based on the movement of fluid in these structures. These are inverted video images of three-dimensional phase contrast MRA images as viewed in the axial plane (**A**) and from the lateral aspect, a sagittal view (**B**). The portion of the anterior cerebral artery (ACA) located between the internal carotid artery and the anterior communicating artery is the A₁ segment (precommunicating). The part of the ACA

immediately rostral to the anterior communicating artery and inferior to the rostrum of the corpus callosum is the **A₂ segment** (infracallosal). The portion of the ACA arching around the genu of the corpus callosum is the **A₃ segment** (precallosal) and the **A₄** (supracallosal) and **A₅** (post-callosal) **segments** are located superior to (above), and caudal to, the corpus callosum. Compare these images with arteries and veins as depicted in Figures 2-18 and 2-19 (p. 21), 2-21 (p. 23), and 2-24 (p. 25).

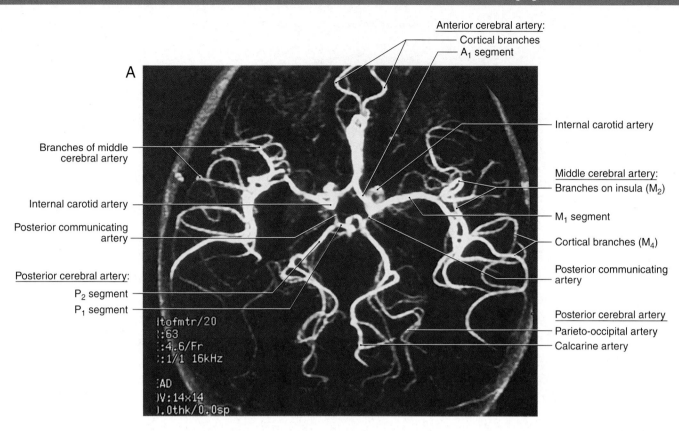

A

Anterior cerebral artery:
— Cortical branches
— A$_1$ segment

Internal carotid artery

Branches of middle cerebral artery

Internal carotid artery

Posterior communicating artery

Posterior cerebral artery:

P$_2$ segment

P$_1$ segment

Middle cerebral artery:
Branches on insula (M$_2$)

M$_1$ segment

Cortical branches (M$_4$)

Posterior communicating artery

Posterior cerebral artery
Parieto-occipital artery
Calcarine artery

ltofmtr/20
:63
:4.6/Fr
:1/1 16kHz

:AD
)V:14x14
).0thk/0.0sp

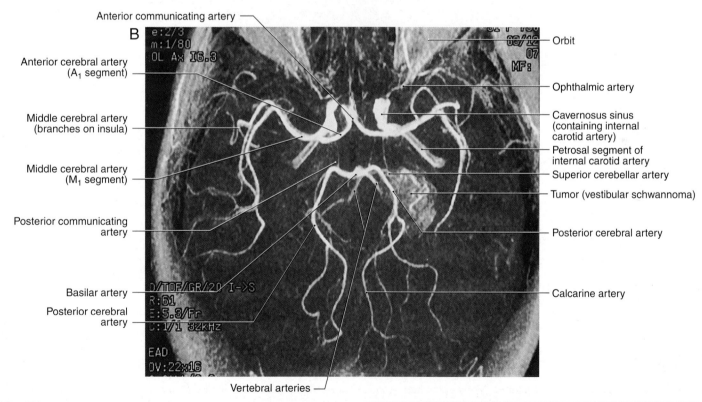

B

Anterior communicating artery

Anterior cerebral artery (A$_1$ segment)

Middle cerebral artery (branches on insula)

Middle cerebral artery (M$_1$ segment)

Posterior communicating artery

Basilar artery

Posterior cerebral artery

Orbit

Ophthalmic artery

Cavernosus sinus (containing internal carotid artery)

Petrosal segment of internal carotid artery

Superior cerebellar artery

Tumor (vestibular schwannoma)

Posterior cerebral artery

Calcarine artery

Vertebral arteries

10-10 MRA images, in the axial plane, of the vessels at the base of the brain forming much of the cerebral arterial circle (of Willis) (**A,B**). Note the anterior, middle, and posterior cerebral arteries as they extend outward from the circle. The upper image is from a normal individual, and the lower image is from a patient with a **vestibular schwannoma**. These tumors are generally slow growing, usually present (95%+ of the time) with **hearing deficits** (**difficulty discriminating** sounds, hearing loss), and, if especially large (generally, >2.5 cm in size), may involve the trigeminal root with a corresponding sensory loss on the face. Additional deficits include **tinnitus, dysequilibrium, headache, facial numbness** (about 30% of cases), and **facial weakness** (interestingly enough, only about 10%–14% of cases). Descriptions of the segments of the anterior, middle, and posterior cerebral arteries are found on pp. 19, 23, 27, 37, and 312.

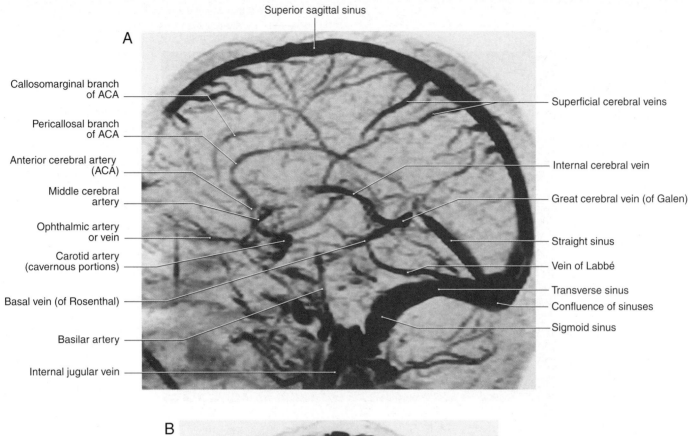

A

Superior sagittal sinus

Callosomarginal branch of ACA

Pericallosal branch of ACA

Anterior cerebral artery (ACA)

Middle cerebral artery

Ophthalmic artery or vein

Carotid artery (cavernous portions)

Basal vein (of Rosenthal)

Basilar artery

Internal jugular vein

Superficial cerebral veins

Internal cerebral vein

Great cerebral vein (of Galen)

Straight sinus

Vein of Labbé

Transverse sinus

Confluence of sinuses

Sigmoid sinus

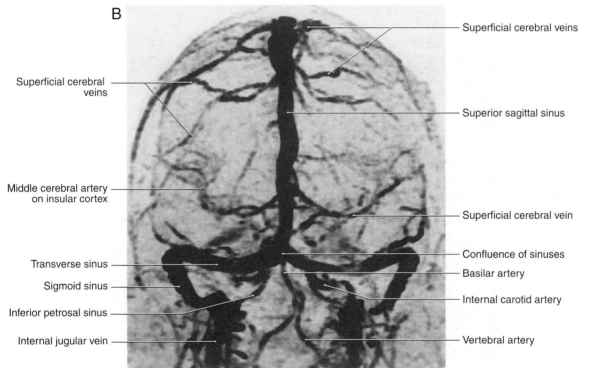

B

Superficial cerebral veins

Superficial cerebral veins

Middle cerebral artery on insular cortex

Transverse sinus

Sigmoid sinus

Inferior petrosal sinus

Internal jugular vein

Superior sagittal sinus

Superficial cerebral vein

Confluence of sinuses

Basilar artery

Internal carotid artery

Vertebral artery

10-11 Magnetic resonance venography (MRV) primarily demonstrates veins and venous sinuses, although arteries (seen in **A** and **B**) will also sometimes be visualized. Many veins and venous sinuses can be seen in this lateral, or sagittal, view (**A**) and in the anterior–posterior, or coronal, view (**B**). Note that the continuation of the superior sagittal sinus is most prominent into the right transverse sinus (**B**, compare with Figure 10-6 on p. 315). Compare with Figures 2-13 (p. 17), 2-16 (p. 19), 2-19 (p. 21), and 2-28 (p. 27).

A

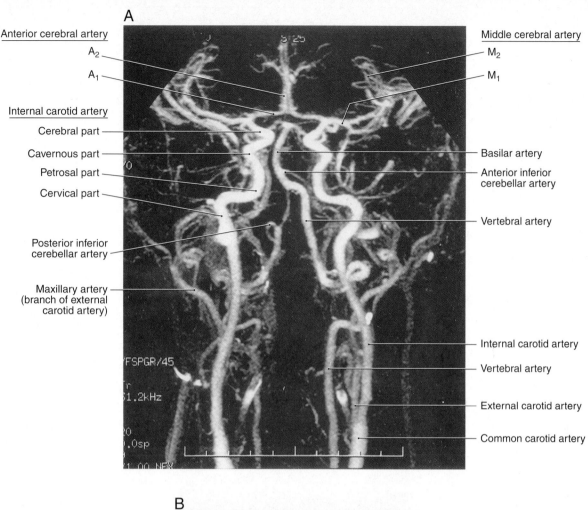

Anterior cerebral artery
- A₂
- A₁

Internal carotid artery
- Cerebral part
- Cavernous part
- Petrosal part
- Cervical part

Posterior inferior cerebellar artery

Maxillary artery (branch of external carotid artery)

Middle cerebral artery
- M₂
- M₁

Basilar artery

Anterior inferior cerebellar artery

Vertebral artery

Internal carotid artery

Vertebral artery

External carotid artery

Common carotid artery

B

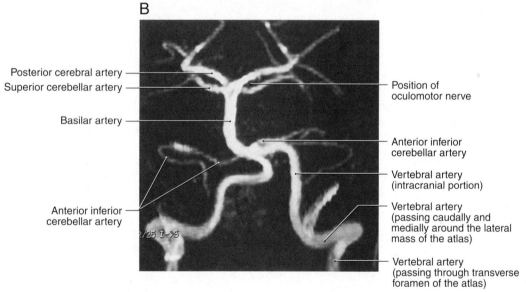

Posterior cerebral artery
Superior cerebellar artery

Basilar artery

Anterior inferior cerebellar artery

Position of oculomotor nerve

Anterior inferior cerebellar artery

Vertebral artery (intracranial portion)

Vertebral artery (passing caudally and medially around the lateral mass of the atlas)

Vertebral artery (passing through transverse foramen of the atlas)

10-12 Overview (**A**) of the arteries in the neck that serve the brain (internal carotid and vertebral) and of their main terminal branches (anterior cerebral artery and middle cerebral artery, vertebro-basilar system) as seen in an MRA (anterior–posterior view). In approx-imately 40%–45% of individuals, the left vertebral artery is larger, as seen here, and in about 4%–7% of individuals, one or the other of the vertebral arteries may be hypoplastic as seen here on the patient's right. The MRI in (**B**) is a detailed view of the vertebrobasilar system from the point where the vertebral arteries exit the transverse foramen to where the basilar artery bifurcates into the posterior cerebral arteries. Com-pare this image with Figure 2-21 on p. 23.

The vertebral artery (VA) is generally described as being composed of four segments sometimes designated as V_1 to V_4. The first segment (V_1) is between the VA origin from the subclavian artery and the entrance of VA into the first transverse foramen (usually C6); the sec-ond segment (V_2) is that part of VA ascending through the transverse foramen of C6–C2; the third segment (V_3) is between the exit of VA from the transverse foramen of the axis and the dura at the foramen magnum (this includes the loop of the VA that passes through the trans-verse foramen of C1/the atlas); the fourth segment (V_4) enters the poste-rior fossa and joins its counterpart to form the basilar artery.

NOTES

Q&As: A Sampling of Study and Review Questions, Many in the USMLE Style, All With Explained Answers

There are two essential goals of a student studying human neurobiology, or, for that matter, the student of any of the medical sciences. The *first* is to gain the knowledge base and diagnostic skills to become a competent health care professional. Addressing the medical needs of the patient with insight, skill, and compassion is paramount. The *second* is to successfully negotiate whatever examination procedures are used in a given setting. These may be standard class examinations, Subject National Board Examination (now used/required in many courses), the USMLE Step 1 Examination (required of all U.S. medical students), or simply the desire, on the part of the student, for self-assessment.

The questions in this chapter are prepared in two general styles. First, there are **study** or **review** questions that test general knowledge concerning the structure and function of the central nervous system. Second, there are single one-best-answer questions in the **USMLE Style** that use a **patient vignette** approach in the stem. These questions have been carefully reviewed for clinical accuracy and relevance as used in these examples. At the end of each explained answer, page numbers appear in parentheses that specify where the correct answer, be it in a figure or the text, may be found. In order to make this a fruitful learning exercise, some answers may contain additional relevant information to extend the educational process.

In general, the questions are organized by individual chapters, although Chapters 1 and 2 are combined. Reference(s) to the page (or pages) containing the correct answer are usually to the chapter(s) from which the question originated. However, recognizing that neuroscience is dynamic and three-dimensional, some answers contain references to chapters other than that from which the question originated. This provides a greater level of integration by bringing a wider range of information to bear on a single question. Correct diagnosis of the neurologically compromised patient may also require inclusion of concepts gained in other basic science courses. In this regard, a few questions, and their answers, may include such additional basic concepts.

This is not an all-inclusive list of questions, but rather a sampling that covers a variety of neuroanatomical and clinically relevant points. There is certainly a much larger variety of questions that can be developed from the topics covered in this atlas. It is hoped that this sample will give the user a good idea of how basic neuroscience information correlates with a range of clinically relevant topics and how questions on these topics may be developed.

Print and Online Q&As

The following is a sampling of Questions and Answers that are random and not divided according to chapters. This sample of 60 Q&As plus about 250 additional (for a total of over 310) are all available online as one of the several Bonus Materials available for this atlas. This entire set of Q&As is organized according to chapter and follows the other general guidelines described above.

1. A 69-year-old woman is brought to the Emergency Department. The daughter reports that her mother suddenly seemed unable to speak but seemed to understand her difficulty. The examination reveals that the woman has a nonfluent (Broca) aphasia. A sagittal MRI would most likely show a lesion in which of the following gyri?

   (A) Angular
   (B) Inferior frontal
   (C) Lingual
   (D) Middle frontal
   (E) Supramarginal

2. A 71-year-old morbidly obese man is brought to the Emergency Department by his son. The son reports that the man complained of a sudden excruciating headache and then became stuporous (difficult to arouse). Suspecting a ruptured aneurysm, the physician orders a CT. Which of the following would specify the appearance of acute blood in the subarachnoid space in this patient?

   (A) Black (hypodense)
   (B) Black to gray
   (C) Light gray
   (D) Medium gray
   (E) White (hyperdense)

3. Which of the following venous structures is found deep in the lateral sulcus on the surface of the insular cortex?

   (A) Anterior cerebral vein
   (B) Basal vein of Rosenthal
   (C) Deep middle cerebral vein
   (D) Superficial middle cerebral vein
   (E) Vein of Labbé

4. A 47-year-old man presents with an intense pain on his face arising from stimulation at the corner of his mouth. The diagnosis is trigeminal neuralgia (tic douloureux). MRI shows a vessel impinging on the root of the trigeminal nerve. Aberrant branches of which of the following vessels would most likely be involved?

(A) Anterior inferior cerebellar artery

(B) Basilar artery

(C) Posterior cerebral artery

(D) Posterior inferior cerebellar artery

(E) Superior cerebellar artery

5. A 22-year-old man is brought to the Emergency Department from the site of a motor vehicle collision. The examination reveals facial lacerations, a dilated right pupil, and loss of most eye movement on the right. He has no other motor or sensory difficulties. CT reveals fractures of the face and orbit. A fracture that traverses which of the following, and damages its contents, would most likely explain this man's deficits?

(A) Foramen ovale

(B) Foramen rotundum

(C) Inferior orbital fissure

(D) Superior orbital fissure

(E) Stylomastoid foramen

6. A 71-year-old woman is diagnosed with a one-and-a-half syndrome resultant to a lesion on the right side of the pons. Movement of which of the following muscles is preserved in this patient?

(A) Left lateral rectus

(B) Left medial rectus

(C) Left superior rectus

(D) Right lateral rectus

(E) Right medial rectus

7. Bacterial meningitis is an inflammation of the meninges that generally is found in which of the following locations?

(A) Epidural space

(B) Subarachnoid space

(C) Subdural space

(D) Subpial space

(E) Ventricular space

8. An 85-year-old woman is brought to the Emergency Department by her family because she suddenly became confused and lethargic. The examination revealed a left homonymous hemianopia. CT shows a hemorrhagic event in the vascular territory serving the medial and lateral geniculate bodies. Which of the following structures would also likely be involved in this vascular lesion?

(A) Anterior thalamic nucleus

(B) Rostral dorsomedial nucleus

(C) Globus pallidus

(D) Pulvinar nucleus(i)

(E) Subthalamic nucleus

9. A 16-year-old boy is brought to the Emergency Department following a diving accident at a local quarry. The initial examination reveals a bilateral loss of motor and sensory function from about T4 down including the lower extremities. At 36 hours after the accident, the boy is able to dorsiflex his toes, slightly move his right lower extremity at the knee, and is able to perceive pinprick stimulation

of the perianal skin (sacral sparing). Which of the following most specifically describes the spinal cord lesion in this patient?

(A) Central cord

(B) Complete

(C) Hemisection

(D) Incomplete

(E) Large syringomyelia

10. A 71-year-old man is brought to the Emergency Department by his wife. She explains that he suddenly became weak in his left lower extremity. She immediately rushed him to the hospital, a trip of about 20 minutes. The examination reveals an alert man who is obese and hypertensive. He has no cranial nerve deficits, is slightly weak on his left side, and has no sensory deficits. Within 2 hours the weakness has disappeared. A CT and MRI obtained within 5 hours shows no lesions. Which of the following most specifically describes this man's medical experience?

(A) Central cord syndrome

(B) Small embolic stroke

(C) Small hemorrhagic stroke

(D) Syringobulbia

(E) Transient ischemic attack

11. An 81-year-old woman is brought to the Emergency Department by her adult grandson. He explains that during dinner she slumped off of her chair, did not lose consciousness, but had trouble speaking. The examination in the ED revealed weakness of the left upper and lower extremities, deviation of the tongue to the right on protrusion, and loss of vibratory sense on the left. Which of the following most specifically describes the deficits in this elderly patient?

(A) Alternating (crossed) hemianesthesia

(B) Hemihypesthesia

(C) Inferior alternating (crossed) hemiplegia

(D) Middle alternating (crossed) hemiplegia

(E) Superior alternating (crossed) hemiplegia

12. Which of the following structures is located immediately internal to the crus cerebri, appears as a dark shade of gray (hypointense) in a sagittal T1-MRI, and when its cells are lost a pill-rolling tremor is seen?

(A) Brachium of the inferior colliculus

(B) Periaqueductal gray

(C) Pretectal area

(D) Red nucleus

(E) Substantia nigra

13. A 15-year-old boy is brought to the Emergency Department after an accident on his father's farm. The examination reveals significant weakness (a hemiparesis) of the left lower extremity. There is a loss of pinprick sensation on the right side beginning at the T8 dermatome (about half way between the nipple and umbilicus), and dorsiflexion of the left great toe in response to plantar stimulation. Based on this examination, which of the following represents the most likely approximate location of this lesion?

(A) T6 on the left side

(B) T6 on the right side

(C) T8 on the left side

(D) T8 on the right side

(E) T10 on the left side

14. The physician is conducting a routine neurological examination of a 16-year-old boy in preparation for summer football camp. As part of this examination, he taps the patellar tendon and elicits a knee-jerk reflex. The functional integrity of which of the following spinal levels is tested by this reflex?

(A) C5–C6

(B) C7–C8

(C) T8–T10

(D) L2–L4

(E) L5–S1

15. During a busy day in the Emergency Department, the neurology resident sees three patients with brainstem lesions. The first is an 83-year-old woman with a lesion in the territory of the midbrain served by the quadrigeminal and lateral posterior choroidal arteries. The second is a 68-year-old man with a posterior inferior cerebellar artery (lateral medullary or Wallenberg) syndrome. The third is a 47-year-old woman with a presumptive glioblastoma multiforme invading the mid to lateral portions of the pontine tegmentum and adjacent portions of the middle cerebellar peduncle. Which of the following would most likely be seen in all three patients assuming a thorough neurological examination?

(A) Claude syndrome

(B) Contralateral hemiplegia

(C) Facial hemiplegia

(D) Horner syndrome

(E) Medial medullary syndrome

16. Somatovisceral reflexes are those in which the afferent limb arises from a cutaneous receptor (a somatic afferent), and the efferent limb is mediated through pre- and postganglionic visceromotor fibers. A grain of sand blown into the eye results in increased secretions of the lacrimal gland in an effort to flush the offending object. In the tearing (or lacrimal) reflex, which of the following represents the location of the postganglionic cell bodies that innervate the lacrimal gland?

(A) Dorsal motor vagal nucleus

(B) Geniculate ganglion

(C) Otic ganglion

(D) Pterygopalatine ganglion

(E) Superior salivatory nucleus

17. A 23-year-old man is brought to the Emergency Department from an accident at a construction site. CT shows a fracture of the left mastoid bone with total disruption of the stylomastoid foramen. Which of the following deficits would most likely be seen in this man?

(A) Alternating hemianesthesia

(B) Alternating hemiplegia

(C) Central seven

(D) Facial hemiplegia

(E) Hemifacial spasm

18. A 59-year-old man, who is a family physician, confides in a neurology colleague that he believes he has early-stage Parkinson disease. The neurological examination reveals a slight resting tremor of the left hand, slow gait, and subtle change in the normal range of facial expression. Which of the following is the most likely location of the degenerative changes, at this stage, of this physician's disease?

(A) Bilateral substantia nigra

(B) Left globus pallidus

(C) Left substantia nigra

(D) Right globus pallidus

(E) Right substantia nigra

19. An inherited (autosomal recessive) disorder may appear early in the teenage years. These patients have degenerative changes in the spinocerebellar tracts, posterior columns, corticospinal fibers, cerebellar cortex, and at select places in the brainstem. The symptoms of these patients may include ataxia, paralysis, dysarthria, and other clinical manifestations. This constellation of deficits is most characteristically seen in which of the following?

(A) Friedreich ataxia

(B) Huntington disease

(C) Olivopontocerebellar degeneration (atrophy)

(D) Parkinson disease

(E) Wallenberg syndrome

20. A 20-year-old man is brought to the Emergency Department from the site of a motorcycle accident. The examination reveals multiple head injuries, facial lacerations, and a broken humerus. Cranial CT shows a basal skull fracture extending through the jugular foramen. Assuming that the nerve, or nerves, that traverse this opening are damaged, which of the following deficits would most likely be seen in this man?

(A) Deviation of the tongue to the injured side on protrusion

(B) Diplopia and ptosis

(C) Drooping and difficulty elevating the shoulder

(D) Drooping of the face on the ipsilateral side

(E) Loss of the efferent limb of the corneal reflex

21. Which of the following represents a relay nucleus of the thalamus?

(A) Centromedian

(B) Dorsomedial

(C) Medial geniculate

(D) Pulvinar

(E) Thalamic reticular

22. A 39-year-old woman presents with sustained and oscillating muscle contractions that have twisted her trunk and extremities into unusual and abnormal postures. This woman is most likely suffering from which of the following?

(A) Dysarthria

(B) Dysmetria

(C) Dysphagia

(D) Dyspnea

(E) Dystonia

23. The concerned mother of a 16-year-old girl brings her to the family physician. The girl explains that she occasionally has drops of a white fluid coming from her breasts. Further examination confirms that the girl is not sexually active and is not pregnant. An MRI reveals a small tumor in the area of the pituitary and hypothalamus. Based on this girl's signs and symptoms, she is most likely suffering from which of the following?

(A) Excessive corticotrophin production

(B) Excessive growth hormone production

(C) Excessive luteinizing hormone production

(D) Excessive prolactin production

(E) Excessive vasopressin production

24. The neurologist on call sees three patients in the Emergency Department. The first is a 61-year-old woman with a superior alternating hemiplegia, the second a 12-year-old boy with an ependymoma of the fourth ventricle that is impinging on the facial colliculus, and the third a 72-year-old man with a vascular infarct in the territory of the paramedian branches of the basilar artery at the pontomedullary junction. Which of the following do all of these patients have in common?

    (A) Aphasia
    (B) Agnosia
    (C) Diplopia
    (D) Dysarthria
    (E) Dysphagia

25. A 44-year-old woman presents to her family physician with the complaint of persistent headache and difficulty seeing out of her left eye. The examination reveals that the woman has significantly impaired vision in her left eye. When a light is shined into her left eye there is no direct or consensual pupillary light reflex; the afferent limb is compromised. Magnetic resonance angiography (MRA) shows a large aneurysm at the origin of the ophthalmic artery. Which of the following represents the likely point of origin of this vessel?

    (A) Cavernous part of the internal carotid artery
    (B) Cerebral part of the internal carotid artery
    (C) First segment (A_1) of the anterior cerebral artery
    (D) First segment (M_1) of the middle cerebral artery
    (E) Petrous part of the internal carotid artery

Questions 26 and 27 are based on the following patient.
A 59-year-old woman presents with the complaint of a sudden severe headache that did not respond to OTC medications, but cleared after several hours. Upon questioning her physician discovers that she had similar prior episodes over the last 3 months and he orders an MRI. This series of images reveals a large fusiform aneurysm of the P_3 segment.

26. Based on its location, which of the following gyri would most likely be impinged upon by this aneurysm?

    (A) Cuneus
    (B) Lingual
    (C) Orbital
    (D) Parahippocampal
    (E) Superior temporal

27. Assuming the neurosurgeon decides that this is a serious vascular lesion that requires treatment, based on its location which of the following deficits might this patient experience?

    (A) Blindness in one eye
    (B) Partial bilateral hearing loss
    (C) Partial bilateral visual loss
    (D) Somatomotor loss on the body
    (E) Somatosensory loss on the body

Questions 28 and 29 are based on the following patient.
A 63-year-old man has hearing loss, tinnitus (ringing or buzzing sounds in the ear), vertigo, and unsteady gait; all of these deficits developed slowly, but progressively, over several years. MRI reveals a large tumor (3 cm in diameter) at the cerebellopontine angle, most likely a vestibular schwannoma (incorrectly called an acoustic neuroma).

28. What additional deficit could this patient also have?

    (A) Anosmia
    (B) Hemianopsia

    (C) Numbness on the face
    (D) Visual field deficits
    (E) Weakness of the tongue

29. In addition to the vestibulocochlear nerve, which of the following structures would most likely also be affected by the tumor in this man?

    (A) Anterior inferior cerebellar artery
    (B) Facial nerve
    (C) Glossopharyngeal nerve
    (D) Posterior inferior cerebellar artery
    (E) Vagus nerve

Questions 30 and 31 are based on the following patient.
A 23-year-old man is brought to the Emergency Department from the site of an automobile collision. The neurological examination reveals weakness of the right lower extremity and a loss of pain and thermal sensations on the left side beginning at the level of the umbilicus. CT shows a fracture of the vertebral column with displacement of bone fragments into the vertebral canal.

30. Damage to which of the following tracts would correlate with weakness of the lower extremity in this man?

    (A) Left lateral corticospinal tract
    (B) Reticulospinal fibers on the right
    (C) Right lateral corticospinal tract
    (D) Right rubrospinal tract
    (E) Vestibulospinal fibers on the right

31. Which of the following represents the most likely level of damage to the spinal cord resulting from the fracture to the vertebral column in this man?

    (A) T6 on the left
    (B) T8 on the left
    (C) T8 on the right
    (D) T10 on the left
    (E) T10 on the right

Questions 32 and 33 are based on the following patient.
A 71-year-old woman presents to her family physician with the complaint that "food dribbles out of my mouth when I eat." The examination reveals a unilateral weakness of muscles around the eye (palpebral fissure) and the opening of the mouth (oral fissure). She also has a loss of pain and thermal sensations on the opposite side of the body excluding the head. CT shows an infarcted area in the lateral portion of the pontine tegmentum.

32. Damage to which of the following nuclei would most likely explain the muscle weakness experienced by this woman?

    (A) Abducens
    (B) Arcuate
    (C) Facial motor
    (D) Hypoglossal
    (E) Trigeminal motor

33. The loss of pain and thermal sensations experienced by this woman would most likely correlate with a lesion involving which of the following structures?

    (A) Anterior (ventral) trigeminothalamic tract
    (B) Anterolateral system
    (C) Lateral lemniscus
    (D) Medial lemniscus
    (E) Spinal trigeminal tract

Questions 34 and 35 are based on the following patient.
A 41-year-old man is brought to the Emergency Department after an accident at a construction site. The examination reveals a weakness (hemiplegia) and a loss of vibratory sensation and discriminative touch all on the left lower extremity, and a loss of pain and thermal sensations on the right lower extremity. CT shows a fracture of the vertebral column adjacent to the T8 level of the spinal cord.

34. Damage to which of the following fiber bundles or tracts would most likely explain the loss of vibratory sensation in this man?
    (A) Anterolateral system on the right
    (B) Cuneate fasciculus on the left
    (C) Cuneate fasciculus on the right
    (D) Gracile fasciculus on the left
    (E) Gracile fasciculus on the right

35. The loss of pain and thermal sensation in this man reflects damage to which of the following fiber bundles or tracts?
    (A) Anterolateral system on the left
    (B) Anterolateral system on the right
    (C) Cuneate fasciculus on the left
    (D) Gracile fasciculus on the left
    (E) Posterior spinocerebellar tract on the left

Questions 36 through 38 are based on the following patient.
An 88-year-old man is brought to the Emergency Department by his daughter. She indicates that he complained of sudden weakness of his "arm" and "leg" (upper and lower extremities) on the right side and of "seeing two of everything" (double vision—diplopia). CT confirms an infarcted area in the medial area of the pons at the pons–medulla junction. The infarcted area is consistent with the vascular territory served by paramedian branches of the basilar artery.

36. Weakness of the extremities on the right can be explained by damage to which of the following structures?
    (A) Corticospinal fibers on the left
    (B) Corticospinal fibers on the right
    (C) Middle cerebellar peduncle on the left
    (D) Rubrospinal fibers on the left
    (E) Rubrospinal fibers on the right

37. The diplopia (double vision) this man is having is most likely the result of damage to which of the following structures?
    (A) Abducens nerve root
    (B) Facial nerve root
    (C) Oculomotor nerve root
    (D) Optic nerve
    (E) Trochlear nerve or root

38. Recognizing that this patient's lesion involves the territory served by paramedian branches of the basilar artery, which of the following structures is also most likely included in the area of infarction?
    (A) Anterolateral system
    (B) Facial motor nucleus
    (C) Hypoglossal nucleus
    (D) Medial lemniscus
    (E) Spinal trigeminal tract

Questions 39 through 42 are based on the following patient.
A 69-year-old man is brought to the Emergency Department with the complaint of a sudden loss of sensation on his face and in his

mouth. The history and examination reveals that the man is overweight, hypertensive, and does not regularly take medication. When the man speaks his voice is gravelly and hoarse. The examination further reveals a loss of pain and thermal sensations on the right side of his body and on the left side of his face. CT shows an infarcted area in the medulla.

39. Damage to which of the following structures would most likely explain the man's hoarse, gravelly voice?
    (A) Facial nucleus
    (B) Gracile nucleus
    (C) Hypoglossal nucleus
    (D) Nucleus ambiguus
    (E) Spinal trigeminal nucleus

40. Injury to which of the following structures in this man is most specifically related to the loss of pain and thermal sensations on the body below the neck?
    (A) Anterolateral system
    (B) Cuneate fasciculus
    (C) Gracile fasciculus
    (D) Medial lemniscus
    (E) Spinal trigeminal tract

41. Damage to which of the following structures would most specifically explain the loss of pain and thermal sensations on this man's face?
    (A) Anterolateral system
    (B) Medial lemniscus
    (C) Medial longitudinal fasciculus
    (D) Solitary tract
    (E) Spinal trigeminal tract

42. The CT shows an infarcted area in the medulla in this man. Based on the combination of deficits experienced by this man, which of the following vessels is most likely occluded?
    (A) Anterior spinal artery
    (B) Posterior spinal artery
    (C) Posterior inferior cerebellar artery
    (D) Anterior inferior cerebellar artery
    (E) Penetrating branches of the vertebral artery

Questions 43 through 45 are based on the following patient.
A 73-year-old man is brought to the Emergency Department after losing consciousness at his home. CT shows a large hemorrhage into the right hemisphere. The man regains consciousness, but is not fully alert. After 3–4 days the man begins to rapidly deteriorate. His pupils are large (dilated) and respond slowly to light, eye movement becomes restricted, there is weakness in the extremities on the left side, and the man becomes comatose. Repeat CT shows an uncal herniation.

43. Based on its location, which of the following parts of the brain is most likely to be directly affected by this herniation, especially in its early stages?
    (A) Diencephalon/thalamus
    (B) Mesencephalon/midbrain
    (C) Myelencephalon/medulla
    (D) Pons and cerebellum
    (E) Pons only

44. Damage to corticospinal fibers in which of the following locations would most likely explain the weakness in this man's extremities?

 (A) Left basilar pons

 (B) Left crus cerebri

 (C) Right basilar pons

 (D) Right crus cerebri

 (E) Right posterior limb of the internal capsule

45. The dilated, and slowly responsive, pupils in this man are most likely explained by damage to fibers in which of the following?

 (A) Abducens nerve

 (B) Corticonuclear fibers in the crus

 (C) Oculomotor nerve

 (D) Optic nerve

 (E) Sympathetic fibers on cerebral vessels

46. A newborn girl baby is unable to suckle. The examination reveals that muscles around the oral cavity and of the cheek are poorly developed and some are absent. A failure in proper development of which of the following structures would most likely contribute to this problem for this baby?

 (A) Head mesoderm

 (B) Pharyngeal arch 1

 (C) Pharyngeal arch 2

 (D) Pharyngeal arch 3

 (E) Pharyngeal arch 4

Questions 47 and 48 are based on the following patient.
A 62-year-old woman presents with tremor and ataxia on the right side of the body excluding the head, and with a loss of most eye movement on the left; the woman's eye is rotated slightly down and out at rest. The left pupil is dilated. There are no sensory losses on her face or body.

47. Based on the deficits seen in this woman, which of the following represents the most likely location of the causative lesion?

 (A) Cerebellum on the left

 (B) Cerebellum on the right

 (C) Medulla on the left

 (D) Midbrain on the left

 (E) Midbrain on the right

48. The dilated pupil in this woman is most likely a result of which of the following?

 (A) Intact parasympathetic fibers on the left

 (B) Intact parasympathetic fibers on the right

 (C) Intact sympathetic fibers on the left

 (D) Intact sympathetic fibers on the right

 (E) Interrupted hypothalamospinal fibers on the left

Questions 49 and 50 are based on the following patient.
A 69-year-old man is diagnosed with dysarthria. The history reveals that the man has had this problem for several weeks. MRI shows an infarcted area in the brainstem on the right side.

49. Damage to which of the following structures would most likely explain this deficit in this man?

 (A) Cuneate nucleus

 (B) Nucleus ambiguus

 (C) Solitary tract and nuclei

 (D) Spinal trigeminal tract

 (E) Vestibular nuclei

50. Assuming that the infarcted area in the brain of this man is the result of a vascular occlusion, which of the following arteries is most likely involved?

 (A) Anterior inferior cerebellar

 (B) Labyrinthine

 (C) Posterior inferior cerebellar

 (D) Posterior spinal

 (E) Superior cerebellar

Questions 51 through 53 are based on the following patient.
An 80-year-old woman is brought to the Emergency Department from an assisted care facility. The woman, who is in a wheelchair, complains of not feeling well, numbness on her face, and being hoarse, although she claims not to have a cold. The examination reveals a loss of pain and thermal sensations on the right side of her face and the left side of her body. CT shows an infarcted area in the lateral portion of the medulla.

51. A lesion of which of the following structures in this woman would explain the loss of pain and thermal sensations on her body excluding the head?

 (A) Anterolateral system on the left

 (B) Anterolateral system on the right

 (C) Medial lemniscus on the left

 (D) Spinal trigeminal nucleus on the left

 (E) Spinal trigeminal tract on the left

52. The hoarseness in this woman is most likely due to which of the following?

 (A) Lesion of the facial nucleus

 (B) Lesion of the hypoglossal nucleus/nerve

 (C) Lesion of the nucleus ambiguus

 (D) Lesion of the spinal trigeminal tract

 (E) Lesion of the trigeminal nucleus

53. Assuming this woman suffered a vascular occlusion, which of the following vessels is most likely involved?

 (A) Anterior inferior cerebellar artery

 (B) Anterior spinal artery

 (C) Posterior inferior cerebellar artery

 (D) Posterior spinal artery

 (E) Superior cerebellar artery

Questions 54 and 55 are based on the following patient.
A 37-year-old-man is brought to the Emergency Department from the site of an automobile collision. He was unrestrained and, as a result, has extensive injuries to his face and head. CT shows numerous fractures of the facial bones and skull and blood in the rostral areas of the frontal lobes and in the rostral 3–4 cm of the temporal lobes, bilaterally. After several weeks of recovery the man is moved to a long-term care facility. His behavior is characterized by: (1) difficulty recognizing sounds such as music or words; (2) a propensity to place inappropriate objects in his mouth; (3) a tendency to eat excessively or to eat nonfood items such as the leaves on the plant in his room; and (4) a tendency to touch his genitalia.

54. Which of the following most specifically describes the tendency of this man to eat excessively?

 (A) Aphagia

 (B) Dysphagia

(C) Dyspnea

(D) Hyperorality

(E) Hyperphagia

55. Based on the totality of this man's deficits he is most likely suffering from which of the following?

(A) Klüver-Bucy syndrome

(B) Korsakoff syndrome

(C) Senile dementia

(D) Wallenberg syndrome

(E) Wernicke aphasia

Questions 56 and 57 are based on the following patient.
A 23-year-old man is brought to the Emergency Department from the site of an automobile collision. CT shows fractures of the facial bones and evidence of bilateral trauma to the temporal lobes including blood is the parahippocampal gyri and hippocampus.

56. As this man recovers, which of the following deficits is likely to be the most obvious?

(A) A bilateral sensory loss in the lower body

(B) A loss of immediate and short-term memory

(C) A loss of long-term (remote) memory

(D) Dementia

(E) Dysphagia and dysarthria

57. Assuming that this man also has sustained bilateral injury to the Meyer-Archambault loop, which of the following deficits would he also most likely have?

(A) Bitemporal hemianopsia

(B) Bilateral inferior quadrantanopia

(C) Bilateral superior quadrantanopia

(D) Left superior quadrantanopia

(E) Right superior quadrantanopia

Questions 58 through 60 are based on the following patient.
A 67-year-old man is brought to the Emergency Department by his wife. She explains that he fell suddenly, could not get out of his bed, and complained of feeling nauseated, but did not vomit. The examination revealed a left-sided weakness of the upper and lower extremities, a lack of most movement of the right eye, and a dilated pupil on the right. MRI shows an infarcted area in the brainstem.

58. The weakness of this man's extremities is explained by damage to the axons of cell bodies that are located in which of the following regions of the brain?

(A) Left somatomotor cortex

(B) Right anterior paracentral gyrus

(C) Right crus cerebri

(D) Right precentral gyrus

(E) Right somatomotor cortex

59. This man's dilated pupil is due to damage to which of the following fiber populations?

(A) Preganglionic fibers from the Edinger-Westphal nucleus

(B) Preganglionic fibers from the inferior salivatory nucleus

(C) Postganglionic fibers from the ciliary ganglion

(D) Postganglionic fibers from the geniculate ganglion

(E) Postganglionic fibers from the superior cervical ganglion

60. Which of the following descriptive phrases best describes the constellation of signs and symptoms seen in this man?

(A) Alternating hemianesthesia

(B) Brown-Séquard syndrome

(C) Inferior alternating (crossed) hemiplegia

(D) Middle alternating (crossed) hemiplegia

(E) Superior alternating (crossed) hemiplegia

Answers

1. **Answer B:** The inferior frontal gyrus consists of the pars orbitalis (Brodmann area 47), pars triangularis (area 45), and pars opercularis (area 44). A lesion located primarily in areas 44 and 45 in the dominant hemisphere will result in a nonfluent (Broca, or motor) aphasia. The supramarginal (area 40) and angular (area 39) gyri represent what is called the Wernicke area, and the middle frontal gyrus contains areas 6 and 8. The lingual gyrus is located below the calcarine sulcus; the superior quadrant of the opposite visual fields is represented in this gyrus (area 17). (pp. 12, 16)

2. **Answer E:** The most common cause of blood in the subarachnoid space is resultant to trauma; the second most common cause is rupture of an intracranial aneurysm. Patients who experience rupture of an intracranial aneurysm frequently complain of an intense, sudden headache ("the most horrible headache I have ever had"). Acute blood in the subarachnoid space will appear white to very white on CT; this blood is hyperdense. This will contrast with the medium gray of the brain and the black of cerebrospinal fluid (CSF) in the ventricles. The degree of white may vary somewhat, based on the relative concentration of blood, from very white (concentrated blood) to white (mostly blood, some CSF), to very light gray (mixture of blood and CSF). (pp. 1–3)

3. **Answer C:** The deep middle cerebral vein is located on the insular cortex and, by joining with the anterior cerebral vein, forms the basal vein of Rosenthal. The superficial middle cerebral vein is located on the lateral aspect of the hemisphere in the vicinity of the lateral sulcus, arches around the temporal lobe, and joins the cavernous sinus. The vein of Labbé drains the lateral aspect of the hemisphere into the transverse sinus. (pp. 17, 19, 21, 311)

4. **Answer E:** Branches of the superior cerebellar artery are most frequently involved in cases of trigeminal neuralgia that are presumably of vascular origin. The posterior cerebral artery and its larger branches serve the midbrain–diencephalic junction or join the medial surface of the hemisphere. The basilar artery serves the basilar pons and the anterior inferior cerebellar artery serves the caudal midbrain, inner ear, and the inferior surface of the cerebellar surface. The basal vein drains the medial portions of the hemisphere and passes through the ambient cistern to enter the great cerebral vein (of Galen). (pp. 23, 49)

5. **Answer D:** This man's deficits, loss of most (but not all) eye movement and dilation of the pupil, are on the right side. These losses, with no other deficits, indicate damage to the oculomotor nerve; this nerve exits the cranial cavity via the superior orbital fissure. This fissure also transmits the ophthalmic nerve. The foramen ovale transmits the mandibular nerve (plus fibers to the masticatory muscles) and the foramen rotundum transmits the maxillary nerve. After the maxillary nerve passes through the rotundum, it shifts course and enters the orbit via the inferior orbital fissure. The facial nerve passes through the stylomastoid foramen. (pp. 22–24, 44–45)

6. **Answer A:** In this patient the pontine lesion is on the right side. This results in a paralysis of the right lateral rectus (abducens lower

motor neurons) and of the right and left medial recti on attempted lateral gaze (damage to the axons of interneurons entering the medial longitudinal fasciculus on both sides). The surviving muscle is the left lateral rectus. (pp. 53–54)

7. **Answer B:** The inflammation in meningitis generally occupies the subarachnoid space and its minute extensions into the sulci; the infection may also extend into cisterns. The commonly used clinical terms leptomeningitis (signifying arachnoid + pia) or pia-arachnitis reflect the fact that this infection is frequently sequestered within the subarachnoid space. Meningitis may involve the dura (pachymeningitis) and, by extension, invade the minute spaces between the pia and brain surface (subpial space). However, these are not the main locations of this disease process. Epidural and subdural spaces are the result of trauma or some pathologic process and, around the brain, are not naturally occurring spaces. (pp. 58–61)

8. **Answer D:** The geniculate bodies are tucked-up under the caudal and inferior aspect of the pulvinar nucleus(i). The groove between the medial geniculate body and pulvinar contains the brachium of the superior colliculus. The geniculate bodies and the pulvinar have a common blood supply from the thalamogeniculate artery, a branch of P_2. None of the other choices have a close apposition with the geniculate bodies. The anterior thalamic, rostral dorsomedial, and subthalamic nuclei do not share a common blood supply with the pulvinar. (pp. 25, 31, 81–83, 175)

9. **Answer D:** Although this patient initially presented with complete motor and sensory losses, some function had returned by 36 hours; in this case, the lesion is classified as an incomplete lesion of the spinal cord. Patients with no return of function at 24+ hours and no sacral sparing have suffered a lesion classified as complete and it is unlikely that they will recover useful neurological function. In a central cord and a large syringomyelia, there is generally sparing of posterior column sensations and in a hemisection the loss of motor function is on the side of the lesion and the loss of pinprick is on the opposite side. (pp. 108–109)

10. **Answer E:** The short-term loss of function, frequently involving a specific part of the body, is characteristic of a transient ischemic attack (commonly called a TIA). The follow-up MRI shows no lesion because there has been no permanent damage. TIAs are caused by a brief period of inadequate perfusion of a localized region of the nervous system; recovery is usually rapid and complete. However, TIAs, especially if repeated, may be indicative of an impending stroke. Hemorrhagic strokes frequently result in some type of long-term or permanent deficit, and the central cord syndrome has bilateral deficits. A small embolic stroke would be visible on the follow-up MRI and, in this patient, would have resulted in a persistent deficit. Syringobulbia (cavitation within the medulla) may include long tract signs as well as cranial nerve signs. (pp. 108–109, 174–175)

11. **Answer C:** Weakness of the extremities accompanied by paralysis of muscles on the contralateral side of the tongue (seen as a deviation of the tongue to that side on protrusion) indicates a lesion in the medulla involving the corticospinal fibers in the pyramid and the exiting hypoglossal roots. This is an inferior alternating (crossed) hemiplegia. Middle alternating (crossed) hemiplegia refers to a lesion of the pontine corticospinal fibers and the root of the abducens nerve, and superior alternating (crossed) hemiplegia specifies damage to the oculomotor root and crus cerebri. Alternating (alternate, or crossed) hemianesthesia and hemihypesthesia are sensory losses. (pp. 124–125)

12. **Answer E:** The substantia nigra is located internal to the crus cerebri and, in T1-weighted MRI, appears as a darker shade of gray (hypointense) than does the crus. Loss of the dopamine-containing cells of the nigra results in characteristic motor deficits, including a pill-rolling (resting) tremor. The red nucleus and the periaqueductal gray are located in the midbrain, but do not border on the crus cerebri. The brachium of the inferior colliculus is found on the lateral surface of the midbrain, and the pretectal area is adjacent to the cerebral aqueduct at the midbrain–diencephalic junction. (pp. 179, 181, 183, 258–259)

13. **Answer A:** The combination of weakness on the left side (corticospinal involvement) and a loss of pain sensation on the right side specifies components of Brown-Séquard syndrome. The motor loss is ipsilateral to the damage and the sensory loss is contralateral; second order fibers conveying pain information cross in the anterior white commissure ascending about two spinal segments in the process. In this patient, the lesion is on the left side at about the T6 level; this explains the left-sided weakness and the loss of pain sensation on the right beginning at the T8 dermatome level. Lesions at T8 or T10 would result in a loss of pain sensation beginning, respectively, at dermatome levels T10 or T12 on the contralateral side. (pp. 196–199, 210–213)

14. **Answer D:** A tap on the patellar tendon stretches the muscle spindles in the quadriceps muscles, results in contraction of the same muscle group of the thigh, and the knee abruptly swings forward; this is mediated through spinal levels L2–L4. This is a monosynaptic reflex (and a muscle stretch reflex) with excitation of the extensor muscles of the leg and, through an interneuron, inhibition of leg flexors. The biceps reflex is mediated through C5–C6, and the triceps through C7–C8. The abdominal reflex is mediated through spinal levels T8–T10; level S1, with contributions from L5 and S2, mediates the ankle reflex. (p. 234)

15. **Answer D:** Lesions in the lateral portions of the brainstem damage descending projections from the hypothalamus to the ipsilateral intermediolateral cell column at spinal levels T1–T4, these being the hypothalamospinal fibers. The result is Horner syndrome (ptosis, myosis, anhydrosis on the face) on the side ipsilateral to the lesion. Horner syndrome also may be seen following cervical spinal cord lesions. A contralateral hemiplegia is not seen in lesions in lateral areas of the brainstem. The other choices are syndromes or deficits specific to medial brainstem areas or to only a particular level. (pp. 124–125, 138–139, 152–153, 262–263)

16. **Answer D:** The afferent limb of the tearing (lacrimal) reflex is via the trigeminal nerve (pain receptors in the conjunctiva and cornea), and the efferent limb travels on the facial nerve; the preganglionic parasympathetic cells are in the superior salivatory nucleus, and the postganglionic cells are in the pterygopalatine ganglion. The dorsal motor vagal nucleus contains preganglionic parasympathetic cells that distribute to ganglia in the thorax and abdomen. The geniculate ganglion contains the cell bodies of somatic afferent (SA) and visceral afferent (VA) fibers that enter the brain on the facial nerve; the otic ganglion contains postganglionic parasympathetic cell bodies that serve the parotid gland. (pp. 230–233, 237)

17. **Answer D:** The paralysis of facial muscles on one side of the face (left in this case) with no paralysis of the extremities is a facial hemiplegia; this is also commonly known as Bell palsy or facial palsy. Hemifacial spasms are irregular contractions of the facial muscles, and a central seven (also called a supranuclear facial palsy) refers to paralysis of muscles on the lower half of the face contralateral to a lesion in the genu of the internal capsule. Alternating (crossed)

hemiplegia describes a motor loss related to a cranial nerve on one side of the head and motor deficits of the extremities on the contralateral side of the body. A similar pattern of sensory losses is called an alternating hemianesthesia. (pp. 230–233)

18. Answer E: Degenerative changes in the dopamine-containing cells of the substantia nigra pars compacta on the right side correlate with a left-sided tremor. The altered message through the lenticular nucleus and thalamus and on to the motor cortex on the side of the degenerative changes will result in tremor on the opposite (right) side via altered messages traveling down the corticospinal tract. The initial symptoms of Parkinson disease appear on one side in about 75%–80% of patients and extend to bilateral involvement as the disease progresses. Bilateral changes in the substantia nigra correlate with bilateral deficits. The globus pallidus does not receive direct nigral input but rather input via a nigrostriatal-striatopallidal circuit. (pp. 254–259)

19. Answer A: This inherited disease is Friedreich ataxia; it initially appears in children in the age range of 8–15 years and has the characteristic deficits described. Huntington disease is inherited, but appears in adults (age range at onset 35–45 years); olivopontocerebellar atrophy is an autosomal dominant disease and gives rise to a totally different set of deficits. The cause of Parkinson disease is unclear, but it is probably not inherited and generally seen in patients 45+ years of age. The Wallenberg syndrome is a brainstem lesion resulting from a vascular occlusion and most commonly characterized by an alternating (crossed) hemianesthesia. (pp. 242–243)

20. Answer C: A fracture through the jugular foramen would potentially damage the glossopharyngeal (IX), vagus (X), and spinal accessory (XI) nerves. The major observable deficit would be a loss of the efferent limb of the gag reflex and paralysis of the ipsilateral trapezius and sternocleidomastoid muscles (drooping of the shoulder, difficulty elevating the shoulder especially against resistance, difficulty turning the head to the contralateral side). The patient would also experience difficulty swallowing (dysphagia) and speaking (dysarthria). Involvement of facial muscles would suggest damage to the internal acoustic or stylomastoid foramina; this would also be the case for the efferent limb of the corneal reflex. Diplopia and ptosis would suggest injury to the superior orbital fissure, as all three nerves controlling ocular movement traverse this space. The hypoglossal nerve (which supplies muscles of the tongue) passes through the hypoglossal canal. (pp. 226–233)

21. Answer C: A relay nucleus is one that receives a specific type of information from a comparatively specific source, and sends this information on to an equally specific cortical target. The medial geniculate nucleus receives mainly auditory information from the cochlear nuclei and brainstem auditory relay nuclei and projects to the transverse temporal gyrus. The dorsomedial, centromedian, and pulvinar are association nuclei; these receive input from diverse sources and project to equally diverse cortical targets. The thalamic reticular nucleus, while not specifically classified as either a relay nucleus or an association nucleus, basically functions as an association nucleus. (pp. 278–279)

22. Answer E: Dystonia is a movement disorder characterized by abnormal, sometimes intermittent, but frequently sustained, contractions of the muscles of the trunk and extremities that force the body into a twisted posture. Dystonia may be seen in patients with diseases of the basal nuclei. Dysmetria, the inability to judge the distance and trajectory of a movement, is a feature of cerebellar disease or lesions. Dyspnea is difficulty breathing; this may result from heart and/or lung disorders as well as from neurological disorders, which

may include central or nerve root lesions. Dysphagia is difficulty swallowing, dysarthria is difficulty speaking, and both may be seen together in several central or peripheral lesions. (pp. 254–255)

23. Answer D: A prolactinoma, a tumor that produces excessive amounts of prolactin (a hypersecreting tumor), may result in milk production in females in the absence of pregnancy. In females, excess luteinizing hormone may disrupt the ovarian cycle but not result in milk production. Overproduction of corticotrophin results in Cushing disease; excessive growth hormone results in either gigantism (before growth plates close) or acromegaly (after growth plates close). Overproduction of vasopressin influences urine excretion. (pp. 294–295)

24. Answer C: These three involve the roots of the oculomotor and abducens nerve and the nucleus of the abducens nerve, all of which innervate extraocular muscles. Each of these patients would experience some form of diplopia, one of their complaints would be seeing "double" or "two of everything." Aphasia and agnosia are usually associated with lesions of the forebrain. Dysarthria and dysphagia are frequently seen in medullary lesions, lesions involving the nuclei or roots of some cranial nerves of the medulla, but may also be seen in patients with large hemispheric strokes. Hemianesthesia may be present in patients with lesions at many levels of the central nervous system, but not in medially located lesions as is the case with these three patients. (pp. 226–229)

25. Answer B: In most instances (approximately 80%–85%), the ophthalmic artery originates from the cerebral portion of the internal carotid artery just after this parent vessel leaves the cavernous sinus and passes through the dura. In a small percentage of cases, the ophthalmic artery may originate from other locations on the internal carotid artery, including its cavernous portion (about 7%). This vessel does not originate from the petrous portion of the internal carotid or from anterior or middle cerebral arteries. (pp. 23, 310, 319)

26. Answer D: The P_3 segment lies along the orientation of, and adjacent to, the parahippocampal gyrus as this part of the posterior cerebral artery courses around the midbrain. Branches of the P_3 segment serve the inferior surface of the temporal lobe, which includes much of the laterally adjacent occipitotemporal gyri, and lower portions of the optic radiations. The lingual gyrus and the cuneus are in the territory of the P_4 segment and the orbital gyri are served by branches of the anterior and middle cerebral arteries. The superior temporal gyrus is served by M_4 branches of the inferior trunk of the middle cerebral artery. (pp. 19, 27)

27. Answer C: Treating fusiform aneurysms (in this case on the P_3 segment) present special considerations and complications and may result in blockage of all blood flow to targets distal to this point. Distal portions of the posterior cerebral artery (the P_4 segment) serve the primary visual cortex. Somatosensory, somatomotor, and auditory regions of the cerebral cortex are served by terminal branches of the middle cerebral artery (M_4 in the case of motor and sensory, M_3/M_4 in the case of auditory). Blindness in one eye would result from a lesion rostral to the optic chiasm; in the case of a vascular cause, this may relate to damage to the ophthalmic branch of the internal carotid. (pp. 19, 27)

28. Answer C: Vestibular schwannomas larger than 2.0 cm in diameter may enlarge rostrally, impinge on the sensory root of the trigeminal nerve and, cause loss of sensation on the same side of the face. Although the other deficits listed (olfactory loss, visual deficits, tongue weakness) are not seen in these patients, diplopia (involvement of

oculomotor, abducens or trochlear nerves, singularly or in combination) may be present, in fewer than 10%, of patients with vestibular schwannoma. (pp. 22–23, 50, 319)

29. Answer B: The internal acoustic meatus contains the vestibulocochlear nerve, the facial nerve, and the labyrinthine artery, a branch of the anterior inferior cerebellar artery. A vestibular schwannoma located at the meatus may affect the facial nerve and result in facial weakness. Large schwannomas usually produce sensory loss on the face (30%+ of the time) while facial weakness may be seen in about 10%+ of cases. The vagus and glossopharyngeal nerves exit the skull via the jugular foramen (along with the accessory nerve). The cerebellar arteries originate within the skull and distribute to structures within the skull. (pp. 24, 44–45, 50, 319)

30. Answer C: In this patient the weakness of the right lower extremity is related to a lesion of lateral corticospinal tract fibers on the right side of the spinal cord. The left corticospinal tract serves the left side of the spinal cord and the left lower extremity. Rubrospinal, reticulospinal, and vestibulospinal fibers influence the activity of spinal motor neurons; however, the deficits related to corticospinal tract damage (significant weakness) will dominate over the lack of excitation to flexor or extensor motor neurons in the spinal cord via these tracts. These latter tracts are dominate in cases of decorticate and decerebrate posturing. (pp. 102–105, 108–109, 210–213)

31. Answer C: The loss of pain and thermal sensations beginning at the level of the umbilicus (T10 dermatome) on the left side results from damage to fibers of the anterolateral system at about the T8 level on the right. These fibers ascend about two spinal levels as they cross the midline. Damage at the T6 level would result in a loss beginning at the T8 level on the contralateral side and damage at the T10 level would result in a loss beginning at about the T12 level. (pp. 102–105, 196–199)

32. Answer C: Weakness of the muscles of the face, particularly when upper and lower portions of the face are involved, indicates a lesion of either the facial motor nucleus or the exiting fibers of the facial nerve; both are located in the lateral pontine tegmentum at caudal levels. The hypoglossal nucleus, which is located in the medial medulla, innervates muscles of the tongue. The trigeminal nucleus innervates masticatory muscles and is present in the mid to more rostral pontine tegmentum. The abducens nucleus is found internal to the facial colliculus and innervates the lateral rectus muscle. These nuclei innervate muscles on the ipsilateral side. The arcuate nucleus is a group of cells located on the surface of the pyramid. (pp. 118–119, 130–135, 226–233)

33. Answer B: The fibers of the anterolateral system are located in the lateral portion of the pontine tegmentum anterior (ventral) to the facial motor nucleus; these fibers convey pain and thermal inputs from the contralateral side of the body. The spinal trigeminal tract and the anterior trigeminothalamic tract also convey pain and thermal input but from the ipsilateral and contralateral sides of the face, respectively. The lateral lemniscus is auditory in function and the medial lemniscus conveys proprioception, vibratory sense, and discriminative touch also from the contralateral body. (pp. 54, 122–131, 138–139, 196–199)

34. Answer D: Damage to the gracile fasciculus on the left (at the T8 level this is the only part of the posterior columns present at this level) accounts for the loss of vibratory sensation (and discriminative touch). Injury to the gracile fasciculus on the right would result in this type of deficit, but on the right side. The level of the cord

damage is caudal to the cuneate fasciculi and the anterolateral system conveys pain and thermal sensations from the contralateral side, not proprioceptive information. (pp. 100–105, 108–109, 192–195)

35. Answer A: The loss of pain and thermal sensations on the right side of the body correlates with a lesion involving the anterolateral system on the left side of the spinal cord. The axons carrying this sensory information cross the midline ascending about two spinal levels as they do so. A lesion of the right anterolateral system would result in a left-sided deficit. The gracile and cuneate fasciculi convey discriminative touch, vibratory sensation, and proprioception from the ipsilateral side of the body. The posterior spinocerebellar tract conveys similar information, but it is not perceived/recognized as such (consciously) by the brain. (pp. 104–105, 108–109, 196–199)

36. Answer A: In this case the weakness of the upper and lower extremities on the right, in association with the diplopia (abducens injury), reflects damage to corticospinal fibers on the left side of the basilar pons. A lesion of these fibers on the right side of the pons would produce a left-sided weakness after they cross in the motor decussation. Rubrospinal fibers are not located in the territory of paramedian branches of the basilar artery. Also, lesions of rubrospinal fibers and of the middle cerebellar peduncle do not cause weakness but may cause other types of motor deficits, particularly in lesions causing decorticate and decerebrate rigidity. (pp. 130–133, 138–139, 220–223)

37. Answer A: The best localizing sign in this case is the diplopia; along with the corticospinal deficit and vascular territory, it specifies a lesion at the pons–medulla junction on the left. The exiting fibers of the abducens nerve (on the left) are in the territory of the paramedian branches of the basilar artery and are laterally adjacent to corticospinal fibers in the basilar pons. Diplopia may result from lesions of the oculomotor and trochlear nerves, but these structures are not in the domain of the paramedian basilar branches. A lesion of the optic nerve results in blindness in that eye and damage to the facial root does not affect eye movement but may cause a loss of view of the external world if the palpebral fissure is closed due to facial muscle weakness. (pp. 53–54, 130–133, 138–139)

38. Answer D: At caudal pontine levels most, if not all, of the medial lemniscus is located within the territory served by paramedian branches of the basilar artery. Penetrating branches of the anterior spinal artery serve the hypoglossal nucleus. The other choices are generally in the territories of short or long circumferential branches of the basilar artery. The hypoglossal nucleus and its root are in the territory of the anterior spinal artery. (pp. 54, 124–125, 138–139)

39. Answer D: The vocalis muscle (this muscle is actually the medial portion of the thyroarytenoid muscle) is innervated, via the vagus nerve, by motor neurons located in the nucleus ambiguus. The gracile nucleus conveys proprioception and vibratory sense from the body and the spinal trigeminal nucleus relays pain and thermal sensory input from the face. The hypoglossal nucleus is motor to the tongue and the facial nucleus is motor to the muscles of facial expression. (pp. 116–121, 124–125)

40. Answer A: Fibers comprising the anterolateral system convey pain and thermal sensations from the body, excluding the face. These fibers are located in lateral portions of the medulla adjacent to the spinal trigeminal tract; this latter tract relays pain and thermal sensations from the face. Both of these tracts are in the territory of the posterior inferior cerebellar artery. The gracile and cuneate fasciculi convey proprioception, discriminative touch, and vibratory sense in the

spinal cord and the medial lemniscus conveys this same information from the medulla to the dorsal thalamus. (pp. 116–121, 124–125)

41. **Answer E:** The loss of pain and thermal sensations on one side of the face correlates with damage to the spinal trigeminal tract; in this case the loss is ipsilateral to the lesion. The anterolateral system relays pain and thermal sensations from the contralateral side of the body, the solitary tract conveys visceral sensory input (general visceral sense and taste), and the medial lemniscus contains fibers relaying information related to position sense and discriminative touch, also from the contralateral side. The medial longitudinal fasciculus does not contain sensory fibers. (pp. 116–121, 124–125)

42. **Answer C:** The posterior inferior cerebellar artery (commonly called PICA by clinicians) serves the posterolateral portion of the medulla, which encompasses the anterolateral system, spinal trigeminal tract, and nucleus ambiguus plus other nuclei. This combination of deficits is variably called the PICA syndrome, lateral medullary syndrome, or Wallenberg syndrome. The anterior and medial areas of the medulla (containing the pyramid, medial lemniscus, and hypoglossal nucleus/nerve) are served by the anterior spinal artery and the anterolateral area of the medulla (the region of the olivary nuclei) is served by penetrating branches of the vertebral artery. The posterior spinal artery serves the posterior column nuclei in the medulla and the anterior inferior cerebellar artery (commonly called AICA) serves caudal portions of the pons and cerebellum. (pp. 53–54, 116–121, 124–125)

43. **Answer B:** The uncus is at the rostral and medial aspect of the parahippocampal gyrus, and, in this position, is directly adjacent to the anterolateral aspect of the midbrain. The diencephalon is rostral to this point and the medulla, the most caudal part of the brainstem, is located in the posterior fossa. Late stages of uncal herniation may, but not always, result in damage to the rostral pons; this is especially the case if the patient becomes decerebrate. The cerebellum is not involved in uncal herniation but may participate in upward or downward cerebellar herniation. (pp. 164–167, 301)

44. **Answer D:** Herniation of the uncus through the tentorial incisura compresses the lateral portions of the brainstem, particularly the midbrain, eventually resulting in compression of the corticospinal fibers in the crus cerebri. Weakness on the patient's left side indicates damage to corticospinal fibers in the right crus. In situations of significant shift of the midbrain due to the herniation, the contralateral crus also may be damaged, resulting in bilateral weakness. Although all other choices contain corticospinal fibers, none of these areas are directly involved in uncal herniation. (pp. 152–153, 164–167, 301)

45. **Answer C:** The root of the oculomotor nerve conveys (general) somatic efferent (SE) fibers to four of the six major extraocular muscles and (general) visceral efferent (VE) parasympathetic preganglionic fibers to the ciliary ganglion from which postganglionic fibers travel to the sphincter muscle of the iris. Pressure on the oculomotor root, as in uncal herniation, will usually compress the smaller diameter, and more superficially located VE fibers first (pupil dilation) followed by eventual compression of the larger diameter motor fibers (muscle weakness). Optic nerve damage results in blindness in that eye, injury to sympathetic fibers to the eye results in constriction of the pupil, and an abducens root injury results in an inability to abduct that eye or in diplopia. A lesion of corticonuclear fibers in the crus results primarily in motor deficits related to the facial, hypoglossal, and accessory nerves. (pp. 152–153, 164–167, 301)

46. **Answer C:** The absence of, or the aberrant development of, muscle around the oral cavity and over the cheek (muscles of facial expression, innervated by the facial [VII] nerve) indicate a failure of proper differentiation of the second pharyngeal arch. Arch 2 also gives rise to the stapedius, buccinator, stylohyoid, platysma, and posterior belly of the digastric. Mesoderm of the head outside of the pharyngeal arches gives rise to the extraocular muscles and muscles of the tongue. The muscles of mastication (plus the tensor tympani, tensor veli palati, mylohyoid, anterior belly of the digastric) arise from arch 1, the stylopharyngeus from arch 3, and striated muscles of the pharynx, larynx, and upper esophagus from arch 4. (pp. 226–233)

47. **Answer C:** The best localizing sign in this patient is the paucity of eye movement and dilated pupil on the left; this indicates a lesion of the midbrain on the left at the level of the exiting oculomotor fibers. The red nucleus is found at the same level and, more importantly, immediately lateral to the red nucleus is a compact bundle of cerebellothalamic fibers. The ataxia and tremor are related primarily to damage these cerebellar efferent fibers. The motor deficit is contralateral to the lesion because the corticospinal fibers, through which the deficit is expressed, cross at the motor (pyramidal) decussation. Lesions at the other choices would not result in a paucity of eye movement, or result in these deficits on the wrong side, and, therefore, are not potential candidates. (pp. 226–229, 248–251)

48. **Answer C:** The lesion on the exiting oculomotor fibers (on the left) damages the preganglionic parasympathetic fibers from the Edinger-Westphal preganglionic nucleus. Activation of these fibers produces pupil constriction; when their influence is removed the pupil dilates. Consequently, the intact postganglionic sympathetic fibers from the ipsilateral superior cervical ganglion predominate, and the pupil dilates. Choices on the right are on the incorrect side. Damage to hypothalamospinal fibers would remove sympathetic influence at the intermediolateral cell column, and the pupil would constrict (parasympathetic domination). (pp. 226–229, 239)

49. **Answer B:** Cell bodies in the nucleus ambiguus innervate muscles of the pharynx and larynx, including what is commonly called the vocalis muscle. One result of damage to this nucleus is dysarthria; another is dysphagia. The solitary tract and nuclei are concerned with visceral afferent information, including taste, and the spinal trigeminal tract is made the central processes of primary sensory fibers conveying (general) somatic afferent (SA) information from the ipsilateral side of the face and oral cavity. Proprioceptive information from the ipsilateral upper extremity is transmitted via the cuneate nucleus; the vestibular nuclei are related to balance, equilibrium, and control of eye movement. (pp. 230–233)

50. **Answer C:** The area of the brainstem that contains the nucleus ambiguus is served by branches of the posterior inferior cerebellar artery (PICA). Occlusion of this vessel usually gives rise to the PICA (lateral medullary or Wallenberg) syndrome. The anterior inferior cerebellar artery (AICA) serves the lateral and inferior cerebellar surface and the superior cerebellar artery serves the superior surface and much of the cerebellar nuclei. The labyrinthine artery, a branch of AICA, serves the inner ear. The posterior spinal artery serves the posterior columns and their nuclei. (pp. 124–125, 138–139)

51. **Answer B:** The lesion in this woman is in the medulla, and the sensory loss on the body (excluding the head) is on her left side; a lesion in the medulla on the right side, involving fibers of the anterolateral system (ALS), accounts for this sensory deficit. The overall sensory deficits in this case may be called an alternate (or crossed) hemianesthesia. A

lesion of the ALS on the left side of the medulla would result in sensory deficits on the right side of the body. The spinal trigeminal tract and nucleus convey pain and thermal sensations from the ipsilateral side (right side in this case) of the face, and the medial lemniscus conveys vibratory and discriminative touch sensations from the contralateral side of the body. (pp.196–199, 202–205)

52. Answer C: The woman is hoarse because the lesion involves the region of the medulla that includes the nucleus ambiguus. These motor neurons serve, via the glossopharyngeal (IX) and vagus (X) nerves, the muscles of the larynx and pharynx, including the medial portion of the thyroarytenoid, also called the vocalis muscle. Paralysis of the vocalis on one side will cause hoarseness of the voice. This patient will, most likely, also experience difficulty swallowing (dysphagia). Hypoglossal nucleus or nerve, or facial nucleus lesions, may cause difficulty with speech (altered movements of the tongue or muscles around the mouth) but not hoarseness. The spinal trigeminal tract conveys sensory input from the ipsilateral side of the face. There are no historical or examination findings to support a diagnosis of upper respiratory viral findings (cold or flu). (pp. 54, 226–233)

53. Answer C: The posterior inferior cerebellar artery (PICA) serves the lateral area of the medulla that contains the anterolateral system, spinal trigeminal tract (loss of pain and thermal sensations from the ipsilateral side of the face), the nucleus ambiguus, and other structures. Many patients that present with a PICA (Wallenberg or lateral medullary) syndrome may also have involvement of the vertebral artery on that side. The posterior spinal artery serves the posterior column nuclei in the medulla, and the anterior spinal artery serves the pyramid, medial lemniscus, and exiting roots of the hypoglossal nerve. The anterior inferior cerebellar artery and the superior cerebellar artery distribute to the pons and midbrain, respectively, plus significant portions of the cerebellum. (pp. 25, 31, 124–125, 196–199)

54. Answer E: Excessive eating (gluttony), which may also include, in the case of this patient, a propensity to attempt to eat things not considered food items, is hyperphagia. Dysphagia is difficulty in swallowing and frequently related to medullary damage. Aphagia is the inability to eat; this may reflect dysfunction of the masticatory apparatus or the lack of desire to eat. Hyperorality is the tendency to put items in the mouth or to appear to be examining objects by placing them in the oral cavity. Dyspnea is difficulty breathing. (pp. 280–285)

55. Answer A: The constellation of deficits experienced by this man is characteristic of the Klüver-Bucy syndrome; this may be seen following bilateral damage to the temporal poles particularly that which includes the amygdaloid complex. The Korsakoff syndrome (psychosis) is seen, for example, in chronic alcoholics, and senile dementia is a loss of cognitive and intellectual function associated with neurodegenerative diseases of the elderly (e.g., Alzheimer disease). Wernicke (receptive or fluent) aphasia is seen in patients with a lesion in the area of the inferior parietal lobule, and the Wallenberg syndrome results from a lesion in the medulla and is characterized by alternating (crossed) hemisensory losses and, depending on the extent of the damage, other deficits. (pp. 280–285)

56. Answer B: Bilateral damage to the temporal lobes, as in this case, may result in damage to the hippocampus by any one of several mechanisms. While remote memory, the ability to recall events that happened years ago, is intact, the man will have difficulty "remembering" recent (last few days/weeks) or immediate (last few minutes/hours)

events. That is, he will find it difficult, if not impossible, to turn a new experience into longer-term memory (something that can be recalled in its proper context at a later time). Dysphagia (difficulty swallowing) and dysarthria (difficulty speaking) are deficits usually seen in brainstem lesions. Bilateral sensory losses of the lower portion of the body could be seen with bilateral damage to the posterior paracentral gyri (falcine meningioma) or to the anterior white commissure of the spinal cord. Dementia is a multiregional symptom that usually involves several areas of the brain, cortical as well as subcortical. (pp. 280–285)

57. Answer C: The Meyer-Archambault loop (sometimes called the Meyer loop) is composed of optic radiation fibers that loop through the temporal lobe; these fibers, on each side, convey visual input from the contralateral superior quadrant of the visual field. Consequently, a bilateral lesion of these fibers results as a bilateral superior quadrantanopia. Bilateral inferior quadrantanopia is seen in bilateral lesions that would involve the superior portion of the optic radiations. Right or left superior quadrantanopia is seen in cases of unilateral damage to, respectively, the left or right Meyer-Archambault loop. A bitemporal hemianopsia results in a lesion of the optic chiasm. (pp. 262–267)

58. Answer C: The combination of eye movement disorders and a contralateral hemiplegia localizes this lesion to the midbrain on the side of the ocular deficits (right side); the best localizing signs are the third nerve deficits. This also specifies that corticospinal fibers on the right (in the crus) are damaged, and places the location of the cells of origin for these fibers in the somatomotor cortex on the right side. The right crus contains the axons of these fibers but not the neuronal cell bodies. The left somatomotor cortex influences the right extremities. The right precentral gyrus does not contain cells projecting to the left lumbosacral spinal cord (left lower extremity), and the right anterior paracentral gyrus does not contain the cells that project to the left cervical spinal cord (left upper extremity). (pp. 210–217)

59. Answer A: The lesion in this man is in the central (brainstem/midbrain) and involves the third nerve and adjacent structures, such as the red nucleus and cerebellothalamic fibers. Consequently, the damage is to the preganglionic parasympathetic fibers in the root of the oculomotor (III) nerve; this removes the parasympathetic influence (pupil constriction) that originates from the Edinger-Westphal preganglionic nucleus. Fibers from the superior cervical ganglion are intact, hence the dilated pupil. Fibers from the geniculate ganglion and inferior salivatory nucleus distribute on the facial (VII) and glossopharyngeal (IX) nerves, respectively. Postganglionic fibers from the ciliary ganglion, although involved in this pathway, are not damaged in this lesion. (pp. 146–149, 226–229)

60. Answer E: The loss of most eye movement on one side (oculomotor nerve root involvement) coupled with a paralysis of the extremities on the contralateral side is a superior alternating (crossed) hemiplegia (this is also known as the Weber syndrome): superior because it is the most rostral of three; alternating (crossed) because it is a cranial nerve on one side and the extremities on the other; and hemiplegia because one-half of the body below the head is involved. A middle alternating (crossed) hemiplegia involves the abducens (VI) nerve root and adjacent corticospinal fibers (Raymond syndrome), and an inferior alternating (crossed) hemiplegia involves the hypoglossal (XII) nerve root and corticospinal fibers in the pyramid (Déjèrine syndrome). Alternating hemianesthesia is a sensory loss, and a Brown-Séquard syndrome is a spinal cord lesion with no cranial nerve deficits. (pp. 226–229)

Index

Note: Page numbers in italics denote figures; those followed by t refer to table; those followed by Q denote questions; and those followed by A denote answers.